# Immunocytochemistry in diagnostic histopathology

*For Churchill Livingstone*

*Publisher:* Timothy Horne
*Project Editor:* Dilys Jones
*Copy Editor:* Delia Malim-Robinson
*Indexer:* Monica Trigg
*Production Control:* P.S.D.
*Sales Promotion Executive:* Douglas McNaughton

# Immunocytochemistry in diagnostic histopathology

**Bharat Jasani** BSc PhD MRCPath
Senior Lecturer and Honorary Consultant in Immunocytochemistry (Histopathology),
Head of Regional Immunocytochemistry Unit, Department of Pathology, University of Wales
College of Medicine, Cardiff, UK

**Kurt W. Schmid** MD
Professor of Pathology, Gerhard-Domagk Institute of Pathology, University
of Münster, Münster, Germany

CHURCHILL LIVINGSTONE
EDINBURGH LONDON MADRID MELBOURNE NEW YORK AND TOKYO 1993

CHURCHILL LIVINGSTONE
Medical Division of Longman Group UK Limited

Distributed in the United States of America by Churchill
Livingstone Inc., 650 Avenue of the Americas, New York,
N.Y. 10011, and by associated companies, branches and
representatives throughout the world.

First published 1993

ISBN 0-443-04018-4

**British Library Cataloguing in Publication Data**
A catalogue record for this book is available from the British
Library.

**Library of Congress Cataloging in Publication Data**
Jasani, Bharat.
    Immunocytochemistry in diagnostic histopathology / Bharat Jasani,
  Kurt W. Schmid
       p.   cm.
    Includes index.
    1. Immunocytochemistry.  2. Cancer—Immunodiagnosis.  3. Cancer—
Cytodiagnosis.  4. Histology, Pathological—Technique.  I. Schmid,
Kurt W.  II. Title.
    [DNLM: 1. Diagnosis, Laboratory—methods.  2. Histological
Techniques.  3. Immunohistochemistry—methods.  4. Immunologic
Tests.  QY 250 J39i]
RC270.3.I44J38  1993
616.07'56—dc20
DNLM/DLC
for Library of Congress                                        92–49842
                                                                    CIP

Produced by Longman Singapore  Publishers (Pte) Ltd.
Printed in Singapore

# Contents

# Preface

This book was commissioned some three years ago to provide a relatively non-specialist text on the role and scope of immunocytochemistry in routine diagnostic histopathology. The target readership was designated to be students and practitioners of histopathology with either academic or service-oriented interests in immunocytochemistry.

Over the past 20 years, immunocytochemistry has become established as an essential adjunct to routine histopathological practice for confirming or improving the accuracy of diagnosis or prognosis deduced on histological grounds. This has been made possible by the capacity of primary antibodies applied in conjunction with suitable enzyme markers to identify a whole variety of cell lineage, cell differentiation as well as cell proliferation-specific antigens in the direct context of conventionally revealed morbid anatomical features.

In order to understand the pivotal role played by immunocytochemistry, it is necessary for the reader to have a basic appreciation of the histopathological approach to diagnostic and prognostic analyses and a working knowledge of human developmental embryology and biochemistry. In addition, it is essential for the reader to appreciate the basis of primary antibody specificity and sensitivity and the mechanics of the secondary enzyme-linked antibody techniques used for disclosing the primary antibody binding to histologically identifiable tissue elements.

To satisfy these demands, the authors have adopted an integrated approach to the overall subject. Thus, each histopathologically definable disease entity is dealt with primarily in terms of its tissue of origin and one or the other of three fundamental biochemically distinct processes underlying the disease activity, viz. neoplasia,

inflammation or degeneration, respectively. According to this scheme, a disease-associated lesion is categorized, for example, as a neoplasm arising from a specific type of epithelial tissue elements, or inflammation principally targeted at the kidney glomerulus, or degeneration selectively affecting the heart muscle, etc. Since the bulk of histopathological analyses are conducted on formalin-fixed, paraffin-embedded tissue sections, emphasis is placed on immunocytochemical markers and techniques most suitable for this type of tissue substrate.

It is to be stressed that the coverage of the subject is by no means comprehensive and the reader is recommended to refer to the general texts and reviews cited in the bibliography for further details.

The work described is based on over 10 years of the authors' collective experience of routine application of immunocytochemistry in diagnostic histopathology and their many research-oriented immunocytochemical investigations. All this work experience would have been impossible without the encouragement and interest of our respective Heads of Department, Professor Sir Dillwyn Williams, Professor Mikuz, Professor Böcker and our respective academic colleagues, and the excellent support of the technical staff, in particular Mr Norman Thomas and Miss Evelyn Gredler.

Finally, without the unswerving moral support of our immediate family members – Annand, Karishma, Maya and Katharina respectively, the book would have failed to reach its finishing mark. The finished product is therefore most gratefully dedicated to them.

Cardiff and Münster,  B.J.
1993  K.W.S.

# PART I

# Introduction: surgical pathology aspects of immunocytochemistry

# 1. Historical perspective – development of detection techniques suitable for routine histopathology

## DEVELOPMENT OF DETECTION TECHNIQUES SUITABLE FOR ROUTINE HISTOPATHOLOGY

The conceptual and technical bases for immunocytochemistry were first laid in the 1940s by Albert Coons in his attempts to localize antigens and antibody responses related to pathogenic microorganisms in tissues of infected and immunized animals. His original aim was to trace streptococcal antigens in diseased tissues taken from patients dying of rheumatic fever.

For detection of the disease-associated antigen, he invented the direct immunofluorescence method utilizing fluorescein-labelled primary antibody directed against the antigen (see Fig. 1.1a). As for tracing plasma cells involved in specific antibody response to the pathogen, he developed the antigen sandwich method. This used unlabelled antigen as the primary probe and fluor-

escein-labelled antibody to the antigen as the secondary detection antibody reagent (see Fig. 1.1b). In both these studies he found frozen tissue sections prepared from unfixed tissue to be an optimum substrate. As elegantly reviewed by Holborrow, the orientation of these pioneering studies by Albert Coons towards microbial immune responses unfortunately prevented an earlier introduction of immunocytochemistry to histopathological practice.

Consequently, several conceptual and technical barriers had to be overcome before the full potential of immunocytochemistry in diagnostic histopathology could be recognized, as discussed below.

### Introduction of unlabelled primary antibody system

The direct immunofluorescence technique had

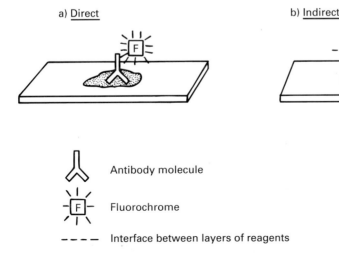

a) Direct          b) Indirect

Antibody molecule

Fluorochrome

Interface between layers of reagents

**Fig. 1.1**  Schematic representation of direct and indirect immunofluorescence methods.

the major drawback of its lack of versatility. Thus for each antigen the relevant specific antibody needed labelling with the fluorochrome, a task technically demanding, labour-intensive and wasteful of the primary antibody reagent.

The introduction of the indirect immunofluorescence technique (see Fig. 1.1b) by Friou et al and Holborrow et al in 1957, helped to overcome this problem in a simple and effective way. Thus instead of using in a single step a direct conjugate of fluorescein-labelled antiserum, a combination of an unlabelled primary antiserum (added in the first step to the section) with a heterologous fluorescein-labelled anti-immunoglobulin secondary antibody reagent (added in the second step) was introduced. This approach was applied in the first instance as a means of detecting anti-nuclear autoantibodies in systemic lupus erythematosus patient sera. The resulting two-step indirect immunofluorescence procedure was found to be more sensitive and more versatile compared to the single step direct immunofluorescence technique. It also helped to pave the way for immunocytochemical study of human tissue antigens not only with disease-associated autoimmune sera but also with heteroimmune antisera raised in animals immunized with human antigens.

## Development of indirect immunoenzyme secondary detection system

Despite its greater versatility and higher sensitivity the indirect immunofluorescence method did not gain the full favour of the routine histopathologists. This was because of certain problems inherent to the signal generated by the fluorescent dye marker. The first and foremost was its lack of capacity to allow the use of a suitable counterstain to reveal the background tissue morphology in relation to the antigen positive cell or tissue components. Secondly, the signal was impermanent both in terms of its fading on exposure to the UV and bright light and its intolerance of permanent mountant systems. Thirdly, its use on formalin paraffin embedded tissue sections was hampered by autofluorescence associated with such preparations.

The development of enzyme-labelled secondary antibody system by Nakane & Pierce in 1967, and

its subsequent improvement over the next 5 years by Avrameas, Mason and Sternberger and co-workers, helped to overcome these disadvantages of the indirect immunofluorescence technique.

Amongst the various immunoenzyme techniques developed, the immunoperoxidase method (see Fig. 1.1a) was found to have the capacity to deposit a coloured product which could be visualized easily with ordinary bright field optics in sections counter-stained with routine histological stains. In addition, its product, based on diaminobenzidine, was found to be permanently stable in that it tolerated dehydration in alcohol and xylene and did not dissolve in the standard permount media.

## Introduction of formalin-fixed paraffin-embedded tissue sections

Despite the advantages accruing from the developing of the indirect immunoperoxidase system, wider acceptance of immunocytochemistry as a useful adjunct to histopathological practice was delayed for almost another decade. Thus the frozen unfixed tissue sections long advocated as the most suitable substrate for immunocytochemical studies were awkward to adapt for routine histological work and did not yield the morphological detail and clarity necessary for histopathological analysis. Unfortunately, for the reasons already stated, formalin-fixed paraffin-embedded tissue sections were considered to be unsuitable for the indirect immunofluorescence technique. This impasse was only overcome when the novel indirect immunoperoxidase method was successfully applied to routine histopathological material by two independent groups, one led by Taylor in Oxford and the other by Nayak in New Delhi.

Almost simultaneously, in 1974, they came to the important conclusion that the indirect immunoperoxidase technique was powerful enough to detect antigens in sections taken from archival formalin-fixed paraffin-embedded material stored for many years. For this momentous realization, Taylor's group had used reactive lymphoid tissue to detect immunoglobulins in plasma cells, in line with the previously successful immunofluorescence studies of Ortega and Mellors (1957) using air-dried frozen sections taken from unfixed tissue sections, and of Sainte-Marie (1962) using cold ethanol-fixed paraffin wax-embedded tissue sections. Nayak's work, on the other hand, was driven by the technical and scientific need to 'complete locational and morphologic identity' between the surface coat antigen of hepatitis B virus and its positivity resulting from the Shikata's orcein stain.

The futuristic significance of these studies was that they emphasized the suitability of the immunoperoxidase method for studying tissue antigens in conventional histopathological material and the possibility of 'mass (immunocytochemical) screening of stored paraffin-embedded' tissue blocks.

However, genuine progress of immunocytochemistry in diagnostic histopathology had to await certain special technical modifications, advent of cell lineage and differentiation-specific primary antibodies, and commercialization of immunocytochemical reagents and techniques.

## Special technical modifications

The initial success of Taylor and Burns in immunostaining of plasma cells with anti-immunoglobulin primary antibodies in formalin-fixed paraffin-embedded sections was largely due to the tissue being fixed in acidic formalin (N D Thomas — personal communication; see also Piris and Thomas (1980)). The systematic studies of Curran and Gregory, which followed in 1978, demonstrated that formalin fixation of tissue at neutral pH is associated with a marked reduction in immunostaining of cytoplasmic immunoglobulin and abolishment of staining due to cell surface and extracellular forms of immunoglobulins. Furthermore, they found that the staining could be restored through short pretreatment of sections with a weak proteolytic enzyme solution (e.g. 0.1% to 0.05% of trypsin solution for 15–30 min at 37°C). The use of acid formalin as a fixative prevented excessive cross-linking of the tissue matrix, thereby allowing sufficient access of the immunocytochemical reagents to the tissue-bound immunoglobulin antigenic sites.

The second special improvement in the technique related to the need to abolish endogenous peroxidatic activity producing potentially distracting tissue staining. An effective method for abolishment of this type of background staining was proposed by Burns and colleagues, based on the original recommendation made by Streefkirk in 1972. It included the use of a methanol/$H_2O_2$ mixture applied for 30 minutes, leading to the inhibition of endogenous peroxidatic activity from many different sources.

Such improvements in tissue treatment prior to immunostaining made it possible to produce immunoperoxidase staining on routine formalin-fixed paraffin-embedded sections which was more consistently reliable and free of endogenous staining (see Heyderman 1979, for an overall appraisal of the technique).

## Development of cell lineage and differentiation-specific antibody markers

The earliest demonstration of the value of cell lineage-specific markers as an aid to histopathological analysis of neoplastic lesions was provided in the seminal observations of Williams on the histogenesis of medullary carcinoma of the thyroid published in 1966. Through very careful histological analysis on many dog and rat spontaneous thyroid tumours and their comparison with a large number of human medullary carcinomas, he showed that a small proportion of the dog and a very large proportion of the rat thyroid tumours had their origin from the parafollicular rather than the follicular cell of the thyroid gland. Most importantly, he went on to suggest that 'medullary carcinoma was derived from parafollicular cell origin and that a proof of this link would help to resolve the discrepancy between the relatively good prognosis and the apparently undifferentiated structure of this tumour'. Thus in a very emphatic way the histopathologist was made aware of the importance of defining the cell lineage origin of the tumour in addition to analysing its usual histopathological characteristics.

This challenge was taken up in the early 1970s by Pearse, Bussolati, Polak and Bloom who set about to exploit the full power of immunocytochemistry in this direction as depicted by their brilliant pioneering analysis of the role of gastro-intestinal neuroendocrine cells in different

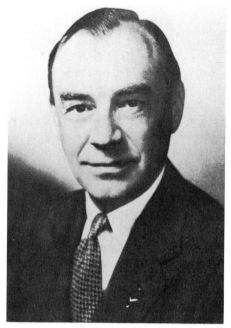

*Albert H. Coons*

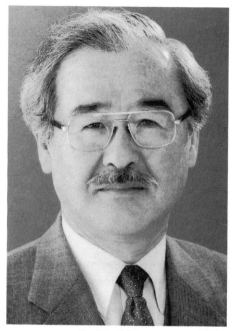

*Paul K. Nakane*

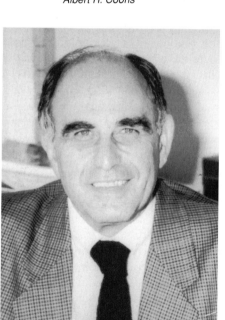

*Stratis Avrameas*

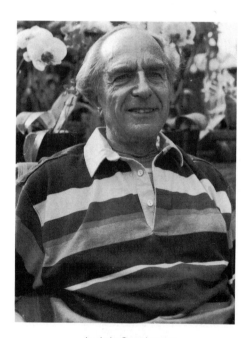

*Ludwig Sternberger*

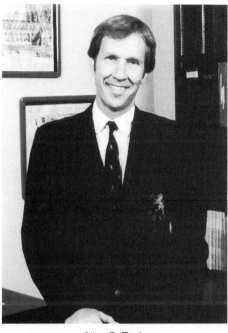

*Clive R. Taylor*

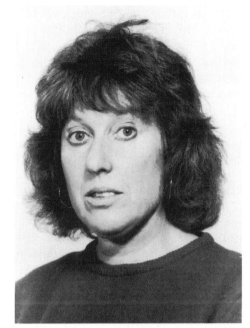

*Julia M. Polak*

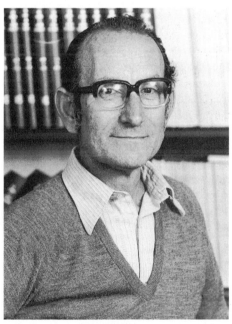

*Cesar Milstein*

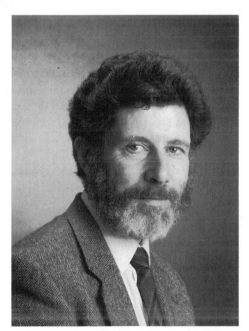

*David Y. Mason*

**Fig. 1.2**   Major contributors to the development and promotion of immunocytochemical technology as an aid to tissue diagnosis: Albert H. Coons (1940)—invention of the immunofluorescence technique and promotion of its applications; Paul K. Nakane (1967)—invention of the immunoperoxidase method; Stratis Avrameas (1969) and Ludwig Sternberger (1970)—improvement and diversification of immunoenzyme technology and promotion of its applications in research and diagnostic fields; Clive R. Taylor (1974)—application of the immunoperoxidase method to diagnostic histopathological analysis (see also Nayak et al 1974); Cesar Milstein (1975)—invention of the monoclonal antibody technology; Julia M. Polak (1986) and David Y. Mason (1987)—promotion of widespread use of the immunocytochemical techniques in diagnostic pathology.

clinical states including the Zollinger–Ellison and the watery diarrhoea syndromes. Around the same time, Wolfe and his co-workers on the other side of the Atlantic used immunocytochemistry to define the significance of hyperplastic C-cells, as detected by calcitonin immunostaining, in familial forms of medullary carcinoma of thyroid.

The earliest exploitation of cell differentiation-specific markers for typing of poorly differentiated neoplastic lesions related to the use of antibodies to myosin for the identification of rhabdomyosarcoma, and to acid phosphatase for the proof of prostatic origin of metastatic adenocarcinoma, as reviewed in 1979 by Bosman and Kruseman's first formal review on the applications of immunoperoxidase methods in diagnostic histopathology.

## Advent of hybrid monoclonal antibody technology

The first major impact of cell lineage-/differentiation-specific primary antibodies, derived from the hybrid monoclonal antibody technology of Köhler and Milstein, was felt in the field of histopathological diagnosis of lymphoreticular tumours as reviewed by Nadler et al in 1981. By the mid-eighties the range of polyclonal and monoclonal primary antibodies to the cell lineage and differentiation had widened sufficiently to allow a fairly comprehensive immunohistochemical approach to identification and classification of malignant undifferentiated neoplasms, as described by Lee and DeLellis in 1987.

## Commercialization of immunocytochemical reagents

The rapid progress of immunocytochemical applications in diagnostic histopathology could not have been achieved without the pioneering, dedicated involvement of commercial firms such as Becton Dickinson of Palo Alto, California and Dakopatts of Copenhagen, Denmark. The early success of both these companies was associated with development of a variety of lymphoreticular cell markers. It involved the employment of first-rate immunologists working in close collaboration with expert lymph node pathologists. This example of a co-operative approach between scientists and pathologists was subsequently taken up by other companies such as the Bionuclears who, together with the Lab Systems, were the first to bring out a comprehensive series of intermediate filament-specific monoclonal antibodies for the typing of epithelial, neural and connective tissue tumours.

In summary, the establishment of immunocytochemistry as a widely practised and useful adjunct to diagnostic histopathological analysis was made possible by a combination of certain specific adjustments of the immunocytochemical technique to suit the routinely processed tissue material and the advent, mass production and commercialization of a wide range of cell lineage- and differentiation-specific polyclonal and monoclonal primary antibodies. Figure 1.2 is a tribute to the major contributors to the development and promotion of immunocytochemical technology as an aid to tissue diagnosis.

REFERENCES AND FURTHER READING

**Development of immunofluorescence method**

Coons A H 1971 The development of immunohistochemistry. Annals of New York Academy of Sciences 177: 5–9
Coons A H, Creech H J, Jones R N 1941 Immunological properties of an antibody containing a fluorescent group. Proceedings of Society for Experimental Biology (New York) 47: 200–202

**Development of immunoperoxidase method**

Avrameas S 1969 Coupling of enzymes to proteins with glutaraldehyde. Use of the conjugates for the detection of antigens and antibodies. Immunochemistry 6: 43–52
Nakane P K, Pierce G B 1967 Enzyme-labelled antibodies: preparation and application for the localisation of antigens. Journal of Histochemistry and Cytochemistry 14: 929–930
Sternberger L A, Hardy P H, Cuculis J J, Meyer H G 1970 The unlabelled antibody enzyme method of immunocytochemistry. Preparation and properties of soluble antigen antibody complex (horseradish peroxidase–anti-horseradish peroxidase) and its use in the identification of spirochaetes. Journal of Histochemistry and Cytochemistry 18: 315–333

**Impact of immunoperoxidase method on histopathology**

Friou G J, Finch S C, Detre K D 1957 Nuclear localisation of a factor from disseminated lupus serum. Federation Proceedings 16: 413

Holborrow E J 1983 The value of immunohistochemistry in diagnosis. In: Filipe M I, Lake B D (eds) Histochemistry in pathology. Churchill Livingstone, Edinburgh, p 26–33

Holborrow E J, Weir D M, Johnson G D 1957 A serum factor in lupus erythematosus with affinity for tissue nuclei. British Medical Journal 2: 732–734

Taylor C R, Burns J 1974 The demonstration of plasma cells and other immunoglobulin containing cells of formalin-fixed paraffin embedded tissues using peroxidase-labelled antibody. Journal of Clinical Pathology 27: 14–20

**Introduction of formalin-fixed, paraffin-embedded tissue sections**

Burns J, Hambridge M, Taylor C R 1974 Intracellular immunoglobulins. A comparative study on three standard tissue processing methods using horseradish peroxidase and fluorochrome conjugates. Journal of Clinical Pathology 27: 548–557

Curran R C, Gregory J 1978 Demonstration of immunoglobulins in cryostat and paraffin sections of human tonsil by immunofluorescence and immunoperoxidase techniques. Effects of processing on immunocytochemical performance of tissues and on the use of proteolytic enzymes to unmask antigens in sections. Journal of Histochemistry and Cytochemistry 31: 974–983

Heyderman E 1979 Immunoperoxidase technique in histopathology: application, methods and controls. Journal of Clinical Pathology 32: 971–978

Nayak N C, Das P K, Bhuyan U N, Mittal A 1974 Localisation of α-feto protein in human and rat fetal livers: an immunohistochemical method using horseradish peroxidase. Journal of Histochemistry and Cytochemistry 22: 414–418

Nayak N C, Sachdeva R 1975 Localisation of hepatitis B surface antigen in conventional paraffin sections of the liver. American Journal of Pathology 81: 479–492

Oretga L G, Mellors R C 1957 Cellular sites of formation of gamma globulin. Journal of Experimental Medicine 106: 627

Piris J, Thomas N D 1980 A quantitative study of the influence of fixation in immunoperoxidase staining of rectal mucosal plasma cells. Journal of Clinical Pathology 33: 361–364

Sainte-Marie G 1962 A paraffin embedding technique for studies employing immunofluorescence. Journal of Histochemistry and Cytochemistry 10: 250–256

Shikata T 1973 Australia antigen in liver tissue: an immunofluorescent and immunoelectron microscopic study. Japanese Journal of Experimental Medicine 43: 231–245

Streefkirk J G 1972 Inhibition of erythrocyte pseudoperoxidase activity by treatment with hydrogen peroxide following methanol. Journal of Histochemistry and Cytochemistry 20: 829–831

Taylor CR, Burns J 1974 The demonstration of plasma cells and other immunoglobulin containing cells in formalin-fixed, paraffin-embedded tissues using peroxidase-labelled antibody. Journal of Clinical Pathology 27: 14–20

**Introduction of immunocytochemistry to diagnostic histopathology**

Bosman F T, Nieuwenhuijzen-Kruseman A C N 1979 Clinical applications of the enzyme labelled antibody method. Immunoperoxidase methods in diagnostic histopathology. Journal of Histochemistry and Cytochemistry 27: 1140–1147

Bloom S R, Polak J M, Pearse A G E 1973 Vasoactive intestinal peptide and watery-diarrhoea syndrome. Lancet 2: 14–16

Pearse A G E, Bussolati G 1970 Immunofluorescence studies of the distribution of gastrin cells in different clinical states. Gut II: 646–648

Polak J M, Stagg B, Pearse A G E 1972 Two types of Zollinger–Ellison syndrome: immunofluorescence, cytochemical and ultra-structural studies of the antral and pancreatic gastrin cells in different clinical states. Gut 13: 501–512

Polak J M, Van Noorden S 1986 Immunocytochemistry: modern methods and applications, 2nd edn. Wright, Bristol.

Taylor C R, Kledzik G 1981 Immunohistologic techniques in surgical pathology — A spectrum of "new" special stains. Human Pathology 12: 590–596

Williams E D 1966 Histogenesis of medullary carcinoma of the thyroid. Journal of Clinical Pathology 19: 114

**Impact of hybrid monoclonal antibody technology**

Köhler G, Milstein C 1975 Continuous cultures of fused cells secreting antibodies of pre-defined specificity. Nature 256: 495–497

Lee A K, DeLellis R A 1987 Immunohistochemical techniques and their applications to tissue diagnosis. In: Spicer S S (ed) Histochemistry in pathologic diagnosis. Marcel Dekker, New York, p 31–76

Mason D Y, Gatter K C 1987 The role of immunocytochemistry in diagnostic pathology. Journal of Clinical Pathology 40: 1042–

Nadler L M, Ritz J, Griffin J D, Todd R F III, Reinherz E L, Schlossman S F 1981 Diagnosis and treatment of human leukemias and lymphomas utilising monoclonal antibodies. Progress in Haematology 12: 187–225

# 2. Current choice of primary reagents and secondary detection systems

## INTRODUCTION

According to a recent Government-sponsored questionnaire survey in the UK conducted by Angel, Heyderman & Lauder (1989), about 80% of the 178 respondents out of a total of 320 histopathology laboratories surveyed, were found to be using immunocytochemistry. Approximately 70% of the district general hospitals appeared to be using immunocytochemistry and 90% of the teaching hospitals. The major areas of application related to the study of lymph node and epithelial malignancies together comprising approximately 50% of all the cases studied. The renal and skin diseases were the second most frequently studied with immunocytochemistry, together accounting for nearly 25% of all the cases, whilst the endocrine tumour studies accounted for the bulk of the remainder.

For these analyses, some 50 different primary antibody reagents (polyclonal and monoclonal) are used routinely, mainly in conjunction with one or other indirect immunoperoxidase method.

The object of this chapter is to review the currently most widely used set of primary antibody reagents and secondary detection techniques in diagnostic histopathology. The more specialist reagents and techniques are described in the chapters dealing with various specialist applications of immunocytochemistry.

## CURRENT CHOICE OF PRIMARY ANTIBODY MARKERS FOR USE IN GENERAL HISTOPATHOLOGY LABORATORIES

Immunocytochemistry has now become an established adjunct to diagnostic histopathology with more than 70% of district general hospital and virtually all teaching hospital pathology departments using the technique on a routine basis. The diagnostic usefulness of immunocytochemistry is primarily determined by the choice of the available antibody markers capable of typing the presence of diagnostically useful antigens in routinely formalin-fixed, paraffin-embedded and dewaxed tissue sections.

## DIAGNOSTICALLY USEFUL ANTIGENS

There are basically nine distinct categories of potentially useful tissue antigens selected on the basis of their capacity to classify diseases in terms of pathologically important cellular features; these are listed in Table 2.1. The first six varieties of antigen have proved valuable in diagnostic and prognostic evaluation of neoplastic diseases, a practice which accounts for the bulk of the applications of immunocytochemistry in diagnostic histopathology. The cell lineage- and cell differentiation-specific antigenic markers have proved most helpful in the diagnosis of histopathologically difficult or poorly preserved tumours, whilst the cell activation-, proliferation- and invasion-

**Table 2.1** Pathologically important cellular features

1. Cell lineage
2. Cell differentiation
3. Cell activation
4. Cell proliferation
5. Cell invasion
6. Cell clonality
7. Cell inflammation
8. Cell infection
9. Cell degeneration

specific markers have the potential for providing more accurate prognostic classification and assessment of tumours. The cell clonality markers offer the promise of differentiation between benign neoplastic and florid reactive lesions.

The cell inflammation markers are used mainly for diagnostic and prognostic typing of immunologically mediated lesions involving the skin, the kidney or the small blood vessels. The cell infection/infestation markers have a potential role in the typing of occult infections mainly of viral origin. Finally, the cell degeneration-specific markers have proved helpful mainly in the diagnosis of amyloid and related disorders.

## DIAGNOSTICALLY USEFUL ANTIBODY MARKERS

The choice of antibodies capable of typing the presence of the above variety of tissue antigens in the context of diagnostic histopathology is governed by a number of constraints listed in Table 2.2. The diagnostic or prognostic specificity of an antibody marker is defined according to the proportion or percentage of true-negative results yielded by it in relation to a class of differential diagnostically relevant lesions expected to be negative for this marker.

The sensitivity on the other hand relates to the proportion or percentage of true-positive results yielded by the antibody in relation to a class of diagnostically homogeneous lesions expected to be positive with the marker.

The ideal marker for diagnostic analysis is the one which possesses both high specificity and high sensitivity for its target antigen. However, in practice this is rarely found to be the case. Most markers with high specificity ( e.g. >90%) are usually of lower sensitivity (e.g. <70%), and vice versa. Nevertheless it has been found feasible to

achieve higher levels of specificity and sensitivity by use of carefully selected panels of high-affinity monoclonal or polyclonal monospecific antibodies directed against diagnostically relevant antigens.

Versatility relates to the capacity of the antibody to work effectively on a variety of tissue substrates, e.g. tissue or cells either unfixed, or freshly frozen and/or fixed in a variety of fixatives, or embedded in a variety of embedding media. Fortunately, an antibody known to work well in formalin-fixed, paraffin-embedded tissue section is usually liable to prove equally effective in a wide variety of tissue substrate settings, including protease treatment, or exposure to decalcifying fluid or mild bleaches, or embedding in plastic media.

Wherever possible the use of commercially available monoclonal antibody markers is recommended for diagnostic work in order to ensure adequate internal and external quality control. However, the choice of antibodies selected for routine application should also be governed by their overall cost-effectiveness in terms of their purchase price, potency and projected shelf-life.

## CURRENT CHOICE OF DIAGNOSTICALLY RELIABLE ANTIBODY MARKERS

On the basis of the criteria of reliability defined above, the following antibody markers are eligible for use in routine diagnostic practice with respect to the applications listed below. Applications of immunocytochemistry for diagnostic and/or prognostic analysis of lesions of uncertain neoplastic or malignant potential, or of an occult immunological, infective or degenerative disease origin, are best restricted to specialist centres because of their generally greater complexity and cost.

### Malignancy of unknown cell lineage

1. Leucocyte common antigen (LCA; CD45) indicative of a lymphoma
2. Carcinoembryonic antigen (CEA) indicative of carcinoma; also, broad-spectrum cytokeratin (CK) if tumour is negative for VIM, or epithelial membrane antigen (EMA) if the tumour is negative for VIM and LCA
3. Vimentin (VIM) indicative of sarcoma,

**Table 2.2** Constraints on the choice of diagnostically useful antibody markers

1. Specificity
2. Sensitivity
3. Versatility
4. Commercial availability
5. Cost-effectiveness

melanoma or mesothelioma, if tumour is negative for LCA, CEA and CK

4. Chromogranin A (ChA) and/or synaptophysin (SYNAP) indicative of neuroendocrine cell origin; also, neurone-specific enolase (NSE) indicative of neural/neuroendocrine cell origin if tumour is negative for VIM and LCA

5. Placental alkaline phosphatase (PLAP) indicative of a germ cell lineage if tumour is negative for CK.

## Malignancy of unknown cell differentiation

1. Lymphoma
   a. T cell: polyclonal CD3+/UCHL-1 (CD45RO)+/L26(CD20)–
   b. B cell: L26(CD20)+/polyclonal CD3–, and UCHL-1– except for immunoblastic B cell lymphomas
2. Carcinoma
   a. Prostatic: prostate-specific antigen (PSA)+ prostatic acid phosphatase (PAPh)+
   b. Thyroid follicular: thyroglobulin (Tg)+
   c. Thyroid medullary: calcitonin (CAL)+
3. Sarcoma
   a. Skeletal muscle: desmin (DES)+/myoglobin (MYG)+
   b. Smooth muscle: alpha smooth muscle actin (α-SMA)+/DES+/MYG–
   c. Endothelium: Factor VIII-related antigen (F-VIII-RAG)+
4. Other tumours
   a. Melanocyte: S-100+/melanoma marker (HMB45)+/CK–
   b. Mesothelial: CEA– and VIM+/CK+
   c. Histiocytic: CD68+/S-100±

The available spectrum of diagnostically reliable sets of immunocytochemical markers is a testimony and a tribute to the tremendous progress, both scientific and commercial, that has been made in the short period of less than two decades towards establishing immunocytochemistry as a diagnostically useful adjunct to conventional histopathological analysis. Review articles by DeLellis, Angel, Norton and Gatter and colleagues are recommended for a more detailed appraisal of the subject.

## CHOICE OF SECONDARY DETECTION METHODS

Amongst the immunoperoxidase methods, the three most widely used in the UK include the peroxidase–antiperoxidase (PAP), the avidin–biotin complex (ABC) peroxidase, and the simple indirect peroxidase techniques respectively. The basic design and the principal advantages and disadvantages of these techniques are briefly considered below under separate subheadings.

### Simple indirect immunoperoxidase method

This method represents the simplest version of all the immunoperoxidase methods in use in diagnostic histopathology laboratories. It is based on the original method designed by Nakane & Pierce and improved later on by Avrameas, and Nakane & Kawaoi.

*Design*

This is a two-layer technique in which an unlabelled primary antibody is added in the first step followed by HRP-linked secondary antibody conjugate directed at the primary antibody reagent animal species and class-specific immunoglobulin determinants (see Fig. 2.1a for schematic representation).

*Advantages*

**Simplicity and wide commercial availability**. The technique involves only two steps based on a straightforward antigen–antibody interaction rather than the more complex bridge principle. Also, many commercial companies have dedicated themselves to production of high-quality immunoperoxidase conjugates of many different specificities to cover the application of a wide variety of primary antibody reagents.

**Lack of Bigbee effect**. No Bigbee effect is observed at the use of higher concentration of a primary antibody agent, since the method does not involve the use of the antibody bridge principle. (See below for a fuller discussion.)

*Disadvantages*

**Relative lack of efficiency**. The two-step

procedure lacks the efficiency of the three- or multilayer technique because of its lower level of intrinsic amplification (see page 15).

There is also the problem of unavoidable loss of enzyme activity inherent to its chemical coupling with the immunoglobulin molecules. Between 20 and 50% of the enzyme activity is likely to be lost as a result of the chemical coupling, as described by Ishikawa and colleagues. The latter group of workers have described chemical methods using heterobifunctional reagents as opposed to the homobifunctional reagent used by Avrameas, i.e. glutaraldehyde, or the periodic acid method of Nakane & Kawaoi (1974). However, despite their proven advantages, these more sophisticated conjugates have not been widely promoted for use in routine immunocytochemistry.

*Endogenous immunoglobulin interference.* This method is based on the use of a secondary antibody conjugate directed against the primary antibody reagent's animal species- and class-specific immunoglobulin determinants. Hence, it suffers from the severe disadvantage of picking up endogenous immunoglobulins as part of the background staining. This is also true of the PAP and the ABC techniques, especially when applied to tissue preparations derived from animal species donating the primary antibody reagent.

Recently, an indirect immunoperoxidase conjugate with specificity directed at DNP–hapten has become commercially available. This is likely therefore to help overcome the problem of endogenous immunoglobulins in very much the same way as described below for the DNP–hapten-labelled antibody bridge technique.

## Peroxidase–antiperoxidase (PAP) procedure

This method was introduced by Sternberger in the late 1960s as an improvement over the simple

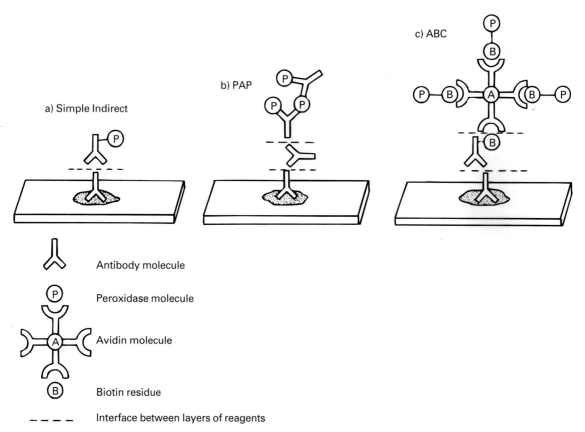

**Fig. 2.1**   Currently popular immunoperoxidase procedures.

two-step indirect immunoperoxidase techniques devised earlier by Nakane and Pierce, and the prototype four-step antibody bridge system of Mason et al (1969).

## Design

The PAP method is a three-layer bridge antibody system in which the unlabelled primary antibody is first applied to the tissue substrate followed by an antibody bridge reagent specific for the primary antibody's species (usually rabbit) and class of immunoglobulins (invariably IgG). This bridge reagent (usually of IgG class) is added in sufficient excess to ensure that it binds to the primary antibody target with only one of its two antigen-binding sites. The free binding sites of the bound bridge molecules are then allowed to interact in the third step with a soluble preformed peroxidase–antiperoxidase (PAP) immune complex. The technique derives its name from the acronym PAP given to this reagent which is prepared using a polyclonal (or monoclonal) antibody specific to horseradish peroxidase (HRP) and is designed to be of the same animal species and immunoglobulin class as the primary antibody reagent.

Thus, as shown in Figure 2.1b, a complex molecular bridge is formed via the bridge antibody (added in the second step) between the primary antibody (added in the first step) and the PAP complexes (added in the third step).

## Advantages

**High specificity**. The bridge formation is exquisitely specific due to the identical specificities of the two binding sites of the bridge antibody reagent. The resulting immunochemically precise one-to-one correspondence between the primary antibody molecules and the PAP complexes is responsible for the technique's renowned capacity to produce very high specificity immunoperoxidase staining.

**High efficiency**. The PAP method is also acknowledged for its high efficiency of antigen detection. This quality is a combined attribute of the PAP complex (capable of delivering three HRP molecules to every bound bridge antibody molecule) and the primary antibody's immunoglobu-

lin structure (capable of accommodating up to 10 antibody bridge molecules to bind to every tissue-bound primary molecule). The overall result is a substantial amplification of the signal at each antigen target site.

## Disadvantages

**Lack of versatility**. According to the design of the PAP technique, for each different species or class of immunoglobulins used as the primary antibody there is a necessity to provide a tailor-made set of bridge antibody and PAP reagents.

This disadvantage can be overcome in principle through the use of hapten-labelled primary antibody and PAP complexes, respectively, in conjunction with an antihapten bridge antibody reagent as originally proposed and described by Jasani et al (1981) (see below, and Fig. 2.2 for illustration of the principle).

**Interference from endogenous immunoglobulins**. Since the bridge antibody's specificity is directed at the antigenic determinants of the primary antibody reagent's animal species and class of immunoglobulins, the use of the PAP procedure on tissues derived from the primary antibody-donating animal species is likely to result in potentially unavoidably high amounts of background staining. This is mainly due to the presence of endogenous immunoglobulins causing direct tissue-binding of the bridge antibody reagent, but also may be due to the binding of the PAP complexes to endogenous Fc receptors. The problem of such non-specific staining is particularly bad in relation to frozen tissue section staining. This disadvantage may also be overcome by the use of any one of the three varieties of the hapten-labelled antibody method (Figs 2.2a, b & c) as successfully attempted recently by Gee et al (1990).

**Bigbee effect**. The bridge antibody reagent, if not added in sufficient excess to fully saturate the amount of the primary antibody bound to the tissue, will tend to bind instead with both its binding sites. Thus the use of supraoptimal primary antibody concentrations is likely to result in a paradoxical drop in the staining intensity, as more and more of the bridge reagent's free valencies are used up in two-site binding. The resulting curve of the intensity of staining versus the primary antibody concentration applied will be bell-shaped instead of the expected rectangular parabola. This phenomenon is true of any bridge system and in the case of the PAP system it is referred to as the Bigbee effect (after Bigbee and his co-workers, who were the first to give a rational explanation of this phenomenon).

This disadvantage has been partly overcome by relegation of the bridge step to one step further beyond the primary antibody step as in the avidin–biotin complex (ABC) immunoperoxidase method described below.

## Avidin–biotin complex (ABC) procedure

This method was introduced by Hsu and co-workers in the early 1980s. It represents a considerable improvement in efficiency compared to the prototype avidin–biotin bridge system originally proposed by Avrameas and co-workers in the early 1970s.

### Design

The ABC is a three-step procedure consisting of an unlabelled primary antibody (added in the first step), an affinity-purified, biotin-labelled anti-immunoglobulin reagent specific to the primary antibody immunoglobulin species (added in the second step) and a preformed avidin–biotin-labelled peroxidase complex with a free valency for biotin (added in the third step). The three layers form a complex of the type shown in Fig. 2.1c at the tissue-binding sites of the primary antibody molecules.

### Advantages

*Higher efficiency*. The preformed avidin–biotin-labelled peroxidase complexes are prepared freshly to give the highest specific activity for HRP enzyme bound to the complex. This is also achieved partly by using biotin-labelled HRP in a form which does not lose its activity on binding to the avidin molecules during the formation of

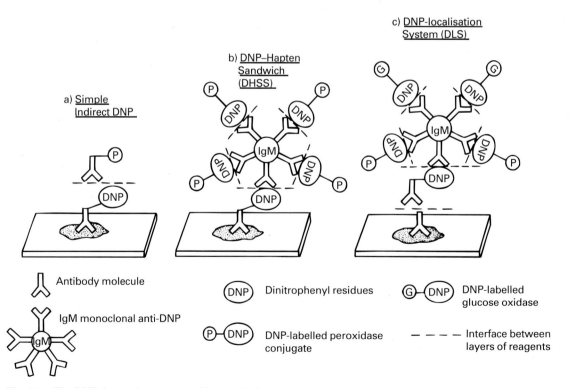

**Fig. 2.2** The DNP–hapten immunoperoxidase methods.

either the avidin enzyme complex in solution or *subsequently* at the tissue antigen site level.

In contrast, the PAP complexes are liable to suffer from a loss in HRP activity from any anti-peroxidase antibody binding too close to the enzyme's active sites. However, this problem again has been overcome recently by Sternberger through use of carefully selected monoclonal per-oxidase antibodies directed at HRP antigen de-terminants located away from the enzyme active site.

*Greater versatility*. The ABC procedure is more versatile than the PAP on the basis that the same ABC enzyme complex may be used for the detection of a variety of primary antibodies belonging to different animal species and immu-noglobulin classes. However, a set of affinity-puri-fied, biotin-labelled secondary antibody reagents directed at the different animal species/classes of immunoglobulin is required to satisfy this condition.

On the other hand, the DNP–hapten-labelled antibody technique allows the use of the same secondary as well as the tertiary layer reagents for virtually any variety of DNP-labelled primary antibodies or other non-antibody primary probes such as those described by Jasani and co-workers.

*Relative abolishment of Bigbee effect*. The ABC procedure has a much-reduced tendency to give paradoxically poor or false-negative results at the higher (i.e. supraoptimal) primary antibody concentrations compared to the PAP technique. This is due to the fact that the bridge complex formation is designed to take place at one step further removed from the primary antibody binding step (see Fig. 2.1c). The same advantage has been successfully introduced recently to the DNP–hapten-labelled antibody technique through the modification of the method into its commer-cially available analogue, the DNP Localization System (Fig. 2.2c).

## Disadvantages

***Interference from endogenous immuno-globulins***. Because the secondary reagent in the ABC procedure is directed at primary antibody immunoglobulin species- and class-specific deter-minants, its use on tissues derived from primary antibody-donating animal species is likely to lead to an unacceptable level of background staining, as already described above for the PAP and the indirect two-step procedures.

Again, the use of the hapten-labelled primary antibodies is probably the most effective way of overcoming this difficulty, as described by Gee et al (1990).

## DNP–hapten sandwich staining (DHSS) procedure

The DHSS procedure was introduced largely to overcome the problem of background staining re-sulting from endogenous immunoglobulins cross-reacting with the secondary detection reagents, as well as any non-specific or unwanted specific pri-mary binding. (See Jasani et al (1981) for dis-cussion of the original rationale and Jasani et al (1992) for the latest review.)

### Design and unique advantages

The prototype technique was based on the PAP method in which the primary antibody and the PAP complexes were introduced in their DNP–hapten-labelled forms. The DNP–hapten-modi-fied PAP technique had the same sensitivity as the conventional PAP method (based on rabbit primary antibody and rabbit PAP immune com-plexes). However, it could be applied to tissues derived from rabbits and other rodents (e.g. rat, mouse or guinea pig) without the fear of endog-enous immunoglobulin-associated background staining. (See Figure 2.3 for a photomicrographic illustration of this advantage.)

The technique proved to have two additional advantages, however, largely accruing from the quality of the DNP-labelling compound and the bridge antibody reagent used in the initial studies.

The DNP-labelled compound was designed to have an imidoester-based chemical coupling func-tional group in order to ensure that the DNP-labelling of immunoglobulins did not lead to any undue inactivation of the antibody activity or in-solubilization of the protein moiety. This was sub-sequently verified by formal studies undertaken by Hewlins et al (1984). Also, it was consistently ob-served that the DNP–imidoester compound could

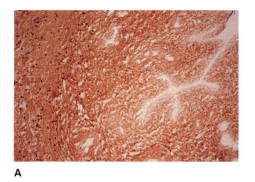

A

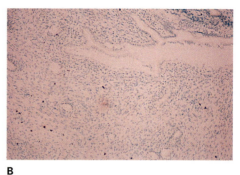

B

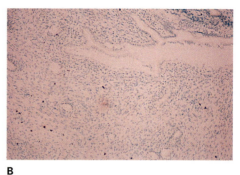

C

**Fig. 2.3** Illustration of the capacity of the DHSS technique to overcome the problem of endogenous immunoglobulin staining affecting the PAP method. (**A**) Application of a rat IgG immunoglobulin-specific PAP reagent system producing marked staining of endogenous immunoglobulins in a frozen section taken from a rat uterus. (**B**) Lack of such staining when applying the DNP–hapten-specific DHSS reagent system. (**C**) Successful detection of rat oestrogen receptors in rat uterine cells (see nuclear staining) obtained using DNP-labelled rat antihuman oestron receptor antibody (H222) applied in conjunction with the DHSS system. DAB–silver enhancement (Amersham) was applied to intensify the staining. (Courtesy of Dr Julia Gee, Tenovus Institute, University of Wales College of Medicine, Cardiff.)

efficiently label a variety of antibody preparations (e.g. polyclonal or monoclonal, IgG or other classes, affinity purified, or in an unfractionated ascites or whole serum state) without any noticeable loss of or difference in their respective immunocytochemical staining activities.

Finally, the compound was found to be capable of labelling non-antibody ligands (e.g. polypeptide hormones) with equal efficacy.

The versatility of the DNP-labelling compound was fully matched by the versatile capacity of the IgM monoclonal anti-DNP bridge antibody reagent to detect DNP groups (covalently linked via the imidoester linkage) on a whole variety of antibody and non-antibody proteins. The result was a highly flexible immunocytochemical detection system capable of detecting any variety of antigens and receptors provided the appropriate DNP-labelled antibodies or receptor ligands were made available. (See Figure 2.2b for a schematic illustration of the basic technique and Schmid et al 1988 for a further discussion of its application for detection of DNP-labelled polypeptide hormone ligand/receptor complexes.)

The uniquely efficient combination of these two

reagents allowed two further advantages of the DHSS procedure to be put into practice. The first related to the technique's alleged capacity to avoid interference from endogenous immunoglobulins. This point was fully put to the test in the recent studies of Gee et al (1991) in which rat monoclonal antibodies to oestrogen receptors were applied to rat tissues to determine their receptor status by immunocytochemical means.

The second advantage resulted from the multivalent character of the IgM anti-DNP bridge reagent. Thus it was initially proposed by Williams (Jasani et al 1985a) that it may be possible to improve the specificity signal generation by the DNP–peroxidase (added in the third step) if it were to receive its obligate substrate, $H_2O_2$ from DNP-labelled glucose oxidase bound to the same set of IgM bridge molecules (Fig. 2.2c).

The application of DNP–glucose oxidase in combination with DNP–peroxidase was found in practice to result in a remarkably high signal intensification without any concomitant increase in the background (Jasani et al 1985b, Kumar et al 1985).

The glucose–oxidase principle has therefore

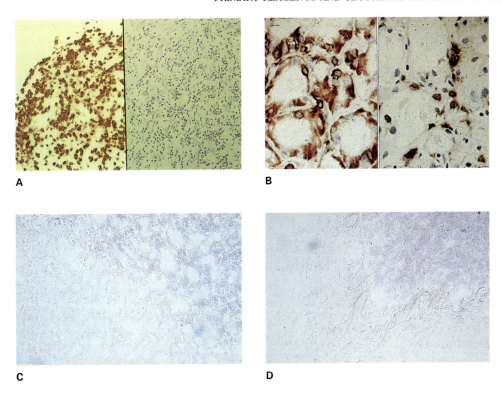

**Fig. 2.4**  Illustration of the non-deleterious nature of the sodium azide/glucose oxidase/glucose method for inhibiting endogenous peroxidase developed by Andrews & Jasani (1987) for frozen sections and subsequently successfully applied by Hittmair & Schmid (1989) to formalin-fixed, paraffin-embedded sections. (**A**) Very strong endogenous peroxidatic staining (left panel) due to a large presence of eosinophils in a case of Hodgkin's lymphoma, completely inhibited (right panel) by the sodium azide method. (**B**) Similar inhibition of endogenous thyroid peroxidase activity with full retention of OKT8 (CD8) staining (DHSS procedure). (**C**) The deleterious effect of the methanol/H$_2$O$_2$ regimen on neurofilament in contrast to (**D**) the non-deleterious nature of the sodium azide system (two-step) indirect immunoperoxidase method).

been adopted as a regular feature of the DHSS procedure (see Jasani et al 1992 for a full review).

*Disadvantages*

The DHSS procedure has been found in practice to suffer from two main disadvantages.

***Instability of DNP–PAP complexes***. The DNP-labelled PAP complexes are less stable than their unlabelled counterparts. Hence, it has been necessary to replace them with a covalently stable conjugate of DNP and horseradish peroxidase (HRP) in which cytochrome C (CC) has been introduced as a relatively small lysine residue-rich carrier to bear the DNP groups (Jasani et al 1983, Newman & Jasani 1984). The resulting enzyme marker, DNP–CC–HRP, is much smaller than its

PAP analogue, with an average molecular weight of around 100 kDa compared to the minimum of 900 kDa for the PAP complexes. The DNP–CC–HRP has therefore proved to be an excellent high-resolution marker for immunoperoxidase labelling under the electron microscope (Newman & Jasani 1984).

***Bigbee effect***. The DHSS procedure, being based on an antibody bridge principle, suffers from the Bigbee effect described for the PAP method. (See above for a further discussion.) An attempt has been made to alleviate this in two possible ways, as follows.

In the first approach, similar to the ABC complex method, an extra reagent intervening between the primary antibody and the enzyme marker has been introduced (Jasani et al 1986).

This has led to the development of the four-layer commercially available DNP Localization System (DLS) by Bioclinical Services Ltd (Cardiff, Wales, UK).

More recently, the introduction of a reliable indirect peroxidase conjugate to DNP by Dakopatts Ltd (Copenhagen, Denmark) has permitted the development of a simple two-step procedure for detecting DNP-labelled primary antibodies. This method, which is entirely free of the Bigbee effect, has proved particularly useful in simultaneous double immunolabelling of antigens (Navabi et al 1990, Nair et al 1991).

The two varieties of commercially available DNP–hapten-directed indirect immunoperoxidase technique are schematically illustrated in Figure 2.2 in comparison with the prototype DHSS procedure.

## Chromogen choice for immunoperoxidase staining

The popularity of the immunoperoxidase method in diagnostic histopathology laboratories is based not only on the advantages of the various techniques described above but also on the high quality of the staining deposited by the peroxidase enzyme. From the very beginning the most favoured chromogen has been diaminobenzidine (DAB). The obligate substrate of the peroxidase enzyme, hydrogen peroxide, $H_2O_2$, oxidatively polymerizes diaminobenzidine to a brown polymeric compound which has the following four virtues making it the first choice chromogen for immunoperoxidase staining reactions:

1. The DAB polymer is a highly tenacious substance which sticks virtually instantaneously and irreversibly to the tissue at the precise site of its generation.

2. The DAB polymer is also very resistant to alkali, acids and various dehydrants such as alcohols and xylene, and is therefore a virtually permanently stable product which does not diffuse or fade in its intensity even after many years of storage.

3. The colour or shade of the DAB deposit varies from smooth yellow amber to dark brown which contrasts well with the blue of the haema-toxylin nuclear counterstain widely used in histopathological practice.

4. The DAB polymer has high affinity for heavy metal salts such as osmium tetroxide, gold chloride, cobalt chloride, etc., allowing its colour intensity and quality to be improved for light as well as electron microscopic viewing.

The last described property of the DAB product has been exploited by Newman, Jasani & Williams (1983a & b) to generate highly specific silver deposition (using a light-insensitive physical development system) to intensify and render visible trace amounts of DAB deposits. The commercial analogue of this is the Amersham DAB Silver Enhancement Kit.

## Endogenous peroxidatic activity

Despite the histochemically ideal quality of the product generated by the immunoperoxidase technique, which largely accounts for its continuing long-standing success in diagnostic histopathology, it carries with it the problem of background staining due to ubiquitously present endogenous peroxidase activity (EPA).

The EPA is expressed by a wide variety of proteins bearing the biochemically active protoporphyrin IX haem group. These include various mammalian cell peroxidases, for example, myeloperoxidase, present in eosinophils and neutrophils, thyroid peroxidase, present in thyroid follicular cells, and lactoperoxidase, associated with breast epithelium. The activity is also exhibited by non-enzymic proteins such as haemoglobin, myoglobin and various cytochromes. The staining resulting from these sources is collectively referred to as endogenous peroxidase staining.

Because of the very wide distribution of the sources of endogenous peroxidase staining, virtually every immunoperoxidase study is subject to interference from this kind of staining. Fortunately, barring a certain variety of myeloperoxidase activity associated with the bone marrow cells and eosinophils, all other types of the EPA are highly susceptible to complete quenching by a simple methanol/hydrogen peroxide ($H_2O_2$) regimen first described by Streefkirk, and later on recommended for use in diagnostic studies by Burns et al (1974).

The methanol/$H_2O_2$ mixture is simple and easy to apply and well tolerated by the vast majority of the antigens preserved in formalin-fixed, paraffin-embedded tissue sections, allowing its inclusion in the routine immunocytochemical staining protocol with minimum inconvenience and negligible loss in the antigen detection sensitivity of the overall technique.

However, for unprotected or delicate antigens (e.g. in lightly fixed cell smears and frozen tissue sections) the methanol/$H_2O_2$ method is seriously damaging to the tissue morphology and the antigens. Hence a number of non-deleterious methods have been devised. The most effective and practical of these for routine application has proved to be the sodium oxide/$H_2O_2$ in a buffered aqueous solution as proposed by Jasani, Schmid and colleagues for use on frozen as well as formalin-fixed, paraffin-embedded tissue sections. (See Figure 2.4 for a photomicrographic illustration of the effectiveness of this reagent system.) For bone marrow specimens alkaline phosphatase has been recommended by Mason and colleagues as the preferred enzyme marker.

More recently there has been a growing interest in avoiding the problem of endogenous staining through the use of a non-enzymatic secondary detection system such as the colloidal gold particle-linked antibody conjugate method. The potential of this novel approach to immunocytochemical staining in diagnostic histopathology remains to be evaluated.

## REFERENCES AND FURTHER READING

### Introduction

Angel C A, Heyderman E, Lauder I 1989 Use of immunocytochemistry in Britain: EQA Forum antibody usage questionnaire. Journal of Clinical Pathology 42: 1012–1017

### Current choice of primary antibody reagents

Bobrow L G, Norton A J 1987 Immunohistology in the identification of tumour types. Cancer Surveys 6: 209

Corwin D J, Gown A M 1989 Review of selected lineage-directed antibodies useful in routinely processed tissues. Archives of Pathological Laboratory Medicine 113: 645–652

Leong A S-Y, Wright J 1987 The contribution of immunocytochemical staining in tumour diagnosis. Histopathology 11: 1295–1305

### Choice of primary reagents

DeLellis R A, Dayal Y 1987 The role of immunocytochemistry in the diagnosis of poorly differentiated malignant neoplasms. Seminars in Oncology 14: 173–192

Gatter K C 1989 Diagnostic immunocytochemistry achievements and challenges. C L Oakley Lecture 1989. Journal of Pathology 159: 183–190

Norton A J, Isaacson P G 1989 Lymphoma phenotyping in formalin-fixed and paraffin wax-embedded tissues: II. Profiles of reactivity in the various tumour types. Histopathology 14: 557–579

### Simple indirect immunoperoxidase method

Avrameas S 1969 Coupling enzymes to proteins with glutaraldehyde: use of conjugates for the detection of antigens and antibodies. Immunocytochemistry 6: 43–52

Bigbee J W, Kosek J C, Eng L F 1977 Effects of primary antiserum dilution on staining of antigen rich tissues with peroxidase–anti-peroxidase techniques. Journal of Histochemistry and Cytochemistry 25: 443–447

Heyderman E 1989 Immunoperoxidase technique in histopathology: application, methods and controls. Journal of Clinical Pathology 32: 971–978

Nakane P K, Kawaoi A 1974 Peroxidase labelled antibody. A new method of conjugation. Journal of Histochemistry and Cytochemistry 22: 1084–1091

Nakane P K, Pierce G B 1966 Enzyme-labelled antibodies: preparation and application for the localisation of antigens. Journal of Histochemistry and Cytochemistry 14: 929–931

### Peroxidase–antiperoxidase (PAP) procedure

Bigbee J W, Kosek J C, Eng L F 1977 Effects of primary antiserum dilution on staining of antigen rich tissues with peroxidase–anti peroxidase techniques. Journal of Histochemistry and Cytochemistry 25: 443–447

Gee J M W, Nicholson R I, Jasani B et al 1990 An immunocytochemical method for localisation of estrogen receptors in rat tissues using a dinitrophenyl (DNP) labelled rat monoclonal primary antibody. Journal of Histochemistry and Cytochemistry 38: 69–78

Jasani B, Wynford-Thomas D, Williams E D 1981 Use of monoclonal anti-hapten antibodies for immunolocalisation of tissue antigens. Journal of Clinical Pathology 34: 1000–1002

Jasani B, Edwards R E, Thomas N D, Gibbs A R 1985 The use of vimentin antibodies in the diagnosis of malignant mesothelioma. Virchows Archiv A, Pathological Anatomy and Histopathology 406: 441–448

Mason T E, Phifer R F, Spicer S S, Swallow R A, Dreskin R B 1969 An immunoglobulin-enzyme bridge method for localising tissue antigens. Journal of Histochemistry and Cytochemistry 17: 563–569

Nakane P K, Pierce G B 1966 Enzyme-labelled antibodies; preparation and application for the localisation of antigens. Journal of Histochemistry and Cytochemistry 14: 929–931

Sternberger L A, Hardy P H, Cuculis J J, Meyer H G 1970

The unlabelled antibody enzyme method of immunocytochemistry. Preparation and properties of soluble antigen–antibody complex (horseradish peroxidase–anti-horseradish peroxidase) and its use in the identification of spirochaetes. Journal of Histochemistry and Cytochemistry 18: 315–333

Wofsy L, Henry C, Cammisulis 1978 Hapten-sandwich labelling of cell surface antigens. Contemporary Topics in Molecular Immunology 7: 215–237

## Avidin–biotin complex (ABC) procedure

Gee J M, Nicholson R I, Jasani B et al 1990 An immunocytochemical method for localisation of estrogen receptors in rat tissues using a clinitrophenyl (DNP)-labelled rat monoclonal primary antibody. Journal of Histochemistry and Cytochemistry 38: 69–78

Guesdon J L, Ternynck T, Avrameas S 1978 The use of avidin–biotin interacting in immunoenzyme techniques. Journal of Histochemistry and Cytochemistry 27: 1131–1139

Hsu S M, Raine L, Fanger H 1981 Use of a avidin–biotin peroxidase complex (ABC) in immunoperoxide technique: a comparison between ABC and unlabelled antibody (PAP) procedures. Journal of Histochemistry and Cytochemistry 29: 577–580

Jasani B, Wynford-Thomas D W, Williams E D 1981 Use of monoclonal anti-hapten antibodies for immunolocalisation of tissue antigens. Journal of Clinical Pathology 34: 1000–1002

Schmid K W, Jasani B, Morgan J M, Williams E D 1988 Light microscopic immunocytochemical demonstration of thyroid-stimulating hormone (TSH) receptors on normal rat thyroid cells. Journal of Histochemistry and Cytochemistry 36: 977–982

## DNP–hapten sandwich staining (DHSS) procedure

Gee J M W, Nicholson R I, Jasani B et al 1990 An immunocytochemical method for localisation of oestrogen receptors in rat tissue using a dinitrophenyl (DNP)-labelled rat monoclonal primary antibody. Journal of Histochemistry and Cytochemistry 38: 69–78

Hewlins M J E, Weeks I, Jasani B 1984 Non-deleterious dinitrophenyl (DNP)-hapten labelling of antibody protein: preparation and properties of some short-chain DNP imido-esters. Journal of Immunological Methods 70: 111–118

Jasani B, Wynford-Thomas D, Williams E D 1981 Use of monoclonal anti-hapten antibodies for immunolocalisation of tissue antigens. Journal of Clinical Pathology 34: 1000–1002

Jasani B, Thomas N D, Newman G R, Williams E D 1983a DNP–hapten sandwich staining (DHSS) procedure: design, sensitivity, versatility and applications. Immunological Communications 12: 50

Jasani B, Edwards R E, Thomas N D, Gibbs A R 1985 The use of vimentin antibodies in the diagnosis of malignant mesothelioma. Virchows Archiv A, Pathologic Anatomy 406: 441–448

Jasani B, Thomas N D, Ludgate M, Williams E D 1986 Adaptation of dinitrophenyl (DNP)–hapten sandwich staining (DHSS) procedure for screening monoclonal antibodies. Proceedings of Royal Microscopical Society 20: 1M7

Jasani B, Thomas N D, Navabi H, Millar D M, Newman G R, Gee J, Williams E D 1992 Dinitrophenyl (DNP) Localisation system: a review of principle reagents and applications developed over past 10 years. Journal of Immunological Methods 50: 193–198

Kumar S, Jasani B, Hunt J S et al 1985 A system for accurate immunolocalization of Tamm–Horsfall protein in renal biopsies. Histochemical Journal 17: 1251–1258

Navabi H, Morgan J M, Jasani B 1990 Simultaneous L and K isotype immunolabelling of plasma cells (PCS) in Graves' disease (GT) for estimation of light chain restriction at individual patient level. Journal of Pathology 160: 152A

Nair S, Navabi H, Jasani B 1991 High frequency of light chain restricted plasma cells in primary B-cell gastric lymphoma demonstrated by double immunolabelling. Journal of Pathology 164: 348A

Newman G R, Jasani B 1984 Post-embedding immunoenzyme techniques. In: Polak J M, Varndell I (eds) Immunolabelling for electron microscopy. Elsevier, Amsterdam, p 53–70

Schmid K W, Jasani B, Morgan J M, Williams E D 1988 Light microscopic immunocytochemical demonstration of thyroid-stimulating hormone (TSH) receptors on rat thyroid cells. Journal of Histochemistry and Cytochemistry 36: 977–982

## Chromogen choice for immunoperoxidase staining

Newman G R, Jasani B, Williams E D 1983a Metal compound intensification of the electron-density of diaminobenzidine. Journal of Histochemistry and Cytochemistry 31: 1430–1434

Newman G R, Jasani B, Williams E D 1983b The visualization of trace amounts of diaminobenzidine (DAB) polymer by a novel gold-sulphide-silver method. Journal of Microscopy 32: RPI–RP2

## Endogenous peroxidatic activity

Andrew S, Jasani B 1987 An improved method for the inhibition of endogenous peroxidase non-deleterious to lymphocyte surface markers. Application of immunoperoxidase studies on eosinophil-rich tissue preparations. Histochemical Journal 19: 426–430

Burns J, Hambridge M, Taylor C R 1974 Intracellular immunoglobulins. A comparative study on three standard tissue processing methods using horseradish peroxidase and fluorochrome conjugates. Journal of Clinical Pathology 27: 548–557

Cordell J L, Falini B, Erber W, Gatter K C, Mason D Y 1984 Immunoenzymatic labelling of monoclonal antibodies using complexes of alkaline phosphatase and monoclonal anti-alkaline phosphate (APAAP) complexes. Journal of Histochemistry and Cytochemistry 32: 219–229

Hacker G W, Springall D R, Van Noorden S, Bishop A E, Grimelius L, Polak J M 1985 The immunogold–silver staining method: A powerful tool in histopathology. Virchows Archiv. (Pathologic Anatomy) 406: 449–461

Hittmair A, Schmid K W 1989 Inhibition of endogenous peroxidase for the immunohistochemical demonstration of intermediate filament proteins (IFP). Journal of Immunological Methods 116: 199–205

Streefkirk J G 1972 Inhibition of erythrocyte pseudoperoxidase activity by treatment with hydrogen peroxide following methanol. Journal of Histochemistry and Cytochemistry 20: 829–831

# 3. Role and scope of immunocytochemistry in routine histopathological analysis

The object of this chapter is to discuss how and to what extent immunocytochemistry is useful in diagnostic histopathology.

In order to appreciate the role and scope of immunocytochemistry in a histopathological approach to diagnostic and prognostic analysis of disease, it is necessary to have a basic understanding of the commonly used tissue preparative methods and histological stains as well as the widely practised approaches to diagnosis and classification of disease on morphological grounds. A comprehensive account of histological tissue preparation and staining techniques is given by Culling et al (1985).

## ROUTINE TISSUE PREPARATIVE METHOD

### Fixation

The most widely used fixative is a 4% solution of formaldehyde in physiological saline (i.e. 0.15 M NaCl solution in water). This fixative, which is also known as 10% formol–saline, is a slowly progressive fixative achieving adequate fixation (aldehyde-mediated chemical cross-linking of proteinaceous amine groups) only after 12 to 24 h, depending upon the size or depth of tissue considered. Ideally, the tissue should be trimmed down to a size no bigger than 1 cm$^3$ for adequate and even fixation. Beyond this critical 1 cm depth, the tissue is progressively more likely to be fixed by subsequent tissue dehydration steps alone.

### Dehydration and embedding

Following fixation, the tissue is dissected if necessary to expose the lesion and take appropriate blocks from it for paraffin wax embedding. The tissue blocks are placed in their proper orientation (whenever possible) in standard plastic cassettes and transferred through a mechanized series of alcohol (absolute ethanol) and xylene changes in order to achieve complete dehydration.

The dehydrated blocks are most commonly embedded in paraffin wax (melting point 55–60°C), again using a standard mechanized system.

### Sectioning

A set of serial sections, usually of 5 μm thickness, are taken from the most representative portion of each tissue block. Individual sections are taken on to plain glass slides, ensuring that they are all in the same orientation with respect to each other. The slides are inscribed permanently with the respective block and case numbers, and incubated in a 60°C oven to allow the sections to dry flat and firmly on to the glass surface.

### Staining

One section from every tissue block is stained with standard haematoxylin and eosin (H&E) stain usually on an automatic staining machine. Additional routine or special stains (listed in Table 3.1) are included depending on the nature of the tissue specimen and tissue elements comprising the target of the main diagnostic inquiry.

### Microscopic examination and evaluation

The H&E-stained sections constitute the primary basis of all morphological analysis. In 90–95% of routinely analysed cases, the morphological features revealed by sections stained with H&E and

**Table 3.1**  Additional routine and special stains for histological identification of various tissue elements

| Tissue | Stain | Target tissue element |
|---|---|---|
| Kidney | PAS | Basement membrane |
| | Methanamine silver | Immune complex deposits |
| | | Mesangium |
| | | Basement membrane |
| Skin | Phloxine–tartrazine | Keratin |
| | Orcein | Elastin |
| | Toludine blue | Mast cells |
| | | Melanin |
| | | Peripheral nerves |
| Diffuse neuroendocrine system | Masson–Hampert argentaffin | EC1 and EC2 cells |
| | Gomori's aldehyde fuchsin | B cells in pancreas |
| | Grimelius' argyrophil | Most cells of the diffuse neuroendocrine system except 'B' and 'D' cells of the pancreatic islets and 'I' cells of the upper small intestine |
| Gastrointestinal tract | Mucus stains | Glandular cells |
| | Acetylcholinesterase | Ganglion cells |
| Lymph nodes | Methyl green pyronin | Plasma cells |
| | Reticular stains | Reticular network |
| | Chloroacetate esterases | Granulocytes |
| | | Promylocytes |
| Bone marrow | May–Grünwald–Giemsa | Haematopoietic cells |
| | Methyl green pyronin | Plasma cells |
| | Perl's | Haemosiderin |
| Muscle | Verhoeff–Van Gieson | Muscle (yellow) |
| | Engel–Cunningham modification of Heidenhaim's iron | Mitochondria, elastic and myelin (black) |
| | Phosphotungstic acid–haematoxylin | Muscle cross-striations |
| | Congo red | Amyloid |
| | Methylene blue | Nerve fibres and endings |
| Anterior pituitary | PAS–orange G | Basophils (magenta) |
| | | Acidophils (orange) |
| | | Chromophobes (pale blue/grey) |

one or more of the additional routine or special stains are sufficient to provide adequate diagnostic and prognostic evaluation. In the remaining 5–10% of cases the help of immunocytochemical staining is usually deemed necessary. The type of primary antibody markers needed will depend on the nature of the underlying disease and the kind of histological difficulty encountered.

There are ultimately three basic varieties of disease process: neoplastic, inflammatory and degenerative. Similarly, there are in essence three principal varieties of histological difficulty encountered. The first two relate to the central need to identify the disease cell population with respect to its lineage and type of differentiation respectively, whilst the third relates to the less frequently encountered need to identify and/or characterize the underlying aetiopathogenic agent or mechanism with the view to making a prognostic or a therapeutic judgement.

The immunocytochemical markers helpful in the identification of cell lineage/differentiation are listed in Table 3.2. The markers useful for aetiopathogenetic analysis of diseases are considered in Chapter 15.

The diagnostic usefulness of immunocytochemical marking derives from the tacit assumption, relevant to every histopathological analysis, that a disease process is usually the result of a single dominant aetiopathogenetic mechanism involving a single tissue or cell lineage-specific target. Thus the more specifically and sensitively the diseased tissue or cell lineage is typed, the greater is likely to be the accuracy of the resultant diagnosis. In this context, immunocytochemical markers, because of their intrinsically greater specificity and sensitivity for tissue or cell lineage parameters, offer a better potential for achieving a diagnosis or prognostic classification with greater certainty than their histological or histochemical counterparts used on their own.

**Table 3.2** Immunocytochemical cell lineage/differentiation markers

| Tissue and cell types | Primary antibody markers |
|---|---|
| *Lymphoreticular tissue* | |
| Leucocytes | CD45 (PD7/26-2B11) |
| B lymphocytes | L26 (CD20-associated); MB2; MT2 |
| T lymphocytes | CD3 (polyclonal); CD45RO (UCHL-1); CD43 (MTI) |
| Natural killer cells | CD57 (Leu7) |
| Mononuclear phagocyte series cells | CD68 (KP1; EBM11); MAC387 |
| *Epithelial tissue* | |
| GROUP 1 | |
| Hepatocellular | Cytokeratin (e.g. CAM5.2) |
| Neuroendocrine | |
| Renal | |
| Endometrial | |
| Colonic | |
| GROUP 2 | |
| Breast | Cytokeratin |
| Pancreatic | Epidermal keratin (e.g. rabbit) |
| | Polyclonal antibody (Dakopatts) |
| Ovarian | |
| Lung | |
| Meso-omental | |
| Transitional thymus | |
| GROUP 3 | |
| Squamous | Epidermal keratin |
| *Connective tissue* | |
| All varieties | Vimentin |
| Muscle | Desmin; α-actin; myosin; myoglobin |
| Fibroplast | Vimentin |
| Endothelium | Factor VIII-related antigen |
| *Neuroendocrine tissue* | |
| All varieties | Neurone-specific enolase |
| Restricted varieties | Chromogranin A; Leu7; synaptophysin |
| *Neural tissue* | |
| All varieties | Neurone-specific enolase |
| Neuronal cells | Neurofilament |
| Schwann cells | Leu7; S-100 |
| Glial cells | GFAP |
| Astrocytes | |
| Ependymal | |
| Oligodendroglial | |
| Microglial cells | CD68 (KP1; EBM11) |
| *Mixed tissue lineage* | |
| Mesothelial cells | Vimentin+/cytokeratin+/CEA– |
| *Germ tissue* | |
| Spermatogenic cells | Placental alkaline phosphatase |
| Chrorionic villus cells | Human chrorionic gonadotrophin |
| *Unclassifiable tissue* | |
| Melanocytes | M3080+/S-100+/Vimentin+/cytokeratin– |

In the next section a brief account is given of the specificity and sensitivity of immunocytochemical marking in relation to histopathological definition and classification of disease.

A formal treatment of the subject is given by Makuch & Muenz (1987) in an excellent review article. A discussion of specificity and sensitivity in relation to individual applications of immunocytochemical marking in histopathology is also to be found in the elegant text compiled by Wick & Siegal (1988).

## SENSITIVITY AND SPECIFICITY OF IMMUNOCYTOCHEMICAL MARKING

The disease specificity and sensitivity of individual primary antibody reagents are defined according to the following two equations, respectively:

$$\text{Specificity} = \frac{\text{number of observed negative results}}{\text{total number of expected negative results.}}$$

$$\text{Sensitivity} = \frac{\text{number of observed positive results}}{\text{total number of expected positive results.}}$$

In essence, specificity and sensitivity of a given marker are both inversely related to the rates of false-positive and false-negative observations respectively, made on a defined set of diseased entities using a particular secondary detection technique. The two parameters are fundamentally dependent upon the affinity and the dilution of the primary and secondary antibodies used, the temperature and the duration of their application to the tissue substrate as well as the relative abundance of the immunoreactive target antigen present in the tissues analysed. Their values also depend on how accurately the diseased specimens chosen to represent the positive and the negative controls have been selected in the first place.

Hence sensitivity and specificity are multifactorial attributes of immunocytochemical markers, the significance of which in relation to a given diagnostic inquiry is likely to vary according to the set of conditions used. In a sense their significance is as variable as the meanings of words or expressions used in the context of a language. They depend upon the syntax and do not have an absolute meaning of their own.

For example, in the context of all varieties of epithelial malignancies studied by Swanson (1988),

the overall specificity and sensitivity of the epithelial cell lineage marker, HMFGII, were determined to be 89.1% and 84.8% respectively. However, the same marker was found to have 100% sensitivity with respect to renal-cell carcinoma, eccrine adnexal carcinoma of the skin, all varieties of breast, pulmonary and gastrointestinal carcinomas except the neuroendocrine variety, and the bladder, uterine, ovarian and thymic carcinomas. Similarly it had 100% specificity in discrimination of melanomas from carcinomas, with 43 out of 43 melanomas examined proving to be uniformly negative.

Of all the markers examined so far, the leucocyte common antigen marker studied by Wick (1988) appears to have demonstrably the highest sensitivity and specificity for recognition of a particular cell lineage in the context of histopathological analysis. Thus all of the 375 non-haematopoietic neoplasms tested proved negative (i.e. 100% specificity), and 284 out of 290 non-Hodgkin's lymphomas proved to be positive (i.e. 98% sensitivity).

Most other markers with high specificity (>90%) for cell lineage/differentiation recognition have proved to have relatively low sensitivity (<70%). In a situation where several independent high-specificity but low-sensitivity markers are available for recognition of a single cell or tissue lineage/differentiation, it is possible to improve the sensitivity of detection through use of a combination of these in the form of a panel of markers.

It is equally possible to use a combination of very high-sensitivity but relatively low-specificity markers to increase the specificity of detection or exclusion of a particular cell lineage/differentiation.

Examples of the use of a panel of primary antibodies to improve either the sensitivity or specificity of immunocytochemical marking are given in the chapters to follow.

## COST-EFFECTIVENESS AND PEDIGREE HISTORY

Other factors which limit the use of immunocytochemical markers in diagnostic histopathology relate to their cost-effectiveness in terms of their purchase price, potency and shelf-life. Their wider acceptability is also dependent on their track record in the hands of expert immunohistopathologists responsible for their introduction and initial testing.

REFERENCES AND FURTHER READING

**Routine tissue preparation and staining**

Culling C F A, Allison R T, Barr W T 1985 Cellular
pathology technique. Butterworth, London

**Sensitivity and specificity of immunocytochemical
marking**

Makuch R W, Muenz L R 1987 Evaluating the adequacy of
tumour markers to discriminate amongst distinct
populations. Seminars in Oncology 14: 89–101
Wick M R, Siegal G P 1988 Monoclonal antibodies in
diagnostic immunohistochemistry. Marcel Dekker,
New York, p 7–12
Swanson P E 1988 Monoclonal antibodies to human milk fat
globule proteins. In: Wick M R, Siegal G P (eds)
Monoclonal antibodies in diagnostic
immunohistochemistry. Marcel Dekker, New York
p 227–283
Wick M R 1988 Monoclonal antibodies to leucocyte common
antigen. In: Wick M R, Siegal G P (eds) Monoclonal
antibodies in diagnostic immunocytochemistry. Marcel
Dekker, New York, p 285–307

# PART II

# Immunocytochemistry in diagnosis of neoplastic diseases

# 4. Lymphoreticular tumours

## INTRODUCTION

Peripheral lymphoid tissue consists of the regional lymph nodes and the spleen, and the lymphocyte-rich extranodal tissue principally associated with the mucosal linings of the gastrointestinal and respiratory tracts.

Proliferative disorders of lymphoid tissue of interest to the histopathologist include a variety of neoplastic and reactive lesions arising mainly from the lymphocyte and myelomonocyte lineage cells normally resident in or infiltrating the lymphoid tissue. These include the B lymphocytes, the T lymphocytes, the mononuclear phagocytes, and their respective developmentally distinct subsets.

## EMBRYOLOGY

The first blood cells are formed in the wall of the yolk sac in close association with the formation of the first blood vessels. Thus, when the blood islands differentiate from the angioblasts, some of the cells at the periphery of the islands form the walls of the blood vessels, whilst other more centrally placed cells remain in the lumina of the blood vessels and produce blood cells. These cells are referred to as the haematopoietic stem cells and give rise to all of the fetal red cells and leucocytes. As blood vessels ramify throughout the connective tissue of the body, certain regions of the intraembryonic connective tissue develop the capacity to generate blood cells. Hence, the main site of blood production switches from the yolk sac first to the liver, then to the spleen, the mesonephros and finally to the bone marrow.

## ANATOMICAL AND IMMUNOPHENOTYPIC FEATURES

The pluripotential haematopoietic stem cells give rise to two restricted potential stem cells: the lymphoid and the myeloid stem cells. The former in turn gives rise to the progenitor cells of the lymphocyte series of cells, whilst the latter is responsible for generating the progenitor cells of the myelomonocyte, the erythroid and the megakaryocyte series of cells.

The development of these progenitor cells into their respective mature cell variants is a multistep process as outlined schematically in Figure 4.1 and described in greater detail below.

### B lymphocytes

The pro-B cells are thought to be the earliest progenitor cells of the B lymphocyte series cells. They give rise to the pre-pre-B cells which are the first cells to express positivity for the B cell lineage-specific antibody marker, CD19 (the CD classification system for numbering cell lineage- and differentiation-specific antibodies is defined in a section to follow).

The pre-pre-B cells undergo the first round of immunoglobulin gene rearrangement involving the immunoglobulin heavy chain genes on chromosome 14, and produce cytoplasmic μ heavy chains, cμ. The cells at this stage are referred to as the pre-B cells and exhibit CD19+, cμ+ status. Further gene rearrangements, this time in the kappa (κ), followed by the lambda (λ), gene loci on chromosomes 22 and 2, respectively, lead to the production of cytoplasmic κ or λ light chains

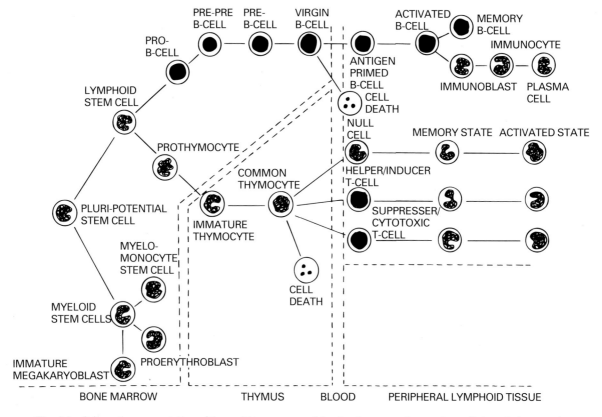

**Fig. 4.1** Schematic representation of the multistep process of the development of progenitor cells into their respective mature cell variants.

which combine with the cell to form the surface receptor immunoglobulin referred to as sIgM. Thus the pre-B cells are converted into virgin immunocompetent B cells possessing the CD19+, sIgM+ marker status.

The virgin B cells leave the bone marrow via the bloodstream to enter the peripheral lymphoid tissue. Here they mature both morphologically and functionally if they encounter an antigen capable of interacting with their surface IgM receptors with high affinity, or die apoptotically if they fail to do so. The immunocytochemically recognizable morphological and functional development of the B cells in the peripheral lymphoid tissue is outlined schematically in Figure 4.2. The virgin B cells are small lymphocyte cells with small, round nuclei and scant cytoplasm. These, under the influence of T helper/inducer (CD4+) and interfollicular dendritic reticulum cells (IDRCS), mature first into as yet unrecognized follicular B cell blasts. In primary immunization, just a few of

these are presumed to act as the precursors of all the centroblasts and centrocytes of the dark and light zones, respectively, of individual secondary B cell follicles. In secondary immunization, they presumably develop from the memory B cells of the mantle zone, and progress to become either the proliferatively active immunoblasts or their end products, the plasma cells.

The progression of the virgin B cells from the centroblast/centrocyte stage to the plasma cell level of maturation also appears to be under the control of the T helper/inducer (CD4+) cells, acting in conjunction this time with the follicular dendritic reticulum cells (FDRCs) as the antigen-presenting cells (APCs).

During this maturation the B cells undergo class switching from IgM to IgG (or IgA or IgE) production as well as somatic point mutations within the variable region genes including the antigen-binding site of the antibody molecule. Thus the cells undergoing immunoblast transformation,

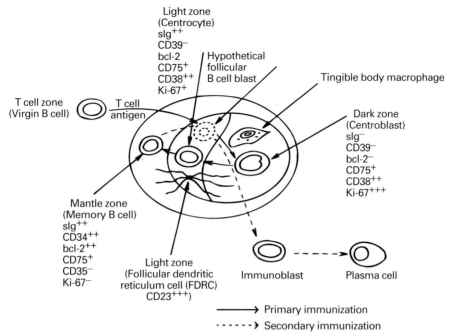

**Fig. 4.2**   Immunocytochemically identifiable micro-anatomy of a secondary lymphoid follicle (after Ling 1988; Liu et al 1992).

as well as the plasma cells resulting from them, are found to be positive predominantly for cytoplasmic IgG or IgA and exhibit relatively unique or private idiotypes reflective of the somatically point-mutated character of the antigen-binding site. The memory B cells which have not undergone all such maturation changes express mainly surface IgM (and the co-translated IgD) and less frequently surface IgG, and show only a scant presence of cytoplasmic immunoglobulin mainly in the perinuclear region.

The morphological and immunophenotypic changes associated with B cell development in the peripheral lymphoid tissue are summarized in Table 4.1 and Figure 4.2.

## T lymphocytes

The lymphoid stem cell gives rise to the T cell progenitor cell, the prothymocyte which is recognizable only on the basis of its expression of cytoplasmic CD3 (cCD3) positivity. The cCD3+ prothymocytes enter the bloodstream from the bone marrow to migrate to the thymus where they undergo maturation in the thymus cortex.

The first stage is the development of an imma-

**Table 4.1**   B cell lineage and differentiation markers in relation to stages of B cell development

| Stage of development | Main markers | Additional markers |
|---|---|---|
| *Bone marrow* | | |
| Stem cell | Nil | |
| Lymphoid precursor | Nil | |
| Pre-pre-B cell | CD19 | cCD22 |
| Pre-B cell | CD19, c | cCD22 |
| Early B cell | CD19, sIgM | CD22 |
| *Peripheral lymphoid tissue* | | |
| *Preantigen challenge* | | |
| Conventional B cells | CD19, sIgM | CD20, CD22 |
| CD5+ B cells | CD5 (low), IgM (low), IgD (low), CD10– | |
| *Postantigen challenge* | | |
| Centroblasts/centrocytes (germinal centre) | CD10+/CD5– | |
| Memory B cells (mantle zone) | CD19, sIgM, sIgD, cIgM | CD20, CD21 CD20 |
| Chronic antigen stimulation (immunoblast to plasma cell) (medullary sinuses) | CD19, cIgM, cIgG, cIgA or cIgE | |
| CD5+ B cells (immunoblasts, rarely plasma cells) (peritoneal cavity; splenic marginal zone) | cIgM mainly, with cλ light chain-predominant expression | |

s = surface; c = cytoplasmic.

ture thymocyte which exhibits cell surface CD3 positivity together with the T cell surface receptor, TCR, capable of recognizing cell surface-associated antigenic or idiotypic determinants. There are three types of TCRs: TCR (αβ), TCR (γδ) and TCR (γγ). The TCR (αβ) is capable of recognizing antigenic peptides strictly in association with cell surface-expressed MHC gene products, whilst TCR (γδ) and TCR (γγ) do so without such restriction. The function of TCR (αβ)+ T cells is that of regulating antigen-specific T cell- and B cell-mediated responses in conjunction with their capacity to recognize Class I and Class II MHC gene products respectively, whilst that of TCR (γδ) cells appears to be related to anti-idiotypic B cell stimulation. The TCR (γγ)+ cells are considered to have the natural killer cell function and, with respect to cell lineage, are related to the large granular lymphocytes.

The cortical CD3+, TCR+ T cells develop into CD3+, TCR+, CD4+, CD8+ cells referred to as the common thymocyte cell population. These cells undergo selective elimination if they happen to bear TCR capable of recognizing self-peptides in conjunction with MHC gene products presented by thymic cortical epithelial cells. Alternatively, they mature into T helper/inducer or T suppressor/cytotoxic if they are reactive against antigenic peptides presented by the thymic variety of APCs, the CD1+ interdigitating dendritic reticulum cells (IDRCs). The T helper/inducer and the T suppressor/cytotoxic cells have the surface immunophenotype of CD3+, TCR+, CD4+, CD8– and CD3+, TCR+, CD4–, CD8+, respectively. These cells, referred to as the memory T cells, migrate into the thymic medulla from where they diffusely infiltrate the peripheral lymphoid systems in the rather loosely defined T cell zones, e.g. parafollicular areas of the lymph nodes. In these regions on encountering the antigen they undergo activation into corresponding T cell subsets bearing positivity for CD25 (interleukin receptors) and CD30 (Ki-1) markers.

On balance, the majority of the CD4+, CD8– T cells accumulate within the B cell-rich areas because of their MHC receptor specificity for the Class II antigens expressed abundantly, for example, by the B cells and the APCs of the FDRC variety. The CD4–, CD8+ T cells, with their MHC receptor specificity directed at the Class I antigens, on the other hand, have a tendency to accumulate near, for example, epithelial cell surfaces expressing abundant amounts of Class I antigens. T cell accumulations are also found in relation to the high endothelial postcapillary venules which seem to be important in allowing their entry into and accumulation within lymphoid and non-lymphoid tissue sites.

T cells of differing functions and immunophenotypes exhibit little or no distinctive morphological features to allow their consistent recognition on histological grounds alone. Immunocytochemical and other methods of marking these cells (e.g. genotypic analysis) are therefore of paramount importance in accurate identification of these cells in their normal and pathological states.

The principal immunocytochemical markers helpful in recognition of the various stages of T cell development are summarized in Table 4.2.

## Mononuclear phagocyte series (MPS) cells

The MPS cells are derived from the myelomonocyte stem cells present in the bone marrow. These in turn are derived from the multipotential CD34+ progenitor cells giving rise to colony- or blood-forming units (CFUs or BFUs) for the generation of granulocyte, eosinophil, mast cells and monocytes (CFU-gemm), megakaryocytes (CFU-m), and erythrocytes (BFU-e), respectively. These CFU-gemm cells express CD33 positivity up to the promyelocyte stage of development.

The promyelocytes diversify into monocytes, granulocytes, eosinophils and basophils all bearing the CD11b positivity. Further maturation of the monocytes converts them into MPS cells bearing the positivity for CD11c as well as the pan-macrophage, CD68 (KP1; EBM11) respectively. At this stage these cells enter the bloodstream, as blood monocytes, and migrate into the tissue to divide and further differentiate into either the scavenger or the accessory type of MPS cells.

Depending on their anatomical site of location and their function, these cells are referred to by different names as shown in Table 4.3 below. All of these cells have been shown to express CD68 positivity which is adequately detectable in trypsinized formalin-fixed, paraffin-embedded sections.

**Table 4.2** T cell lineage and differentiation markers in relation to stages of T cell development

| Stage of development | | Main markers | Additional markers |
|---|---|---|---|
| *Bone marrow* | | | |
| Stem cell | | Nil | |
| Lymphoid precursor cell | | Nil | |
| T cell progenitor (prothymocyte) | | cCD3 | |
| *Thymus* | | | |
| | Immature thymocyte | CD3, TCR (αβ or γδ or γγ) | CD1, CD7 |
| Cortical T cells | | | |
| | Common thymocyte | CD3, TCR, CD4, CD8 | CD1, CD7 |
| Medullary T cells | T helper/inducer | CD3, TCR, CD4 | CD2, CD5 |
| | T suppressor/cytotoxic | CD3, TCR, CD8 | CD2, CD5 |
| *Peripheral lymphoid tissue* | | | |
| Preantigen challenge | | CD3, TCR, CD4 or CD8 CD45RO | CD2, CD5 |
| Postantigen challenge | | CD3, TCR, CD4 or CD8 CD25, CD30 | CD2, CD5 |

TCR = T cell receptor; TCR (αβ) = antigen specific/MHC restricted; TCR (γδ) = idiotype specific (MHC non-restricted); TCR (γγ) = natural killer cell function related (MHC non-restricted); cCD3 = cytoplasmic expression only.

The antigen-presenting Langerhans cells and the IDRC in addition express positivity for S-100 and CD1 markers whilst the FRDCs express low amounts of S-100 and are negative for the CD1 marker. Another form of APC, the dermal dendrocyte, has recently been shown to be S-100 and CD1 negative but positive for the coagulation Factor XIIIa. This cell seems to express both the accessory and the scavenger functions.

The immunocytochemical markers helpful in the identification of the MPS cells and their categorization into scavenger and/or accessory functional types are summarized in Table 4.3.

## The spleen

The spleen is divided up into three anatomically and functionally distinct components—the white pulp, the marginal zone and the red pulp.

The white pulp consists of a central arteriole bearing a sheath of mature T lymphocytes next to which, at an eccentric location, are the B cell follicles either in their primary follicle stage of development (young children) or as secondary follicles identical to the reactive follicles found in the lymph nodes.

The marginal zone and the sinus separate the

**Table 4.3** Functional anatomy of mononuclear phagocytic series (MPS) cells

| Scavenger function | Accessory function |
|---|---|
| *Lung lining:* Alveolar macrophages, CD68+ | *Squamous epithelium:* Langerhans cells, CD68+, S-100+, CD1+ |
| *Liver sinusoids:* Kupffer cells, CD68+ | |
| *Lymph node sinuses:* Sinus histiocytes, CD68+ | *Lymphoid tissue* |
| *Bone margins:* Osteoclasts, S-100+, CD68+ | *B zone:* Follicular dendritic reticulum cells (FDRCs), CD68+, S-100+, CD1– |
| | *T zone:* Interdigitating dendritic reticulum cells (IDRCs), CD68+, S-100+, CD1+ |
| *Dermis:* Dermal dendrocytes, CD68+, Factor XIIIa+ | |
| *CNS:* Microglial cells, CD68+ | |
| *Kidney glomerulus:* Mesangial cells, CD68+ | |
| *Thymus:* Cortical and medullary histiocytes, CD68+ | |
| *Follicular centre:* Tingible body macrophages, CD68+ | |

white pulp from the red pulp and represent the functionally important sites of antigen trapping, antigen–antibody interaction, as well as heavy T cell traffic in and out of the spleen.

The red pulp function is fundamentally that of phagocytosis with venous sinuses and cords as the main sites of the scavenger-type macrophage location and function.

The predominant immunophenotypic character of cells seen in the normal white pulp, red pulp and marginal zone is summarized in Table 4.4.

## CD classification of antibody specificity

This system has been deliberately designed to clear the problem created by the apparently endless variety of monoclonal antibodies produced in the wake of Kohler and Milstein's discovery in 1975 of the monoclonal antibody technology capable of recognizing leucocytes and their various precursors and more mature variants.

Four international workshops have been organized so far for the formal categorization of some 2000 monoclonal antibodies according to their specificity for human leucocyte surface antigens. This has resulted in the definition of 80 or so unique monoclonal antibody categories or clusters designated according to their specificities tested on the basis of three principal techniques:

1. immunofluorescence cell surface labelling of leucocyte preparations using single and double labelling techniques and the fluorescence-activated cell sorter (FACS) system
2. immunoprecipitation of surface-labelled cell antigens followed by SDS–PAGE/Western blotting analysis of their respective molecular weights
3. immunofluorescence/immunoenzyme staining of frozen and/or formalin-fixed, paraffin-embedded tissue sections derived from a wide variety of normal and neoplastic lymphoid and non-lymphoid tissues.

On the basis of these tests performed by independent laboratories it has been found possible to designate to each category of leucocyte surface-specific monoclonal antibodies a unique CD number.

If an antibody is found to have a new specificity which has not been previously defined then it can only be designated a new CD number if at least one other independently produced and tested monoclonal antibody is found with the same specificity characteristics. It should be noted here that the CD number is assigned to a group of antibodies defining an antigen, rather than to the antigen itself. The antibodies of defined CD status with established value in immunohistopathological typing of peripheral lymphoid tissue-proliferative lesions are listed in Table 4.5.

The most useful of the CD-classified antibodies in diagnostic histopathology are those which work well on formalin-fixed, paraffin-embedded tissue. They include the leucocyte common antigen marker, LCA (CD45), L26 (CD20 cytoplasmic domain pan B cell marker), UCHL-1 (CD45RO, marker of mainly early memory T cells), polyclonal CD3 (pan T cell antigen) and KP1 (CD68, pan-macrophage marker). The reactivities of these in formalin-fixed, paraffin-embedded human tonsil section (the most widely used positive control tissue) are photomicrographically illustrated in Figure 4.3.

Two additional useful markers include CD4 (T helper/inducer cell specific) and CD8 (T suppressor/cytotoxic cell specific). These function best in acetone-fixed frozen tissue sections and are occasionally required as aids in the diagnosis of skin lymphomas. Their reactivities in acetone-fixed human tonsil frozen sections (the most popularly used positive control tissue) and in re-

**Table 4.4** Immunophenotypic character of splenic white pulp, red pulp and marginal zone cells

| Splenic area | Predominant types of cells |
| --- | --- |
| *White pulp:* | |
| periarteriolar sheath | *T lymphocytes* (CD4+, CD8–) |
| | IDRC (CD68+, CD1+, S-100+) |
| follicular — | *B lymphocytes* (sIgM+, sIgA+) |
| | FRDCs (CD68+, CD1–, S-100 weak+) |
| *Marginal zone:* | *T lymphocytes* (CD4+, CD8– and CD4–, CD8+ cells) |
| | *B lymphocytes* (sIgG+, sIgM+ or sIgA+ cells) |
| | *Centrocyte-like* (CD5+, CD10–) |
| | *MPS cells* (CD68+, CD1–, S-100–) scavenger type only |
| *Red pulp:* | *MPS cells (no lymphocytes)* (CD68+, CD1–, S-100) scavenger type only |

**Table 4.5** CD classified antibodies of value in diagnostic histopathology

| CD designation | Antibodies | Specificity/usefulness |
|---|---|---|
| CD1 | T6, OKT6, Leu6, NA1/34, Dako 6 | Cortical thymocytes, Langerhans cells in histiocytosis X |
| CD2 | T11, OKT11, Leu5, Dako T11, lyt3 | Normal, activated and neoplastic T cells; peripheral T cell lymphomas |
| CD3 | T3, OKT3, Leu4, UCHT-1 | Immature and mature thymocytes; peripheral T cells |
| CD4 | T4, OKT4, OKT4A, Leu3 a and b, Dako T4 | T helper/inducer cells (some mononuclear phagocytes; mycosis fungoides T cells) |
| CD5 | T1, OKT1, Leu1, RFT1, Dako T1 | T lymphocytes 5–20% of circulating B cells; T cell lymphomas/leukaemias; centrocytic B cell lymphomas; B cell lymphocytic lymphoma/leukaemia |
| CD7 | Leu9, Dako T2, RFT2, 3A1 | Immature/mature T cells; T lymphoblastic lymphoma/leukaemia |
| CD8 | T8, OKT8, OKT5, Leu2, Dako T8 | T suppressor/cytotoxic cells; large-granular-cell lymphocytosis/leukaemia |
| CD10 | CALLA, Dako CALLA | Common acute lymphoblastic leukaemia antigen; non-T, non-B ALL; B lymphoblastic, Burkitt's and centroblastic/centrocyte lymphomas |
| CD15 | LeuM1, 3c4, Dako M1 | X hapten on mature granulocytes and monocytes; Sternberg–Reed cells; some T and B cell lymphomas and many epithelial tumours |
| CD20 | B1, RFB7, Leu16, L27 | B cells (not plasma cells); Ig+ and Ig– B cell lymphomas |
| CD22 | TO15, Dako pan B, TFB4 | Non-activated B cells (not plasma cells); high proportion of B cell lymphomas |
| CD25 | IL2R1, Tac | Interleukin-2 receptor; activated T or B cells; hairy cell leukaemia; HTLV-1 adult T cell lymphomas |
| CD30 | Ki-l, Dako RSC1, BerH2 | Sternberg–Reed cell associated antigen; L and H cells of Hodgkin's disease; Ki-1 lymphomas; lymphomatoid papulosis |
| CD35 | | Follicular dentric cells |
| CD43 | MT1 | T cells and granulocytes; 55–100% of T cell lymphomas; some B cell lymphomas |
| CD45 | Many leucocyte common antigen (LCA, T200) specific antibodies | Pan-leucocyte, i.e. all cells of haematopoietic lineage, not cells of other lineages; high-grade lymphomas versus poorly differentiated non-lymphoid tumours |
| CD45RO | UCHL-1 | Memory T cells (mainly CD4+), granulocytes and some histiocytes (membrane) variety of other tissues (cytoplasm) 50–80% T cell lymphomas |
| CD57 | Leu7, HNK1 | Large granular lymphocytes, natural killer cell subset; neuroendocrine tissue; prostatic epithelium; large-granular-cell leukaemia/lymphomas (CD8+); nerve sheath tumours and gliomas |
| CD68 | KP1, EBM11 | Pan-mononuclear phagocyte series cells; histiocyte proliferations and malignant histiocytes |
| CD74 | LN2 | Germinal centre and mantle zone; HLA-DR B cells; 50–90% B cell lymphomas IDRCs (lymph nodes only) |
| MT2 | Nil others | T cells and mantle zone B cells; 0–10% T cell lymphomas; neoplastic but not reactive B cell follicular centre cells |
| MB2 | Nil others | B cells and wide variety of other tissues; 90–100% B cell lymphomas, 16–18% T cell lymphomas |
| L26 | Nil others | CD20-like; 85% B cell lymphomas (highly specific) Sternberg–Reed cells in Hodgkin's disease |
| LN3 | Nil others | Non-polymorphic HLA-DR germinal centre mantle zone B cells; monocytes/macrophages; IDRCs early to late B cell-derived lymphomas |

lation to lymphoproliferative disorders of the skin, are illustrated in Figure 4.4.

## Role of immunocytochemistry

Histopathologically important proliferative disorders of the peripheral lymphoid tissue include the lymph node- and/or spleen-based varieties of Hodgkin's or non-Hodgkin's lymphomas, the extranodal lymphomas and benign and malignant lesions involving histiocyte proliferation as a major component.

Widely acknowledged and practised systems for histological identification and classification of various forms of lymphomas according to their prognostic grouping are available. These are summarized in Tables 4.6, 4.7 and 4.8.

There is no general classification of the histiocytic

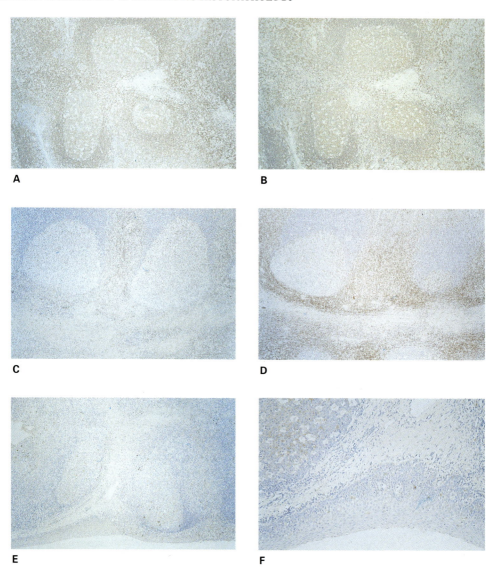

**Fig. 4.3**    Illustration of the reactivities in formalin-fixed, paraffin-embedded human tonsil section of (**A**) the leucocyte common antigen (LCA) marker, CD45; (**B**) L26 (CD20) cytoplasmic domain pan B cell marker; (**C**) UCHL-1 (CD45RO, marker of mainly early memory T cells); (**D**) polyclonal CD3 (pan T cell marker); and (**E**) KP1 (CD68, pan-macrophage marker). The latter marker fails to stain the antigen-presenting cells (the Langerhans cells) in the surface squamous epithelium. S-100 is used instead for this purpose as illustrated in panel **F** (simple two-step indirect immunoperoxidase method).

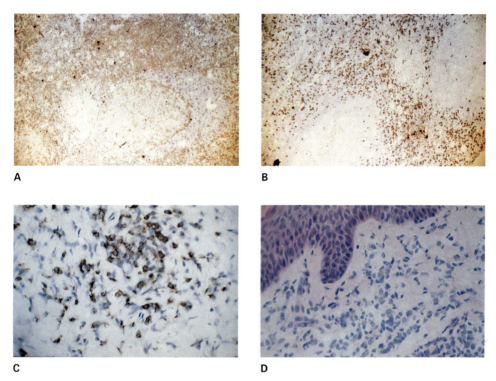

**Fig. 4.4** Illustration of the reactivities in acetone-fixed human tonsil frozen sections of (**A**) CD4 (T helper/inducer cell marker) and (**B**) CD8 (T suppressor/inducer cell marker). In the other two panels the value of CD4 (panel **C**) is illustrated in the diagnosis of a probable T cell skin lymphoma (panel **D**, H&E stain). The vast predominance of CD4-positive cells in the lymphoid infiltrate is consistent with a T cell lymphoma in this location (DHSS immunoperoxidase method).

proliferations but they can be considered rationally according to the categories listed in Table 4.9.

The purpose of immunocytochemical analysis in relation to all these disorders is to aid diagnostic and prognostic analysis of lesions in which the available morphological information is either unhelpful or confusing.

The unhelpful situation usually relates to lesions in which the morphological features of the diseased cell population are either poorly preserved or poorly differentiated (i.e. high-grade lymphomas/anaplastic tumours) or both.

The confusing situation, on the other hand, is mainly related to the difficulty in distinguishing low-grade lymphomas from florid reactive lymphoid hyperplasia and where the neoplastic cell population is distributed in a relatively occult non-clustered manner, or is present in a very scant amount within the lesion.

Regardless of the morphological status of the lesion, T cell lymphomas in general are difficult to identify and categorize accurately because of the lack of any clear-cut histological or cytological features characteristic of these cells or their individual subsets. Hence, immunocytochemical analysis has gradually become almost a compulsory adjunct to all histopathological analysis of T cell disorders.

The value and the applications of immunocytochemistry in relation to individual lymphoproliferative lesions are discussed next. This is followed by an account of combined morphological and immunocytochemical approaches available for dealing with the problems related to distinguishing the high-grade poorly preserved and/or undifferentiated lymphoid neoplasms from each other and various non-lymphoid malignancies, on the one hand, and that of differentiating reactive from low-grade neoplastic proliferations of lymphocytic cells, on the other.

**Table 4.6** Rye classification of Hodgkin's lymphomas

| Type | Prognosis |
| --- | --- |
| Lymphocytic predominant | Good |
| Mixed cellularity | Intermediate |
| Nodular sclerosing | Intermediate |
| Lymphocyte depletion | Poor |

## IMMUNOCYTOCHEMICAL MARKERS FOR INDIVIDUAL PERIPHERAL LYMPHOID TISSUE-RELATED PROLIFERATIVE DISORDERS

### Non-Hodgkin's lymphomas

The vast majority of the non-Hodgkin's lymphomas are of the B cell origin, with fewer than 10 to 15% being of the T cell origin, very few of the natural killer variety, and virtually none of the MPS cell variety.

**Table 4.7** Updated Kiel classification of non-Hodgkin's lymphomas

| B cell | T cell |
| --- | --- |
| *Low-grade* | *Low-grade* |
| Lymphocyte-chronic, lymphocytic and prolymphocytic leukaemia, hairy cell leukaemia | Lymphocyte-chronic, lymphocytic and prolymphocytic leukaemia, small, cerebriform cell mycosis |
| Lymphoplasmacytic/cytoid (LP immunocytoma) | fungoides, Sezary's syndrome Lymphoepithelioid |
| Plasmacytic | (Lennert's lymphoma) |
| Centroblastic/centrocyte | Angioimmunoblastic (AILD, LgX) |
| – follicular and diffuse | |
| – diffuse alone | |
| | *T zone* |
| | Pleomorphic, small cell (HTLV-1+) |
| *High-grade* | *High-grade* |
| Centroblastic | Pleomorphic, medium and large cell (HTLV-1+) |
| Immunoblastic | Immunoblastic (HTLV-1+) |
| Large-cell anaplastic (Ki-1+) | Large-cell anaplastic (Ki-1+) |
| Burkitt's lymphoma | |
| Lymphoblastic | |
| | Lymphoblastic |
| Rare types | Rare types |

Reproduced with permission from Stansfeld AG, Diebold J, Noel H et al 1988 Updated Kiel classification for lymphomas. Lancet 1: 292.

**Table 4.8** Principal categories of extranodal (gastrointestinal) lymphomas

*B cell*
1. Low-grade B cell lymphoma of mucosa-associated lymphoid tissue (MALT)
2. High-grade B cell lymphoma of MALT, with or without evidence of low-grade component
3. Mediterranean lymphoma (immunoproliferative small intestinal disease), low grade, mixed or high grade
4. Malignant lymphoma centrocyte (lymphomatos polyposis)
5. Burkitt-like lymphoma
6. Other types of low- or high-grade lymphoma corresponding to peripheral lymph node equivalents

*T cell*
1. Enteropathy-associated T cell lymphoma (EATCL)
2. Other types associated with enteropathy

Reproduced with permission from Isaacson PG, Spencer J, Wright DH 1988 Classification of primary gut lymphomas. Lancet 2:1148.

## B cell lymphomas

The various morphological types are considered individually according to their order given in the updated Kiel classification system (see Table 4.7).

A summary of the most useful cell lineage and cell differentiation markers for B cell disorders is given in Tables 4.11 and 4.12.

### Hairy cell leukaemia

This is usually diagnosed without difficulty on the basis of clinical grounds and cytological data. More difficulties arise if either the typical 'hair-like' cytoplasmic projections are absent, the malignant cells are present in the blood in very small numbers, or if the diagnosis has to be made in tissue sections.

**Table 4.9** Major categories of histiocytic proliferation

| Association | Type |
| --- | --- |
| *Neoplasia* | Monoblastic leukaemia (rare), histiocytosis X (rare), malignant histiocytic lymphoma (very rare), fibrous histiocytoma (tumour of the mesenchymal cell origin) |
| *Infection* | Intracellular pathogen included (TB, leprosy), abnormal host response (malakoplakia, Whipple's disease) |
| *Foreign Material* | |
| *Storage diseases* | Gaucher's disease |
| *Idiopathic* | Sinus histiocytosis (Rosai–Dorfman disease) |

The diagnostically important markers include TO15 and S-HCL3 monoclonal antibodies. These have a very high sensitivity and specificity except for their cross-reactivity with macrophages. The markers are negative for malignant cells of all other non-Hodgkin's varieties of lymphoid neoplasia.

*Lymphoplasmacytic/cytoid (LP immunocytoma)*

Malignant cells are usually a mixture of monotypic cIg-positive and -negative lymphoplasmacytic/plasmacytoid cells which do not resemble the mantle zone or germinal centre B cell. Their closest resemblance is to the B cells in the splenic red pulp and lymph node medullary cords, both of which are very active sites of plasma cell generation.

*Centroblastic–centrocytic lymphoma (CLB–CC)*

This imitates the reactive follicle patterns of growth and cytological features with follicular organization of centroblast, centrocytic and follicular dendritic (FDC)-like cells.

The centroblasts and centrocytes are TO15+, CD10+, CD5– and monotypic sIg+. The CALLA antigen is weakly expressed and is absent on FDRC (unlike the reactive FDRCs). The associated FDRCs bear the C3b receptors but do not seem to express any binding of immune complexes.

*Centrocytic lymphoma (CL)*

Pure centrocytic lymphoma shows morphological similarities with CB–CC lymphoma, with mainly small and large cleaved cells associated with FDRC meshwork. However, immunocytochemically they differ from CB–CC as summarized in Table 4.10.

*Centroblastic and immunoblastic lymphoma*

Malignant cells are variably positive for HLA-DR, various B cell antigens and sIg with no cells simultaneously positive or negative for all these antigens. The antigen differences between centroblasts and immunoblasts are minor ones and it is not certain whether they represent products of distinct cell origin or intraclonal diversity. The tumours are accompanied by a variable number of MPS cells and T cells.

*Lymphoblastic lymphomas (LB)*

Morphologically and histochemically these are classifiable as Burkitt's, non-Burkitt's, or unclassifiable subtypes. Immunocytochemistry is useful in subclassification of LB in the following manner. The Burkitt's lymphoma cells exhibit HLA-DR, B cell antigens, F8-11-17, sIg and strong expression of CALLA and are negative for Leul, Tü1 and Tü33 markers. The cell of origin appears to be a small non-classed germinal centre cell or early B cell. In contrast, the pre-B cell and pre-pre-B cells have immunophenotypes of HLADR+/sIg–/cIgM+/B cell Ag+ and HLADR+/sIg–/cIg–/CALLA+/B cell Ag+, respectively.

*Low-grade vs high-grade B cell lymphomas*

Because of their high specificity and sensitivity in marking B cells of differing maturity, the following B cell lineage (pan B cell) and B cell differentiation (restricted B cell) markers have been shown to be helpful for typing, confirming or excluding low-grade and high-grade B cell lymphomas, respectively. A small proportion (~10%) of the high-grade B cell lymphomas, in particular the

**Table 4.10** Immunophenotypic differences between centrocytic (CC) and centroblastic–centrocytic (CB–CC) types of B cell lymphomas

| CC | CB–CC |
| --- | --- |
| Always sIgM+ with an unusual λ+ predominance | sIgM, sIgD or sIgG with the usual κ+ predominance |
| Pure culture of single light chain-predominant B cells | Mixture of malignant and reactive B cells |
| High frequency of CD5 expression | Very low frequency or nil CD5 expression |
| CD10– | CD10+ |
| Mantle zone B cells absent | Mantle zone present |
| T cells very few or absent | T cells frequent |
| Bc1-1 gene (t11:14) translocation | Bc1-2 gene (t14:18) translocation |

**Table 4.11** Summary of immunocytochemical markers for typing of B cell lymphoproliferative disorders

| Marker type | Low grade | High grade |
|---|---|---|
| Pan B cell | CD19 (the best) (F) CD20(L26)(next best) (F/P) CD23 (Bu38) (F/P) | CD22 (the best) (F) CD37 (next best) (F) CD20, CD19 (occasional value) (F/P) |
| Restricted B cell | CD5 for CC; CD10 for CB/CC(F) CD32 (FcIIr receptor) LP immunocytomas (F) CD38 lymphoblastic lymphomas (F) CD76 hairy cell leukaemia (F/P) | |

**Table 4.12** Summary of useful B and T cell markers for use on frozen and paraffin sections

| | Frozen | Paraffin |
|---|---|---|
| Pan B cell | CD22 CD37 | L26 (CD20) MB2 |
| Pan T cell | CD2 CD3 | Poly CD3 CD45RO (UCHL-1) CD43 (MTI) BFI (T cell receptor β chain) |
| Restricted B cell | CD5 CD10 | CD23 |
| Restricted T cell | CD1a CD7 CD4 CD8 | CD4 (OPD4) |

immunoblastic variety, have the tendency to express the restricted pan T cell markers UCHL-l (CD45RO) and MTI (CD43).

## T cell disorders

For recognition of lymphomas and their categorization into distinct morphological entities, it is necessary to identify morphologically definable neoplastic cell types and subtypes fairly consistently associated with them. For this, it is necessary to identify the neoplastic cell variant in terms of its normal counterpart and know its level of differentiation and maturation in terms of the sequence of development known for the lymphoid cells in question.

For the B cell lymphomas, a fairly complete and workable morphological classification system is available. The T cells, on the other hand, because of the extreme diversity in histological appearances of both their normal as well as the neoplastic cell variants, have proved very difficult to identify in various types of T cell lymphomas on morphological grounds alone. Immunophenotyping has therefore come to assume a fairly central position in the diagnostic and prognostic classification of T cell neoplasia.

Below, immunocytochemical markers of proven usefulness (see Tables 4.12 and 4.13 for a summary) in this direction are discussed in relation to individual types of T cell proliferative lesions

listed in the updated Kiel classification (see Table 4.7).

### Low-grade T cell lymphomas

***Chronic lymphocytic leukaemia and prolymphocytic leukaemia.*** There are few morphological subsets based on the shape, size and/or tinctorial properties of the neoplastic cell nuclei. These are referred to as the knobby, the round/azurophilic, the pleiomorphic and the large-nucleus-with-a-single-prominent-nucleolus varieties, respectively. The immunophenotypic characteristics of the corresponding neoplastic cells are as summarized in Table 4.14.

***Small, cerebriform cell (mycosis fungoides/Sezary's syndrome).*** Morphologically, the neoplastic cells of this variety of T cell neoplasm are small lymphocytic cells with extreme degrees of nuclear convolution. The mycosis fungoides and the Sezary's syndrome cells are referred to as

**Table 4.13** Summary of immunocytochemical markers for typing of T cell lymphoproliferative disorders

| Lineage or pan T cell | Differentiation or restricted T cell |
|---|---|
| CD2; CD3 (80–90% sensitivity) (F) CD5 (slightly less sensitive) (F) | CD4 (F) CD8(F) CD1a (F) CD7 (F) |
| Polyclonal CD3 (P) (best) CD45RO (UCHL-1) (70% sensitivity; memory T cell specific) (P) CD43 (MTI) (P) | |

**Table 4.14** Relationship between T cell nuclear morphology and immunophenotype

| Nucleus type | | | Immunophenotype |
|---|---|---|---|
| T cell chronic lymphocytic leukaemia | { | Knobby | CD3+/CD4+/CD8– |
| | | Round/azurophilic | CD3+/CD4–/CD8+ |
| | | Pleiomorphic | CD3+/CD4–/CD8+ |
| T cell prolymphocytic leukaemia | { | Large/prominent CD7+ nucleolus } and/or | CD3+/CD4+/CD8– CD3+/CD4–/CD8– CD3+/CD4+/CD8+ (rare) |

Lutzner and Sezary cells, respectively. The histological diagnosis is based on the recognition of these cells in intraepidermal Pautrier's microabscesses in which these cells are expected to be CD3+/CD4+/CD8–.

*Lymphoepithelioid (Lennert's) lymphoma.* Morphologically the neoplastic cells are small lymphocytic cells with very scant cytoplasm and a slightly irregular nucleus. These cells form small clusters of large epithelioid cells (larger than those seen in sarcoidosis) as a result of lymphokine release by activated T cells.

Immunophenotypically, these cells are consistently CD4+/Ki-1 (CD30), indicative of a lymphoma of the helper/inducer subset origin. The main differential diagnosis is LP immunocytoma which has an immunophenotype of CD19/CD32.

*Angioimmunoblastic type.* This appears to be some form of an abnormal immune reaction resulting in a malignant clone of cells with the immunophenotype of CD3+/CD4–/CD8+ in contrast to that of the Lennert's lymphoma which is CD3+/CD4+/CD8–. The neoplastic cells are accompanied by very few reactive cells and associated with a large number of interdigitating dendritic reticular cells (IDRCs) which are Ki-M4 antibody positive. The neoplastic cells also have a tendency to be associated with the high endothelial venules.

*T zone lymphoma.* These occur with or without associated prominent reactive B cell follicles. The T cell zone normally consists of T lymphocytes, IDRCs and high endothelial venules. The neoplastic cells are normally small to intermediate in size with scant cytoplasm and have Lennert's lymphoma cell immunophenotype, CD3+/CD4+/CD8–, and possess a high number of Ki-67+ nuclei, a marker which helps to distinguish these from the reactive counterpart cells.

*Pleiomorphic small type.* These consist of small cells with irregular nucleus morphology and have an immunophenotype of CD3+/CD4+/CD8–/CD1–. Skin and lymph node involvement is an early event.

*High-grade T cell lymphomas*

*Pleiomorphic medium/large size.* HTLV-1 serum antibody positivity constitutes an important practical aid in the diagnosis of this type of T cell lymphoma. Histologically, it resembles mycosis fungoides and has a similar immunophenotype of CD3+/CD4+/CD8–/CD1–. The cells show considerable variation in the cell size, anisocytosis, e.g. 5–9 to 10–12 μm in diameter.

*Immunoblastic.* The cells are uniformly large in size with relatively regular round/oval nuclei and an immunophenotype of CD3+/CD4+/CD8–/CD1–. The condition affects people of younger age, i.e. less than 20 years.

*Large-cell anaplastic.* This is a T cell lymphoma with an immunophenotype of an activated T cell characterized by CD3+ or CD2+ or null type combined with strong expression of the Ki-1 (CD30) antibody-specific antigen in virtually every cell. The cells form cohesive sheets often resembling a carcinoma or a melanoma. In the lymph nodes they have a T zone distribution with the sparing of the B cell follicles.

## Immunocytochemical markers for large granular lymphocytes/natural killer cell proliferative disorders

These arise mainly as large granular lymphocyte (LGL) leukaemia but may present as splenomegaly alone with marked splenic red pulp lymphocytosis suggestive of a primary splenic lymphoma.

The diagnosis may then depend initially on the recognition of LGL immunophenotype amongst the suspected neoplastic cells.

The most common neoplastic LGL immunophenotype appears to be CD3+, CD57+, CD8+. In addition to these markers, abnormal LGL may express CD2 (E-rosette receptor) and CD16 (IgGFc receptors) positivity. Very rarely they are CD4+ instead of CD8+. In about 15% of cases, the neoplastic LGL also present as CD3–, CD57+ cell population which corresponds more closely to the phenotype of the normal circulating natural killer (NK) cells.

The antibody markers for NK cells include CD43 (MTI), CD44 (HK23, L60), CD45 (many varieties), CD45RO (UCHL-1), RA (F8-11-12), RB (PD7/26), CD48 (J4-5) and CD57 (Leu7, HNK-1), respectively.

Since normal LGL have a variety of immunoregulatory functions, including NK activity, antibody-dependent cell-mediated cytotoxicity and B cell regulation, LGL-related proliferative disorders are often accompanied by haematopoietic and/or autoimmune disorders (especially rheumatoid arthritis).

## Hodgkin's lymphoma

The pathognomonic neoplastic cells of Hodgkin's lymphoma have long been considered to the Sternberg–Reed (RS) cells. Finding of two or more RS cells per section of the lesion is taken to be diagnostic of Hodgkin's disease. Furthermore, unlike the non-Hodgkin's lymphomas, the morphological classification of Hodgkin's disease is widely agreed upon and fairly straightforward. The system which is used almost universally is based on a scheme initially proposed by Lukes and Butler in 1966 and later modified at the Rye Conference of 1966. Since then, it has been known simply as the Rye Classification System. It divides the Hodgkin's lymphomas into four categories: lymphocytic predominance (incorporating the nodular and diffuse variants of lymphocytic and/or histiocytic proliferation), mixed cellularity, nodular sclerosis and lymphocytic depletion (incorporating the diffuse fibrosis and reticular categories).

Problems may arise in distinguishing the following:

1. Small-cell lymphoma from lymphocyte-predominant Hodgkin's disease especially when Sternberg–Reed cells are very difficult to find. Use of the pan B and pan T cell reagent combined with the 'clonality' markers may be very helpful in identifying the presence of B or T cell reactive or neoplastic proliferation.

2. Sternberg–Reed-like cells may be seen in follicular lymphomas leading to a confusion with the nodular variant of the lymphocyte-predominant Hodgkin's disease. Pan B cell and monotypic immunoglobulin staining may again help to resolve the difficulty.

3. Sternberg–Reed-like cells have also been noted in myocosis fungoides both in its skin and lymph node variants. Use of pan T and CD4 antibodies in combination with Ki-67 may help to decide the issue. The same applies to the distinction between cutaneous Hodgkin's disease and lymphomatoid papulosis, a chronic skin disease characterized by the appearance of self-healing papulonodular or plaque-like lesions.

4. Lymphocyte- and histiocyte-predominant Hodgkin's disease containing granulomata may be confused with the Lennert's lymphoma.

5. Many large-cell lymphomas contain multinucleated cells resembling Sternberg–Reed cells. The use of pan leucocyte, pan T cell and pan B cell reagents may help to resolve the difficulty. Occasionally, however, an odd Hodgkin's cell may express cytoplasmic CD3 to confuse the issue somewhat.

6. Neoplastic cells of non-lymphoid malignancies, e.g. nasopharyngeal carcinomas, involving lymph nodes in a non-cohesive manner, may resemble Hodgkin's disease. The use of the epithelial markers should help in confirming the presence of a carcinomatous lesion.

8. Finally, non-neoplastic conditions with a predominance of mononuclear Hodgkin's cells may cause a diagnostic confusion. Immunoblasts and cells induced by virus and other types of infections, e.g. toxoplasmosis, may be mistakenly identified to be mononuclear Hodgkin's cells. In these cases, the use of pan-leucocyte, pan B cell, pan T cell and the relatively specific marker of Hodgkin's cell, Ki-1 (CD30), may prove useful.

The cell lineage of Hodgkin's cells still remains

a matter of controversy although the latest work of Stein et al suggests that in at least 40% of the cases these cells seem to be derived from B cells at the pre-pre-B cell stage of genotypic development. Hence, although they lack reaction with virtually all the lymphoid markers except perhaps the pan B cell, the malignant phenotype appears to be fairly mature in character as indicated by the positivity observed for the cell activation markers Ki-1 (CD30) and Taq 1 (CD25).

## Immunocytochemical markers in extranodal lymphomas

The vast majority of these are of B cell origin and constitute between 24 and 36% of all lymphomas. Of these, 50% are gastrointestinal, the bulk of which originate in the stomach. Other sites less commonly involved include skin, bone marrow, salivary glands, thyroid and lungs. These types of lymphomas usually have a long history, are associated with autoimmune disease and have a tendency to recur but have good survival.

The lymphomas arise in close association with the lymphoid tissue resident below the surface epithelium. They have therefore been referred to as mucosa-associated lymphoid tissue lymphomas or MALTOMAS.

Histologically, the lymphoepithelial lesion consisting of a destructive accumulation of centrocyte-like cells in and around the epithelium (particularly the glands epithelium of the gastrointestinal tract) is considered to be diagnostically a very important finding. The cell lineage of these cells seems to be shared by the B cells found in the marginal zone of the splenic white pulp.

Immunocytochemical markers are useful mainly for identifying high-grade varieties of extranodal B cell lymphomas and the differentiation of the very early low-grade variety of B cell lymphomas from reactive autoimmune B cell hyperplasia. For the latter, the clonality typing based on the λ and κ light chain exclusion principle may be paramount. As for the enteropathy-associated T cell lymphomas the use of pan T cell markers (poly CD3, UCHL-1 and/or MTI) is useful. These lymphomas are CD4–, CD8– in status and express HML-1 antibody positivity indicative of their intraepithelial or mucosal T cell origin.

## Poorly differential lymphoid vs non-lymphoid neoplastic lesions

### Mononuclear phagocyte series (MPS) cell disorders

The true neoplastic lesions of the MPS cells appear to be very rare. They include the histiocytosis X syndrome associated with the genetically linked Langerhans cell hyperplasia/neoplasia, and the malignant histiocytosis also referred to as histiocytic medullary reticulosis or histiocytic sarcoma.

The diagnosis depends on the histopathologist's capacity to recognize the histological nature of the proliferating cells. This is relatively straight-forward in the well-differentiated cases but may cause confusion with large malignant cells of lymphoid or non-lymphoid origin associated with Hodgkin's disease, diffuse large-cell lymphoma and anaplastic carcinoma.

In such circumstances, positive identification of the histiocytic nature of the neoplastic cells using a combination of conventional morphological, histochemical and ultrastructural criteria with immunocytochemical features may help to resolve the diagnostic difficulty.

The recent availability of a monoclonal antibody, CD68 (EBM11; KP1), with a high specificity for cells of the human MPS, has eased the burden considerably in this direction. This is especially so because of this antibody's capacity to identify these cells in formalin-fixed, paraffin-embedded sections.

A combination of CD68 with pan-leucocyte (CD45), pan B cell (CD20, L26; MB2), pan T cell (CD3; CD45RO, UCHL-1; MTI) and Hodgkin's cell (LeuMI; CD30, Ki-1) and pan-epithelial cell (e.g. cytokeratin; epithelial membrane antigen) marker-specific antibodies may help to resolve diagnostic difficulty in which a malignant proliferation of the MPS cell is considered as part of the differential diagnosis.

In the case of histiocytosis X, additional studies with S-100 and/or CD1 markers are warranted because of the origin of this condition from the Langerhans cells which belong to the MPS cell group.

## High-grade lymphomas vs undifferentiated non-lymphoid malignancies

Poorly differentiated and/or poorly morphologi-

**Table 4.15**   Panel of antibodies for immunocytochemical differentiation of anaplastic non-lymphoid cell tumours from non-Hodgkin's lymphomas

| Antibody specificity | Results | | | |
|---|---|---|---|---|
| | Non-Hodgkin's lymphoma | Carcinoma | Melanoma | Sarcoma |
| Pan-leucocyte | + | – | – | – |
| Cytokeratin | – | + | – | – |
| Vimetin | + | – | + | + |
| S-100/M3080 | – | +/– | + | – |

cally preserved non-Hodgkin's lymphomas present a specially vexing problem to the histopathologist, since he or she is often unable to decide anything at all on morphological grounds about the lineage or the differentiation character of the underlying diseased cell population. For this reason, immunocytochemistry has become gradually the *tour de force* for making the vital diagnostic and prognostic judgements about such lesions.

The first and foremost emphasis is very much on the identification of the cell lineage of the neoplastic cell. For this the pan-leucocyte antigen, CD45, antibody applied in combination with pan T cell and pan B cell antibody reagents is often chosen as the front-line strategy. The specificity and the sensitivity of the CD45 antibody reagent are both so remarkably high (i.e. approximately 100%) that a positive or a negative result based on it alone is highly instructive. Thus if it is positive then a diagnosis of a non-Hodgkin's lymphoma is confirmed unless proven otherwise. Additional marking with pan B cell and pan T cell reagents is

likely to help to subclassify the neoplastic lesion giving prognostically valuable information.

If the CD45 antibody result is negative then an anaplastic small- or large-cell tumour of non-lymphoid lineage is suspected. The predominant varieties likely to be involved include melanomas and poorly differential tumours of epithelial and connective tissue origin. For this the application of melanoma markers (S-100 and M3080), pan-epithelial cell marker (cytokeratin) and pan-connective tissue marker (vimentin), as a panel of antibodies is likely to provide a sufficiently discriminating and sensitive analysis as depicted in Table 4.15. Figure 4.5 illustrates the use of a combination of CD45 and cytokeratin (CAM5.2) in diagnosis of a large-cell anaplastic tumour.

## Reactive vs neoplastic lymphoproliferations

Some of the early and low-grade lymphoproliferative lesions have a tendency to present with

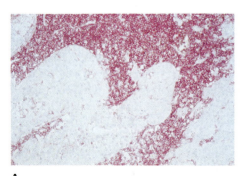
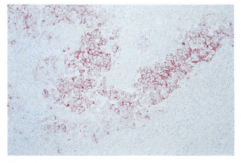

A                                              B

**Fig. 4.5**   Illustration of the value of CD45 in diagnosis of anaplastic large-cell tumour. (**A**) CD45 staining uniformly positive for the background lymphocytic cells in a lymph node and uniformly negative for the large-cell tumour infiltrate. (**B**) Cytokeratin (CAM5.2) giving positive for the tumour cells and negative for the lymphocytic cells, a result indicative of a probably anaplastic carcinoma (APAAP technique).

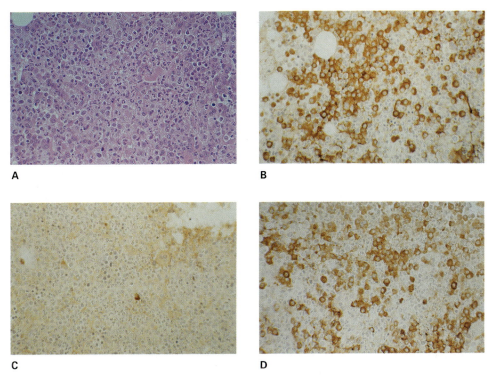

**Fig. 4.6**   Illustration of the use of immunoglobulin light and heavy chain isotype-specific markers in diagnosis of a clonal B cell proliferation. (**A**) An expansion of plasmacytic cells in bone marrow in conjunction with neutrophilic leukaemia (H&E). (**B**) A vast predominance of lambda light chain-positive plasmacytic cells with virtually no kappa-positive cells (panel **C**); the cells were also found to be restricted to a single heavy chain isotype, IgG (panel **D**). The overall findings helped to confirm the presence of a neoplastic plasmacytic proliferation (DHSS immunoperoxidase method).

morphological features which are difficult to distinguish from reactive lymphoid hyperplasias. The histopathologist in these circumstances is forced to resort to alternative methods capable of analysing differences between neoplastic and reactive lymphocytic cells that are more subtle than the morphological ones.

The available approaches include clinical follow-up of the disease entity combined with immunocytochemical, immunogenetical and/or cytogenetical analysis of the lesion with phenotypic and genotypic markers indicative of monoclonality, high proliferative activity, and/or any other intrinsic tumour-cell likeness of the diseased cell population.

*Clonal markers*

Immunocytochemical markers indicative of mono-

clonality of a given B and T cell population principally include the products of immunoglobulin and T cell receptor gene rearrangements, respectively. These may have to be complemented, whenever possible, with immunogenetic and cytogenetic analysis of immunoglobulin and T cell receptor gene rearrangements and/or lymphoma-associated chromosomal translocations, respectively.

For the B cells these relate to the constant light and heavy chain determinants associated with lambda ($\lambda$), kappa ($\kappa$), gamma ($\gamma$), mu ($\mu$), and alpha ($\alpha$) isotypes, or the idiotypic determinants associated with the variable regions of the immunoglobulin molecule. The basic notion behind the use of these determinants as markers of B cell monoclonality is the exclusion prinpciple which states that a given lymphocyte or a clone of cells arising from it, is involved in the production of immunoglobulins bearing a unique combination of a single light chain isotype/idiotype with a single heavy chain isotype/idiotype. The same exclusion principle applies to the T cells with respect to the isotypic/idiotypic markers associated with the α and β chains of the T cell surface receptors.

Thus a B cell population derived from a single clone, barring very few exceptions, is likely to be immunophenotypically positive for λ or κ light chain isotype combined with a single variety of heavy chain isotype (μ, γ, α) only. In addition, this combination is likely to be associated with a unique idiotype borne by the hypervariable region (e.g. CDRIII segment) of the immunoglobulin molecule.

Immunocytochemically, these are most easily detectable on the cell surface in unfixed or very lightly fixed (e.g. acetone treated) cell or frozen tissue section preparations. In routinely prepared tissue sections the surface immunoglobulin markers are not detectable at all and one is left to analyse either (i) the cytoplasmic immunoglobulin associated with the perinuclear region of, for example, memory B lymphocytes, visible usually with the aid of a high magnification oil immersion lens in the mantle zone in sections stained with a highly sensitive secondary detection system, or (ii) the endoplasmic reticulum or storage vacuoles in immunoblasts or plasma cells, respectively. Small clusters and especially large aggregates or sheets of single light chain and single heavy chain positive B cells are considered as presumptive evidence of a monoclonal B cell population as illustrated photomicrographically in Figure 4.6. Diagnosis of a truly monoclonal, neoplastic B cell population needs exclusion of clonal B cell proliferations associated with autoimmune, viral or transplantation aetiopathogenesis, and a study of alternative markers of neoplastic B cell proliferation is discussed next.

B cell idiotypic markers, despite their obvious potential in marking B cell clonality, have not been part of diagnostic use mainly because of their uniqueness to an individual patient. Recently, a number of more public or cross-reactive idiotypes have been discovered and these are likely to find some use in B cell clonality typing in the future, especially those which work on formalin-fixed, paraffin-embedded tissue sections.

The T cell clonality typing is even more difficult to put into diagnostic practice because of a lack of suitable isotypic markers of T cell receptors. Nevertheless, efforts have been made to produce variable region-specific monoclonal antibodies to β chain determinants which are limited to a small percentage (4–8%) of usually individually dispersed T cells. Detection of small or large clusters of T cells positive for these vβ determinants may be considered as presumptive evidence of a monoclonal T cell proliferation.

Mature T cells are also endowed with either CD4 or CD8 related antigens only. Because normal and reactive T cells usually occur as a mixture of individually dispersed CD4+/CD8– and CD8+/CD4– T cells, any unusually large and continuous clusters or sheets of CD4+/CD8– or CD8+/CD4– found in a suspiciously neoplastic lymphoproliferative lesion may be considered as presumptive evidence of monoclonal T cell proliferation. But again, as in the case of the B cells, it is necessary to confirm such a suspicion with other markers of neoplastic T cell proliferation.

*Cell proliferation markers*

Another immunocytochemically exploitable difference between neoplastic and reactive lymphocytes is the generally greater proliferation potential of the neoplastic cells. Thus neoplastic cell populations fairly consistently exhibit a larger growth fraction compared to normal or reactive cells. This means that a greater proportion of the neoplastic cells are essentially in their cell replication phase of the cycle which collectively includes the synthesis phase (S), the Gap 2 ($G_2$) phase and the mitoses (M) phase.

The Ki-67 and the more recently proposed proliferating cell nuclear antigen (PCNA) antibodies represent two independent markers of cell replication phase which have become available for differentiation of neoplastic cell proliferation from the reactive type.

The Ki-67 marker works well only on lightly fixed (i.e. acetone treated) cell or frozen section preparations, whilst the PCNA-specific antibody is effective on alcohol, methacarn and, to a lesser extent, formalin-fixed, paraffin-embedded tissue sections.

A morphologically suspicious T or B cell population showing an increased fraction of Ki-67-positive cells may be considered as evidence in favour of its possible neoplastic origin.

Where the morphological distribution is difficult to interpret, a double immunolabelling approach may be helpful. Thus immunostaining of the lesion with the cell lineage or cell differentiation series of markers in combination with the Ki-67 antibody has been used in an attempt to identify neoplastic T cells in morphologically difficult lesions. This approach has recently been used successfully by Motley et al (1992) in the study of the neoplastic potential and cell lineage of individual lesions in a case of atypical regressing histiocytosis. (See Figure 4.7 for a photomicrographic illustration of the typical findings.)

*Tumour-specific markers*

Tumour cell markers refer to antigens which are more or less uniquely expressed by the neoplastically transformed cells. A great deal of research has been devoted to identifying such antigens but mostly in vain. Recent advances in the molecular biology of tumour formation have revealed that neoplastic cell transformation is constantly associated with an alteration in the function of oncogene products. Oncogenes are a group of growth-regulatory genes involved in the regulation of normal cell growth. Their principal function is to encode the synthesis of positive or negative growth factors and their respective cell-bound receptors. They all belong to a unique class of polypeptides referred to as growth regulins or simply as oncogene products.

The oncogene products are normally produced in quite small amounts and often only in certain phases of the cell cycle. In tumour cells this pattern of expression is disrupted, leading to an over- or underexpression of one or more of various oncogene products.

Thus a tumour cell population is more likely to give a stronger and more widespread, or weak, focal or negative immunocytochemical staining for certain selected series of oncogene products compared to its normal or reactive counterpart.

As far as lymphomas are concerned, the vast majority of these seem to involve oncogene activation related to translocational events involving the immunoglobulin or T cell receptor genes. Recently, it has been possible to identify a consistent (up to 85%) involvement of the bcl oncogene translocation in the formation of follicular B cell lymphoma. Production of antibodies capable of detecting the bcl oncogene protein in formalin-fixed, paraffin-embedded tissue has led to the possibility of immunocytochemical identification of a selective overexpression of this protein in neoplastic as opposed to reactive follicular centres. Hence, this type of immunocytochemical marking offers a novel approach for distinguishing very low-grade follicular B cell lymphomas from florid reactive follicular hyperplasia. Curiously, the pan T cell marker, MT2, has been recently shown on empirical grounds to give the same results as a tailor-made antibody directed at the translocated bcl oncogene product.

## SPECIALIST TECHNIQUES COMPLEMENTARY TO IMMUNOCYTOCHEMISTRY IN THE DIAGNOSIS OF OCCULT LYMPHOMAS

These include in the main flow cytometry and cytogenetic and genotypic analyses.

### Flow cytometry

Flow cytometry or immunofluorescent cell sorter analysis of single-cell suspensions prepared from fresh lymphoid tissue allows more precise quantification of both the numbers and the intensity of staining of cells positive for various lymphoid cell surface markers. It is particularly useful in providing fairly precise kappa:lambda light chain ratios for determination of monoclonality in B cell lesions suspected of undergoing neoplastic transformation or process. Thus a kappa:lambda ratio greater than 3:1, or a lambda:kappa ratio greater than 2:1 is considered to be presumptive evidence of B cell monoclonality and/or neoplasia.

### Cytogenetic analysis

This involves chromosomal studies to reveal chromosomal abnormalities consistently associated with malignant transformation of lymphoid and other types of bone marrow-derived cells. For

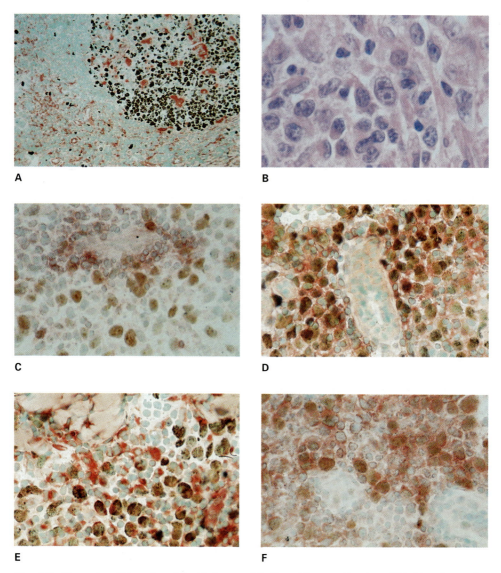

**Fig. 4.7** Illustration of the value of double immunolabelling with a combination of Ki-67 nuclear and leucocyte cell surface markers. (**A**) Ki-67 and KP1 (CD68) staining showing the virtual restriction of Ki-67 immunostaining (black) to the B cell nuclei in the germinal centre and no overlap with KP1 immunostaining (red) of the follicular and interfollicular histiocytic cells. The Ki-67 and KP1 markers were applied using a sequential double immunoperoxidase (DHSS) method. The black staining due to Ki-67 was developed using a DAB–silver enhancement kit (Amersham International), while the red colour due to KP1 was developed using a combination of ethylcarbazole/glucose substrate (DNP Localisation System kit, Bioclinical Services Ltd, Cardiff, Wales, UK). Panels **B–F** illustrate the application of this technique to cell lineage analysis of the culprit pathological cell in a lesion from a case of atypical regressing histiocytosis. (**B**) H&E staining showing Reed–Sternberg-like binucleate giant cells. (**C**) Staining using a combination of Ki-67 and RFTI (CD5) showing no overlap. (**D**) and (**E**) Combinations of Ki-67/CD4 and Ki-67/KP1 showing a partial overlap, and (**F**) a combination of Ki-67/Ki-1 (CD30) showing an almost complete overlap indicative of the main proliferative cell pool (see Motley et al 1992 for further details).

example, the chromosomal translocations t(14;18) and t(17;14) are useful as cytogenetic markers for confirmation of the CB–CC and the CC varieties of B cell lymphomas, respectively. Similarly, t(8;14) and t(15;17) have been found to be pathognomonic of B cell acute lymphocytic leukaemia and acute promyelocytic leukaemia, respectively.

## Genotypic analysis

Since each B cell (or T cell) undergoes a unique set of Ig (or T cell receptor) gene rearrangements, it has been found possible to employ this as a marker of monoclonality using molecular biological techniques such as Southern blot analysis and polymerase chain reaction (PCR), or a combination of these techniques. The Southern blot method has been used extensively for detection of occult B cell or T cell malignancies, or minimal residual disease following treatment of these malignancies. The technique has been recorded to be sensitive enough to reliably detect a minimum clonal T cell population of about 5%, and a minimum clonal B cell population of approximately 1%, of the total lymphoid cell population present in the biopsy material.

The PCR technique is able to detect and amplify clonal gene rearrangements with reliability in several hundred to a few thousand cells.

The amplified rearranged gene segments may be further used as clone-specific markers in Southern blot analysis on follow-up biopsies from treated lymphoma cases. Unlike the other specialist techniques, PCR has the added advantage of being applicable to formalin-fixed, paraffin-embedded tissues.

REFERENCES AND FURTHER READING

**Embryology**

Harrison R G 1978 Clinical embryology. Academic Press, London, p 150–151

**Anatomical and immunophenotypic features**

*B lymphocytes*

Caligaris-Cappio F 1988 B-lymphoproliferations and B-cell differentiation. In: Bird G, Calvert J C (eds) B lymphocytes in human disease. Oxford Medical, Oxford
Ling N 1988 The relationship of B-lymphocyte surface marker phenotype to cell differentiation. In: Bird G, Calvert J C (eds) B lymphocytes in human disease. Oxford Medical, Oxford, p 174–192
Liu Y-J, Johnson G D, Gordon J, MacLennan C M 1992 Germinal centres in T-cell dependent antibody responses. Immunology Today 13: 17–21

*T lymphocytes*

Feller A C, Parwaresch M R, Stein H et al 1986 Immunophenotyping of T-lymphoblastic lymphoma/leukaemia correlation with normal T-cell maturation. Leukaemia Research 10: 1025–1031

*Mononuclear phagocyte series (MPS) cells*

Hogg N 1987 Human mononuclear phagocyte molecules and the use of monoclonal antibodies in their detection. Clinical and Experimental Immunology 69: 687–694
Kelly P M A, Bliss E, Morton J A, Burns J, McGee J O'D 1988 Monoclonal antibody EBM11: high cellular specificity for human macrophages. Journal of Clinical Pathology 41: 510–515
Pulford K A F, Rigney E W, Micklem K T et al 1989 A new monoclonal antibody that detects a monocyte/macrophage associated antigen in routinely processed tissue sections. Journal of Clinical Pathology 42: 414–421

*The spleen*

Van Krieken J H J M, Te Velde J 1986 Immunohistology of the human spleen: an inventory of the localization of lymphocyte sub-populations. Histopathology 10: 285–294

*CD classification of antibody specificity*

Chan J K C, Ng C S, Hui P 1988 A simple guide to the terminology and application of leucocyte monoclonal antibodies. Histopathology 12: 461–480
Deegan M J 1989 Membrane antigen analysis in the diagnosis of lymphoid leukaemias and lymphomas. Archives of Pathological Laboratory Medicine 113: 606–618
Knapp W, Dorken P, Rieber R E et al 1989 CD antigens 1989 American Journal of Pathology 135: 420–421

*Role of immunocytochemistry*

Bennett J M, Catovsky D, Daniel M T et al 1989 Proposals for the classification of chronic (mature) B and T lymphoid leukaemias. Journal of Clinical Pathology 42: 567–584
Isaacson P G, Spencer J, Wright D H 1988 Classification of primary gut lymphomas. Lancet 2: 1148–1149
Jaffe E S 1985 Malignant histiocytes and true (only) histiocytic lymphomas. In: Jaffe E S, Bennington J L (eds) Surgical pathology of lymph nodes and related organs. WB Saunders, Philadelphia, p 381–411
Lukes R J, Cramer L F, Hall T C, et al 1966 Report of the nomenclature committee. Cancer Research 26: 1311
Stansfeld A G, Diebold J, Noel H, Kapanci Y, Rilke F et al 1981 Update of Kiel Classification for lymphomas. Lancet 1: 292–293

*B cell lymphomas*

Cartun R W, Coles F B, Pastuszak W T 1987 Utilization of monoclonal antibody L26 in the identification and confirmation of B-cell lymphomas. A sensitive and specific marker applicable to formalin and B5-fixed, paraffin embedded tissues. American Journal of Pathology 129: 415–421

Hall P A, d'Ardenne A J, Butler M G, Habeshaw J R, Stansfeld A G 1987 New marker of B lymphocytes MB2: comparison with other lymphocyte subset markers active in conventionally processed tissue sections. Journal of Clinical Pathology 40: 151–156

Mason D Y, Comans-Bitter M, Cordell J L et al 1990 Antibody L26 recognises an intracellular epitope on the B-cell associated CD20 antigen. American Journal of Pathology 136: 1215–1222

Norton A J, Isaacson P G 1987 Monoclonal antibody L26: an antibody that is reactive with normal and neoplastic B lymphocytes in routinely fixed and paraffin wax embedded tissues. Journal of Clinical Pathology 40: 1405–1412

Norton A J, Isaacson P G 1989 Lymphoma phenotyping in formalin-fixed and paraffin wax-embedded tissues: II Profiles of reactivity in the various tumour types. Histopathology 14: 557–579

Poppema S, Visser L 1987 Preparation and application of monoclonal antibodies: B cell panel and paraffin tissue reactive panel. Biotest Bulletin 3: 131–139

Poppema S, Hollema H, Vissen L, Vos H 1987 Monoclonal antibodies (MT1, MT2, MB1, MB2, MB3) reactive with leukocyte subsets in paraffin-embedded tissue sections. American Journal of Pathology 127: 418–429

Stein H, Mason D Y, Gerdes J et al 1985 The expression of the Hodgkin's disease associated antigen Ki-1 in reactive and neoplastic lymphoid tissue. Blood 66: 848–858

*T cell disorders*

Feller A C, Parwaresch M R, Stein H, Ziegler A, Herbst H, Lennert K 1986 Immunophenotyping of T-lymphoblastic lymphoma/leukaemia correlation with normal T-cell maturation. Leukaemia Research 10: 1025–1031

Mason D Y, Krissansen G W, Davey F R, Crumpton M J, Gatter K J 1988 Antigens against epitopes resistant to denaturation on T3 (D3) antigen can detect reactive and neoplastic T cells in paraffin embedded tissue biopsy specimens. Journal of Clinical Pathology 41: 121–127

Ng C S, Chan J K C, Hui P K et al 1988 Application of a T-cell receptor antibody BF1 for immunophentypic analysis of malignant lymphomas. American Journal of Pathology 132: 365–371

Norton A J, Ramsay A D, Smith S H, Beverley P C L, Isaacson P G 1986 Monoclonal antibody (UCHL-1) that recognises normal and neoplastic T cells in routinely fixed tissues. Journal of Clinical Pathology 39: 399–405

Stross W P, Warnke R A, Flavell D J et al 1989 Molecule detected in formalin fixed tissue by antibodies MTI, DF-T1, and L60 (Leu22) corresponds to CD43. Journal of Clinical Pathology 42: 953–961

Suchi T, Lennert K, Tu L-y et al 1987 Histopathology and immunohistochemistry of peripheral T cell lymphomas: a proposal for their classification. Journal of Clinical Pathology 40: 995–1015

Yoshino T, Mukuzono H, Aoki H et al 1989 A novel monoclonal antibody (OPD4) recognising a helper/inducer T cell subset. Its application to paraffin-embedded tissues. American Journal of Pathology 134: 1339–1346

*Large granular cell/natural killer cell disorders*

Griffiths D F R, Jasani B, Standen G R 1989 Pathology of the spleen in large granular lymphocyte leukaemia. Journal of Clinical Pathology 42: 885

Loughran T P, Starkebaum G 1987 Large granular lymphocyte leukaemia medicine. Medicine 66: 397–405

*Hodgkin's lymphoma*

Chittal SM, Caverivière P, Schwarting R et al 1988 Monoclonal antibodies in the diagnosis of Hodgkin's disease. The search for a rational panel. American Journal of Surgical Pathology 12: 9–21

Cibull M L, Stein H, Gatter K C, Mason D Y 1989 The expression of CD3 antigen in Hodgkin's disease. Histopathology 15: 597–605

Jack A S, Cunningham D, Soukop M, Liddle C N, Lee F D 1986 Use of Leu M1 and antiepithelial membrane antigen monoclonal antibodies for diagnosing Hodgkin's disease. Journal of Clinical Pathology 39: 267–270

Lee FD 1989 Hodgkin's disease revisited. In: Anthony PP, MacSween RNM (eds.) Recent advances in histopathology. Churchill Livingstone, Edinburgh, ch 5, p 79–96

Nicholas D S, Harris S, Wright D H 1990 Lymphocyte predominance Hodgkin's disease — an immunohistochemical study. Histopathology 16: 157–165

Pallesen G 1990 The diagnostic significance of the CD30 (Ki-l) antigen. Histopathology 16: 409–413

Stein H, Mason D Y, Gerdes J et al 1985 The expression of the Hodgkin's disease associated antigen Ki-1 in reactive and neoplastic lymphoid tissue: evidence that Reed–Sternberg cells and histiocytic malignancies are derived from activated lymphoid cells. Blood 66: 848–858

*Extranodal lymphomas*

Chan J K C, Ng C S, Isaacson P G 1990 Relationship between high-grade lymphoma and low-grade B-cell mucosa-associated lymphoid tissue lymphoma (MALToma) of the stomach. American Journal of Pathology 136: 1153–1164

Myhre M H, Isaacson P G 1987 Primary B-cell gastric lymphoma. A reassessment of its histogenesis. Journal of Pathology 152: 1–11

*Mononuclear phagocyte series (MPS) cell disorders*

Kelly P M A, McGovern M, Gatter K C et al 1988 EBM/11 reactivity in malignant histiocytosis. Journal of Clinical Pathology 41: 1305–1309

Pulford K A F, Rigney E W, Micklem K T et al 1989 A new monoclonal antibody that detects a monocyte/macrophage associated antigen in routinely processed tissue sections. Journal of Clinical Pathology 42: 414–421

Pulford KAF, Sipos A, Cordell J L et al 1990 Distribution of the CD68 Macrophage/myeloid associated antigen. International Immunology 2: 973–980

*Poorly differentiated lymphoma vs non-lymphoid lineage lesions*

Pizzolo G, Sloane J, Beverly P et al 1980 Differential diagnosis of malignant lymphoma and nonlymphoid tumours using monoclonal anti-leucocyte antibody. Cancer 46: 2640–2647

*Reactive vs neoplastic lymphoid lesions*

*Clonal markers*

Clark D M, Boyston A W 1989 T-cell antigen receptor beta chain variable region families. A study of their distribution in normal and reactive tissue. Journal of Pathology 158: 9

Davey M P, Waldman T A 1986 Clonality and lymphoproliferative lesions. The New England Journal of Medicine 315: 509–511

Levy R, Warnke R, Dorfmann R F, Haimovich J 1977 The monoclonality of human B-cell lymphomas. Journal of Experimental Medicine 145: 1014–1028

Ling N R 1983 Immunoglobulin as a differentiation and clonal marker. Journal of Immunological Methods 65: 1–25

*Cell proliferation markers*

Garcia R L, Coltrera M D, Gown A M 1989 Analysis of proliferative grade using anti-PCNA/cyclin monoclonal antibodies in fixed embedded tissues. American Journal of Pathology 134: 733–739

Feller A C, Griessen G H, Mak T W, Lennert K 1986 Lymphoepithelioid lymphoma (Lennert's lymphoma) is a monoclonal proliferation of the helper/inducer T cells. Blood 68: 663–667

Gerdes J, Lemke H, Baisch H et al 1984 Cell cycle analysis of a cell proliferation-associated human nuclear antigen defined by the monoclonal antibody Ki67. Journal of Immunology 133: 1710–1715

Godde-Salz E, Feller A C, Lennert K 1976 Cytogenetic and immunohistochemical analysis of lymphoepithelial cell lymphoma (Lennert's lymphoma): further substantiation of its T-cell nature. Leukaemia Research 10: 313–323

Motley R J, Jasani B, Ford A M, Poynton C H, Calonje-Daly J E, Holt P J A 1992 Regressing atypical histiocytosis — a regressing cutaneous phase of Ki-1 positive anaplastic large cell lymphoma: immunocytochemical, nucleic acid and cytogenetic studies of a new case in view of current opinion. Cancer 70: 476–483

Namikawa R, Suchi T, Ueda R et al 1987 Phenotyping of proliferating lymphocytes in angioimmunoblastic lymphadenopathy and related lesions by the double immunoenzymatic staining technique. American Journal of Pathology 127: 279–287

Stein H, Lennert K, Feller A C, Mason D Y 1984 Immunohistological analysis of human lymphoma correlation of histological and immunological categories. Advances in Cancer Research 41: 67–147

*Tumour-specific markers*

Chilosi M, Mombello A, Menestrina F et al 1990 Immunohistochemical differentiation of follicular lymphoma from florid reactive follicular hyperplasia with monoclonal antibodies reactive on paraffin sections. Cancer 65: 1562–1569

Ngan B-Y, Chen-Levy Z, Weiss L M et al 1988 Expression in non-Hodgkin's lymphoma of the bcl-2 protein associated with the t(14;18) chromosomal translocation. New England Journal of Medicine 318: 1638–1644

Norton A J, Rivos C, Isaacson P G 1989 A comparison between monoclonal antibody MT2 and immunoglobulin staining in the differential diagnosis of follicular lymphoid proliferations in routinely fixed wax-embedded biopsies. American Journal of Pathology 134: 63–70

**Specialist techniques complementary to immunocytochemistry**

*Flow cytometry*

Parker J W 1983 Flow cytometry in lymphoma/leukaemia diagnosis. In: Paatengale J, Luke C, Taylor C (eds) Lymphoproliferative disease: pathologic diagnosis, therapy. Martinus Nijhoff, Boston, p 126–142

Poncelot P, Carayon P 1985 Cytofluorometric quantification of cell surface antigens by indirect immunofluorescence using monoclonal antibodies. Journal of Immunological Methods 85: 65–74

*Cytogenetic analysis*

Rowley J D 1988 Chromosome abnormalities in leukaemia. Journal of Clinical Oncology 6: 194–202

*Genotypic analysis*

Arnold A, Cosman J, Bakhshi A et al 1983 Immunoglobulin gene rearrangements as unique clonal markers in human lymphoid neoplasms. New England Journal of Medicine 309: 1593–1599

Foroni L, Mason P, Luzzatto L 1991 Immunoglobulin and T-cell receptor gene analysis for the investigation of lymphoproliferative disorders. In: Catovsky D (ed) Methods in haematology — the leukaemic cell. Churchill Livingstone, Edinburgh, 13, p 341–391

O'Connor N T J, Wainscoat J S, Weatherall D J 1985 Rearrangement of the T cell receptor beta-chain gene in the diagnosis of lymphoproliferative disorders. Lancet 1: 1295–1297

Papadopoulos K P, Bagg A, Bezwoda W R, Mendelow B V 1989 The routine diagnostic utility of immunoglobulin and T-cell receptor gene rearrangements in lymphoproliferative disorders. American Journal of Clinical Pathology 91: 633–638

Wan J H, Trainor K J, Brisco M J, Morley A A 1990 Monoclonality in B cell lymphoma detected in paraffin wax embedded sections using the polymerase chain reaction. Journal of Clinical Pathology 43: 888–890

Williams M E, Innes D J, Borowitz M J et al 1987 Immunoglobulin and T cell receptor gene rearrangements in human lymphoma and leukaemia. Blood 69: 79–86

Shibata D, Martin W J, Arnheim N 1988 Analysis of DNA sequences in forty-year-old paraffin-embedded thin-tissue sections: A bridge between molecular biology and classical histology. Cancer Research 48: 4564–4566

# 5. Epithelial tumours

## INTRODUCTION

Epithelial tissue consists of a single or a multiple layer of cells. It covers the entire external surface of the body as well as the internal surfaces of the alimentary, respiratory and urogenital tracts and constitutes the parenchyma of their respective organs including the lobules and ducts of all varieties of minor secretory and excretory glands.

The object of this chapter is twofold: firstly, to provide a brief review of embryological, anatomical and biochemical criteria and knowledge usually adopted by the histopathologist for diagnostic analysis of neoplastic diseases of individual types of epithelial tissues; secondly, to summarize the role played by immunocytochemical markers in more specific and sensitive typing of these diseases.

## EMBRYOLOGICAL AND ANATOMICAL BACKGROUND

Epithelial tissues are collectively derived from all the three germ layers (Harrison 1978).

**Table 5.1** Endoderm-derived epithelial tissues

---

*Gut endoderm*
1. Epithelial lining covering the alimentary canal from the oesophagus to the sigmoid colon
2. Epithelial lining of the gallbladder and the pancreatic, bile and cystic ducts
3. Epithelial cell components of liver and pancreas

*Pharynx*
1. Epithelium lining auditory tube, tympanic cavity and intratonsillar cleft
2. Sensory epithelium of the vestibular-cochlear organ
3. Epithelial elements of the parathyroid, thyroid and thymic glands including thyroid C cells derived from the ultimobranchial body

*Tracheobronchial groove*
1. Tracheal and bronchial epithelial linings
2. Alveolar epithelial cells of the lung

---

The endoderm forming the roof lining of the yolk sac gives rise to the gut endoderm, the pharynx and the tracheobronchial groove. These in turn give rise to various epithelial tissues listed in Table 5.1.

The ectoderm forming the floor of the amniotic cavity, on the other hand, gives rise to the epidermis covering the entire external surface of the body, as well as its various derivatives including hair, hair follicles, nails, sebaceous glands, sweat glands and the mammary glands as well as their respective ductal epithelium. At the cephalic and the caudal ends of the early embryos the fusion of endoderm and ectoderm germ layers gives rise to the buccopharyngeal and the cloacal membranes, respectively, which in turn give origin to the epithelial tissues listed in Table 5.2.

At an early stage of embryo development, the ectodermal cells at the caudal end of the embryonic plate assume pluripotential properties giving rise not only to new ectoderm and endoderm but also to intraembryonic mesoderm. The latter grows in between the ectoderm and the endoderm and splits into three parts of which the part designated as the immediate mesoderm is ultimately

**Table 5.2** Epithelial tissues derived from endoderm/ectoderm fusion

---

*Buccopharyngeal membrane*
1. Epithelium lining the mouth, nasal cavities and parts of the teeth
2. Olfactory epithelium
3. Epithelial elements of anterior pituitary gland

*Cloacal membrane*
1. Epithelium lining the urethra, most of the bladder, the vagina, the rectum and the upper two-thirds of the adult anal canal
2. Epithelial elements of the anterior, posterior and lateral lobes of the prostate gland

---

responsible for giving rise to virtually all the epithelial structures associated with the urogenital system (see Table 5.3).

At the microscopic level, epithelial linings are classifiable into three morphologically distinct varieties: simple, stratified and transitional. These entities seem to relate more specifically to their respective functions than to their embryological or anatomical origins. The simple epithelium consists of a single layer of cells which may appear flattened as in the pavement lining typical of the alveolar lining of the lungs. Alternatively it may consist of taller columnar cells characteristic of the epithelium lining the whole length of the gastrointestinal tract including the various types of glands. A specialized variety of stratified columnar epithelium is associated with the linings of the respiratory tract, the tympanic cavity, the uterine cavity and fallopian tubes, the seminiferous tubules of the testes, the lobules of the epididymis and the first part of the vas deferens.

The stratified epithelium occurs either in keratinized or non-keratinized forms depending upon the degree of risk of abrasion injury, whilst the transitional epithelium is restricted more or less to the bladder and the ureters where the epithelium is subject to various degrees of stretching.

From a histopathological viewpoint it is important to stress that the morphological type of an epithelial lining not only fails to relate in any uniform way to a particular germ layer or anatomical setting but is also liable to undergo metaplasia to other morphological types under pathological stress. This ephemeral morphological character of epithelia has forced the histopathologist to rely upon histochemical and immunohistochemical techniques as more specific means of analysing

their origins and background. The latter has proved possible because, as discussed next, the biochemical properties of epithelial cells are in general more stable and more specific markers of the cell lineage, differentiation character and anatomical site of origin of epithelial tumours.

## BIOCHEMICAL BACKGROUND

From the point of view of cell function, simple epithelium is fairly uniformly concerned with either secretion, excretion, absorption or transport of molecules across biological barriers. On the other hand the stratified and the transitional varieties are associated with the mechanical function of protection against abrasive or stretching types of tissue stresses or injuries, respectively.

To comply with these diverse functions individual types of epithelial linings are equipped with distinct varieties of metabolic machinery and cytoskeletal infrastructure. As discussed below, the various biomolecules intimately concerned with these have proved sufficiently stable and accurate correlates of particular types of epithelial cells. This has resulted in the development of reasonably reliable cell lineage-, cell differentiation- and organ-specific markers.

### Cytoskeletal markers

At least 20 distinct varieties of human epithelial cytokeratins have been described on the basis of their positions on two-dimensional gels (Moll et al 1982 and 1992). They are thought to be encoded by 20 different genes, and are further distinguishable on the basis of their molecular weights and isoelectric points.

The Moll catalogue numbers, together with the corresponding molecular weights and isoelectric points of the various cytokeratins, as well as the main variety of epithelial tissue expressing them, are listed in Table 5.4.

In any given type of epithelial tissue the cytokeratins are expressed as pairs of the acidic and basic variants, the basic member always being approximately 8 kDa heavier than the acidic member in molecular weight. Hence, every epithelial cell expresses at least two distinct varieties of cytokeratin.

In general, the various types of epithelial tissues

**Table 5.3** Intermediate mesoderm-derived epithelial tissues

*Urinary system*
Epithelium lining the trigone of bladder, the ureter, the renal pelvis, the minor and major calyces, the collecting ducts and the nephron unit including the Bowman's capsule, proximal and distal convoluted tubules and the loop of Henle

*Genital system*
**Male** – Epithelium lining the medial lobe prostatic glands and ducts, the ejaculating ducts, the seminal vesicles, the vas deferens, the epididymis, ductus efferentes, rete testis, seminiferous tubules and Sertoli cells
**Female** – Epithelium lining part of the vagina, the cervix, the uterine cavity, fallopian tubes, and the ovarian granulosa cells

**Table 5.4** Molecular characteristics and cell distribution specificity of cytokeratins

| Moll catalogue no. | Isoelectric point | Molecular weight | Specificity |
|---|---|---|---|
| 1, 2 | 6–8 (basic) | 65–67 | Stratified/ductal |
| 3 | 7.5 (basic) | 64 | Stratified/ductal |
| 4 | 7.3 (basic) | 59 | Stratified/ductal |
| 5 | 7.4 (basic) | 58 | All varieties |
| 6 | 7.8 (basic) | 56 | All varieties |
| 7 | 6.0 (basic) | 54 | Simple/glandular |
| 8 | 6.1 (basic) | 52 | Simple/glandular |
| 9 | — | — | — |
| 10 | 5.3 (acidic) | 56.5 | Stratified/ductal |
| 11 | — | — | — |
| 12 | 4.9 (acidic) | 55 | Stratified/ductal |
| 13 | 5.1 (acidic) | 51 | Stratified/ductal |
| 14 | 5.3 (acidic) | 50 | All varieties |
| 15 | 4.9 (acidic) | 50 | All varieties |
| 16 | 5.1 (acidic) | 48 | All varieties |
| 17 | 5.1 (acidic) | 41 | All varieties |
| 18 | 5.7 (acidic) | 45 | Simple/glandular |
| 19 | 5.2 (acidic) | 40 | Simple/glandular |
| 20 | Least acidic | 46 | Simple/glandular |

express two to four distinct varieties of cytokeratins in their normal state but may gain additional cytokeratin pairs, or even lose them, e.g. in hyperproliferative or de-differentiated states, respectively. The latter has been found to be true particularly of the stratified variety of epithelia.

As indicated in Table 5.4 the cytokeratins corresponding to the Moll catalogue numbers 5, 6, 14, 15, 16 and 17 are expressed fairly extensively by both the simple and the stratified varieties of epithelia. On the other hand, regardless of the proliferative or differentiation status, selective expression of cytokeratins numbers 1–4 and 10–12 is fairly consistently associated with stratified/ductal type epithelium, whilst selective expression of cytokeratins 7, 8, 18 and 19 is similarly related to simple/glandular epithelia.

**Functional markers**

These include specific enzymes, secretory products and molecules concerned specifically with secretory, excretory, absorption or transport functions of epithelial cell populations.

As discussed in the following sections, some of the cytoskeletal and functional molecules have proven useful targets for immunocytochemical differentiation of epithelial cells and tumours arising from them.

**Immunocytochemical markers**

A battery of primary antibodies directed at cytokeratins, tissue-specific enzymes and secretory products, and antigens associated with membrane functions or embryonic/developmental origins of epithelial tissues have been developed to provide a fairly comprehensive immunocytochemical basis for identification and subtyping of epithelial tumours.

*Cytokeratin-specific antibodies*

For recognition of an epithelial lineage in an undifferentiated tumour or a small biopsy specimen taken from a poorly differentiated tumour mass, a number of broad-spectrum cytokeratin-specific monoclonal antibodies have been developed. For example, an anticytokeratin monoclonal antibody designated KG8.13, directed at an epitope shared by cytokeratins 1, 5, 6, 7, 8, 10, 11 and 18, has proved eminently successful for this purpose.

Cocktails or combinations of monoclonal antibodies to different types of cytokeratins have proved equally or even more effective in covering the whole range of carcinomas arising from a diverse variety of epithelial tissues. These include combinations of monoclonal antibodies AE1 with AE3, KA-4 with UCD/PR-10, 11 (MAK6), and 35BH11 with 34BE12, respectively. The cytokeratin combinations detected by these cocktails are listed in Table 5.5. Relating these data with those included in Table 5.4 it becomes evident why these cocktails have proved so successful as pan-epithelial markers.

As for identifying epithelial tumours arising from simple as against stratified epithelia, monoclonal antibodies CK1, CK2, CK3 and CK4 (Debus et al 1982, 1984), all directed at a single

**Table 5.5** Cytokeratin profiles detected by pan-cytokeratin antibody reagents

| Antibody reagent | Cytokeratin specificity |
|---|---|
| KG8.13 | 1, 5, 6, 7, 8, 10, 11 and 18 |
| AE1 | 7, 10, 14, 15 and 19 |
| AE3 | 1, 2, 3, 4, 5, 6 and 8 |
| KA-4 | 14, 15 and 19 |
| UCD/PR-10,11 | 6, 8 and 18 |
| 35BH11 | 7 |
| 34BE12 | 1, 2 and 10 |

cytokeratin, namely cytokeratin 18 of the Moll catalogue, as well as another monoclonal antibody, CAM5.2 directed at cytokeratins 8, 18 and 19 (Makin et al 1984), have proven particularly useful.

On the contrary, monoclonal antibodies such as 34BE12 raised against normal stratum corneum cytokeratins with molecular weights of 65–67, 64, 59, 56.5, 55 and 51 kDa, respectively, have proven eminently useful for identification of malignant tumours arising from stratified epithelia (McNutt et al 1988).

### Tissue-specific enzymes

Despite a wide variety of enzymes expressed by epithelial tissues, only two types of enzyme have proved sufficiently reliable markers for routine identification of epithelial tumours on a tissue-specific basis. These include prostatic acid phosphatase and placental alkaline phosphatase which act as very reliable antigenic markers in the identification of prostatic tumours and seminomas (and other germ-cell tumours), respectively.

### Secretory function-related markers

These relate to the secretory function itself, on the one hand, and to the secretory products on the other.

***Markers of secretory function.*** Human milk fat globulin (HMFG) is a heavily glycosylated macromolecular complex membranous component of all secretory epithelia. It is generally not expressed by normal and many varieties of neoplastic germ, lymphoreticular, haematopoietic, neuronal, neuroglial and mesenchymal cells. However, certain epineural and perineural fibroblasts and histiocytes and plasma cells have been found to be capable of expressing HMFG. Also certain malignant tumours such as leiomyosarcoma, a variable proportion of Hodgkin's and non-Hodgkin's lymphomas, and malignant fibrous histiocytoma have been found to express HMFG (Swanson 1988).

Two distinct sets of monoclonal antibodies directed against HMFG have been developed. One set is directed at the carbohydrate component and is popularly referred to as the epithelial membrane antigen (EMA), whilst the other set relates to the protein core component of the HMFG complex. This set is referred to as the HMFGII marker.

***Secretory product-specific markers.*** Apart from hormonal products associated with endocrine organs of epithelial origin which are dealt with mainly in Chapter 7, a limited number of other types of secretory products of epithelial origin are available for immunocytochemical analysis. These are listed in Table 5.6 together with the target epithelial tissues identified by these.

### Embryonic/developmental antigens

A monoclonal antibody OC125 directed against CA125, a high molecular weight glycoprotein antigen expressed by coelomic epithelium during its development (Kabawat et al 1983) has proved relatively effective in differentiating Müllerian tissue-derived adenocarcinomas from other types of adenocarcinoma. Thus, for example, the OC125 stains adenocarcinomas related to the ovarian, fallopian tube, endometrium and endocervical epithelia, but not those derived from the breast or the colon.

In contrast, a monoclonal antibody, CA19.9, reactive against the carbohydrate antigen CA19.9, identified to be a sialated lacto-N-fucopentanose which is closely related to the active epitope of the epithelial membrane antigen (EMA), has been shown to exhibit relative specificity for adenocarcinomas of the gut endoderm-derived tissues.

Carcinoembryonic antigen (CEA), though initially considered to be specific for embryonic

**Table 5.6**   Specific epithelial markers

| Secretory product | Target epithelial tissue |
| --- | --- |
| Thyroglobulin (Tg) | Thyroid follicular epithelium |
| Parathyroid hormone (PTH) and parathyroid hormone-related peptide (PTHrp) | Parathyroid gland |
| Prostate-specific antigen (PSA) | Prostatic epithelium |
| Gross cystic disease fluid protein-15 (GCDFP-15) | Breast glandular epithelium |
| Alpha-fetoprotein (AFP) | Hepatocytes |
| β-subunit of human chorionic gonadotrophin | Placental trophoblast neoplastic germ cells |

tissues and colonic carcinomas, has since been shown by many studies to be expressed by a wide variety of epithelial tumours. Interestingly, according to a detailed study reported by Wick (1988), the expression of CEA seems to be more or less restricted to tumours of endoderm and ectoderm origins, as shown in Table 5.7.

## DIAGNOSTIC APPLICATIONS

Epithelial markers are helpful in resolving two important types of histopathological difficulties: the first relates to the need to recognize epithelial differentiation in an undifferentiated malignancy or inadequately preserved or represented neoplastic tissue in a small biopsy; and the second is concerned with the difficulty of resolving the organ of origin of a disseminated epithelial malignancy.

### Epithelial differentiation markers

Three main varieties of epithelial markers, with differing degrees of sensitivity and specificity towards recognition of epithelial differentiation in an undifferentiated malignancy, have been exploited. They include the pan-cytokeratin (PCK) antibodies; the antibodies to the human milk fat globulin antigens, HMFGII and EMA; and those against carcinoembryonic antigen, CEA.

The PCK markers have proved by far the most sensitive and specific reagents in typing of epithelial differentiation.

Thus, as shown in Table 5.8, they exhibit virtually 100% sensitivity for epithelial malignancies regardless of the type of tumour. As far as their

**Table 5.7** Embryological background of tumours generally positive or negative for carcinoembryonic antigen

| Tumour tissue origin | CEA status | Embryological origin |
| --- | --- | --- |
| Colon | + | Endoderm |
| Stomach | + | Endoderm |
| Biliary tree | + | Endoderm |
| Lung | + | Endoderm |
| Urinary bladder | + | Endoderm/ectoderm |
| Cervix | + | Endoderm/ectoderm |
| Sweat glands | + | Ectoderm |
| Kidney | − | Intermediate mesoderm |
| Endometrium | − | Intermediate mesoderm |
| Serosa | − | Mesoderm |
| Lymph node | − | Mesoderm |
| Soft tissues | − | Mesoderm |

specificity is concerned they appear to be 100% specific with respect to exclusion of all varieties of lymphomas and the vast majority of CNS and soft-tissue tumours. The important exceptions include mesotheliomas, epithelioid and synovial sarcomas, glandular variants of malignant schwannomas, choroid plexus tumours and seminomas. In the latter, usually only a few scattered positive cells are noted to be present.

The HMFG-related markers exhibit a slightly lesser degree of sensitivity (85%) and specificity (90%) compared to the PCK reagents (see Table 5.8). False-negative results include hepatocellular, embryonal and basal-cell carcinomas. On the other hand there is a long series of uncommonly encountered tumours which are likely to be falsely positive. The staining characteristics of cytokeratin, HMFGII and CEA are photomicrographically illustrated in Figure 5.1.

### Organ-specific markers

These are useful for two basic purposes. The first relates to the need to identify the primary source of a disseminated epithelial malignancy presenting as a tumour of undetermined origin. The second is concerned with resolution of different diagnoses relating to a poorly differentiated primary tumour.

*Disseminated epithelial malignancy of undetermined origin*

Approximately 10–15% of referred patients with solid tumours are found to have metastatic malignant disease with unresolved site of primary tumour. Of these, over 80% are likely to be epithelial malignancies of one type or the other (Altman & Cadman 1986). About half of these are eventually found through extensive antemortem and/or postmortem investigations to be arising from specific epithelial organs (Stewart et al 1979) with calculated relative frequencies as listed in Table 5.9.

Determination of the primary site of a disseminated malignancy is important because it is often indicative of the nature of the underlying neoplastic process. This in turn is indicative of the possibility of extended survival or cure and/or treatability of the tumour. If the tumour is found to be

**Table 5.8**   Sensitivity and specificity of non-organ-specific epithelial markers

| Marker | Sensitivity | Specificity |
|---|---|---|
| *Pan-cytokeratin (PCK)* *antibody reagents* AE1/AE3 MAK6 35BH11/34BW12 | 100% (No false-positive expected) | 100% with respect to lymphomas and majority of CNS and sarcomatous tumours |
| | | *False-positive tumours* Mesotheliomas; epithelioid and synovial sarcomas; glandular variant of malignant schwannomas; choroid plexus tumour; seminoma |
| *HMFG* *antibody reagents* HMFGII EMA | 85% *False-negative tumours* Hepatocellular carcinoma; embryonal carcinoma; basal-cell carcinoma | 90% *False-positive tumours* Mesotheliomas; synovial and epithelial sarcoma; chordomas; choroid plexus tumours; meningiomas; lymphocyte-predominant Hodgkin's disease; certain T cell and killer cell lymphomas; plasma cell tumours; leiomyosarcomas; malignant fibrous histiocytomas; and some B cell lymphomas |
| *CEA* *antibody reagents* HMA6 CEA | 42% *False-negative tumours* Prostate; kidney; liver; endometrium; nasopharynx; squamous-cell carcinomas; basal-cell carcinomas | 100% *With respect to* Germ-cell tumours; melanomas; mesotheliomas; lymphomas; sarcomas *except* epithelioid sarcoma |

of the untreatable type then it is equally important to know that in advance so as to avoid the toxic side-effects of otherwise useless treatment.

Disseminated epithelial tumours which are amenable to treatment with significant beneficial effect include those arising from prostate, ovary, thyroid, breast and germ cells. Early diagnosis or exclusion of these tumours with the help of immunocytochemical markers is likely therefore to be of considerable benefit to the patient. The relative effectiveness of the various markers available for diagnosis of an epithelial malignancy on an organ-

**Table 5.9**   Relative frequencies of organ-related epithelial malignancies presenting as tumours of undetermined origin

| Organ of origin | Relative frequency of epithelial malignancies |
|---|---|
| Lung | 23.3 |
| Colon | 16.7 |
| Ovary | 13.3 |
| Stomach | 10.0 |
| Prostate | 6.6 |
| Thyroid | 6.6 |
| Germ cell | 6.6 |
| Kidney | 6.6 |
| Hepatoma | 6.6 |
| Pancreas | 3.3 |
| Breast | Rare |

specific basis is discussed next under individual organs.

**Prostatic tumours.** Two prostatic epithelial markers, prostate-specific antigen (PSA) and prostatic acid phosphatase (PAPh) have consistently proved both highly sensitive and specific in diagnosis of prostatic origin of disseminated epithelial malignancy.

Thus, on the basis of 109 cases studied collectively by Nadji et al (1981) and Ellis et al (1984), PSA and PAPh were found to have specificity of 100% and sensitivity of 99.1% and 87.2%, respectively.

**Germ-cell tumours.** These include choriocarcinomas, testicular seminomas, embryonal carcinomas and endodermal sinus tumours. For all these types of tumours, polyclonal antibody reagents specific for β chain of human chorionic gonadotrophin (β-HCG) have proved eminently effective in conjunction with the application of the immunoperoxidase method on formalin-fixed, paraffin-embedded tissues.

The sensitivity of anti-β-HCG is to be judged on the basis of differing patterns of staining produced by it in different types of germ-cell tumours. In choriocarcinomas the positivity is seen in all cells, whilst in the other type of tumours it is often

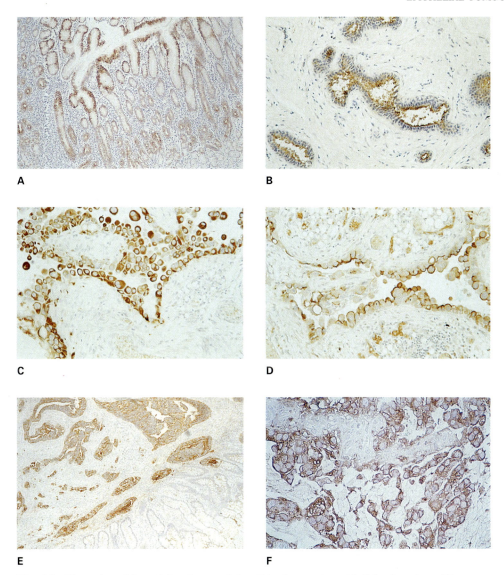

**Fig. 5.1**   Illustration of the staining characteristics of the three major epithelial cell markers. (**A**) Cytokeratin (CAM5.2) staining of normal small-bowel mucosal epithelium. (**B**) Epithelial membrane antigen (HMFGII) staining of normal breast duct epithelium. Note the luminal surface orientation of the staining. **C** and **D** show the cytoplasmic and luminal orientation of the staining due to cytokeratin (CAM5.2) and epithelial membrane antigen (HMFGII), respectively, in an epithelial malignancy. **E** and **F** depict the membrane orientation of staining due to CEA in a carcinoma of the colon and an anaplastic epithelial malignancy. Note the absence of staining of the background colonic epithelium. (DHSS immunoperoxidase method.)

restricted to scattered syncytiotrophoblastic giant cells (Heyderman & Neville 1976). Immunoreactivity for this hormone may also be found in intratubular neoplastic germ cells and large mononuclear cells probably representative of the neoplastic counterpart of the 'intermediate trophoblast' of the normal placenta and trophoblastic neoplasms (Marivel et al 1987).

As for the specificity of anti-β-HCG, it is virtually 100% specific for germ-cell tumours except for the occasional cases of breast, lung, gastrointestinal tract, ovary, uterus and salivary gland tumours in which β-HCG immunoreactivity has been recorded (Marivel 1988).

*Thyroid/follicular tumours*. Thyroglobulin is a 100% specific marker for thyroid follicular epithelial tumours but its sensitivity seems to vary according to the degree of differentiation state of the tumour. Thus the more anaplastic the tumour, the less sensitively antithyroglobulin is likely to stain the tumour (Jasani & Newman 1988).

*Breast tumours*. Whilst human milk fat globulin-related antigens, EMA and HMFGII, are highly sensitive markers of breast tumours of all varieties, they are totally lacking in specificity as they are virtually pan-epithelial tumour markers (see above).

Recently, a major protein antigen of gross cystic disease fluid, GCDFP-15, has proved to be a virtually 100% specific marker of over 50% of breast carcinomas of varieties taken together (Mazoujian 1988). The sensitivity is, however, 100% for infiltrating lobular carcinoma with signet-ring cell diferentiation, and falls to 70% for intraductal carcinomas, 58% for infiltrating ductal tumours, and as low as 5% for the medullary variant.

*Ovarian tumours*. CA125, a high molecular weight glycoprotein originally isolated from an ovarian carcinoma and subsequently found to be expressed by coelomic epithelium and its derivatives (Bast et al 1981) has proved to be a highly effective marker of non-mucinous carcinomas of the ovary. Studies by Ellis & Hitchcock (1988) have shown positive staining in about 95% of serous adeno-carcinomas of the ovary and none in metastatic adenocarcinoma deposits from non-Müllerian sites.

Mucinous ovarian cancers are less amenable to accurate definition with immunocytochemical markers. Thus, although another tumour-related antigen, CA19.9 (lacto-N-fucopentanose II), a sialated derivative of the Lewis A blood group, is consistently expressed by this type of ovarian cancer, there are also a number of alimentary tract tumours which express this antigen. To overcome this handicap, Ellis & Hitchcock (1988) have promoted the use of a panel of antibodies with the expected patterns of staining of the main competitive tumours as summarized in Table 5.10.

*Resolution of differential diagnoses of primary tumours*

There are two main applications of epithelial markers for this purpose as described below.

**Bladder vs prostatic primary**. In resolving bladder vs prostatic primary, three markers have proved quite effective. Thus CEA in combination with PSA and PAPh is sufficient to resolve the majority of the differential diagnostic problems. In a study reported by Wick (1988), 89% (40 out of 45) of bladder tumours and none (0 out of 35) of the prostatic tumours exhibited CEA. In a bigger study, however (Ellis et al 1984), 4 out of 60 cases of prostatic malignancies were found to express CEA positivity, making the overall specificity of CEA to be 95.8% (4 out of 95) in favour of bladder cancer. PSA and PAPh, as already described above, were found to be virtually 100% specific for the prostatic cancers.

**Pulmonary adenocarcinoma vs mesothelioma**. Mesothelioma has the potential of mimicking pulmonary adenocarcinoma on histological

**Table 5.10**  Panel of immunocytochemical markers for differentiation of ovarian tumours from alimentary tract neoplasms

| Tumour type | Immunocytochemical markers | | | |
|---|---|---|---|---|
| | CA125 | CA19.9 | EMA | CEA |
| Ovary (mucinous) | P | O | O | P |
| Ovary (non-mucinous) | O | P | O | O |
| Large bowel | O | O | O | PP |
| Pancreas | O | O | O | O |
| Small bowel | O | O | O | N |
| Stomach | N | N | O | P |
| Gallbladder | O | P | P | P |
| Bile duct | O | PP | O | PP |

EMA = epithelial membrane antigen; CEA = carcinoembryonic antigen; PP = consistent extensive positivity; P = consistent focal positivity; O = inconsistent positivity; N = consistently negative.

**Table 5.11**   Observed CEA positivity rates: pulmonary adenocarcinoma vs mesothelioma

| Case study | CEA positivity rate (%) | |
|---|---|---|
| | *Adenocarcinoma* | *Mesothelioma* |
| Wang et al (1979) | 100 (12/12) | 0 (0/12) |
| Battifora & Kopinsky (1985) | 65 (65/100) | 17 (2/12) |
| Gibbs et al (1985) | 89 (24/27) | 0 (0/29) |
| Pfaltz et al (1987) | 100 (22/22) | 4 (2/47) |
| Wick (1988) | 89 (24/27) | 0 (0/29) |
| Overall sensitivity and specificity, respectively | 84 (202/241) | 3 (4/151) |

grounds on such a scale that it has proved almost mandatory to depend upon immunocytochemistry to resolve the differential diagnosis. Mesothelioma being an occupational disease, there are obvious medico-legal reasons for making sure that the correct diagnosis is reached. The other complication of this kind of lung tumour is that often the diagnosis is made on poorly preserved post-mortem lung tissue.

A considerable effort has therefore been devoted to obtaining a reliable set of markers for differentiating pulmonary adenocarcinoma from lung mesothelioma. Of many markers attempted, only CEA has proved to be both sensitive and specific for pulmonary adenocarcinoma (see Table 5.11 for a summary of data obtained in five independent studies).

Unfortunately, because the sensitivity of CEA for pulmonary adenocarcinoma is not 100%, and because there are no reliable positive markers for lung mesothelioma, a negative CEA result is considered to be highly unreliable. Donna et al (1986)

have proposed an antibody to a cytoplasmic protein unique to primary tumours of mesothelial origin, as a reliable positive marker of lung mesotheliomas. However, the relevant antibody is not yet commercially available and it has not been tested on a large series of lung tumours.

In order to provide a partial solution to the problem, Jasani et al (1985) have proposed a strong immunostaining for both cytokeratin and vimentin as a useful positive discriminant marker combination for identifying mesothelioma. In this study, 75% of a mixed variety of mesotheliomas were found to express a strong positivity for these markers. In comparison, only 6% of the pulmonary adenocarcinomas showed double positivity, though with the vimentin staining was significantly on the weaker side. The strong tendency for mesothelium to express both cytokeratin and vimentin is consistent with its embryological origins.

Thus mesothelium is closely related to the coelomic epithelial tissue arising from the intermediate mesoderm and giving rise to various tissues of the urogenital system including the secretory epithelium of the kidney and the lining of various serous cavities (see the section on the Embryology of Epithelial Tissues, p. 56).

In current practice it is hence recommended to use a panel of antibodies including those against CEA, pan-cytokeratin antigens and vimentin, to most effectively resolve the differential diagnosis between pulmonary adenocarcinoma and lung mesothelioma.

## REFERENCES AND FURTHER READING

### Embryological and anatomical background

Cooper D, Schermer A, Sun T-T 1985 Biology of disease. Classification of human epithelia and their neoplasms using monoclonal antibodies to keratins: strategies, applications and limitations. Laboratory Investigation 52: 243–256

Gould V E 1986 Histogenesis and differentiation: a re-evaluation of these concepts as criteria for classification of tumours. Human Pathology 17: 212–215

Harrison R G 1978 Clinical embryology, Academic Press, London p 68–109, 160–181

### Biochemical background and diagnostic applications

Altman, E, Cadman E 1986 An analysis of 1539 patients with cancer of unknown primary site. Cancer 57: 120–124

Bast R C Jr, Feeney M, Lazarus H et al 1981 Reactivity of a monoclonal antibody with human ovarian carcinoma. Journal of Clinical Investigation 8: 1331–1337

Battifora H, Kopinsky M I 1985 Distinction of mesothelioma from adenocarcinoma. Cancer 55: 1679–1685

Debus E, Weber K, Osborn M 1982 Monoclonal antibodies that distinguish simple from stratified squamous epithelia: characterisation on human tissues. EMBO Journal 1: 1641–1647

Debus E, Moll R, Franke W W et al 1984 Immunocytochemical distinction of human carcinomas by cytokeratin typing with monoclonal antibodies. American Journal of Pathology 114: 121–130

Donna A, Betta P G, Bellingeri D, Marchesini A 1986 New marker for mesothelioma: an immunoperoxidase study. Journal of Clinical Pathology 39: 961–968

Ellis I O, Hitchcock A 1988 Tumour marker

immunoreactivity in adenocarcinoma. Journal of Clinical Pathology 41: 1064–1067

Ellis D W, Leffers S, Davies J S, Ng A B P 1984 Multiple immunoperoxidase markers in benign hyperplasia and adenocarcinoma of the prostate. American Journal of Clinical Pathology 81: 279–284

Gibbs A R, Harach R, Wagner J C, Jasani B 1985 Comparison of tumour markers in malignant mesothelioma and pulmonary adenocarcinoma. Thorax 40: 91

Heyderman E, Neville A M 1976 Syncytiotrophoblasts in malignant testicular tumours. Lancet 1: 103

Jasani B, Newman G R 1988 Application of immunocytochemistry to thyroid tumours. In: Wynford-Thomas D, Williams E D (eds) Thyroid tumours: molecular basis of pathogenesis. Churchill Livingstone, Edinburgh, p 140–147

Jasani B, Edwards R E, Thomas N D, Gibbs A R 1985 The use of vimentin antibodies in the diagnosis of malignant mesothelioma. Virchows Archiv. (Pathologic Anatomic) 406: 441–448

Kabawat S E, Bast R C, Bhan A K et al 1983 Tissue distribution of a coelomic-epithelium-related antigen recognised by the monoclonal antibody OC125

McNutt M A, Bolen J W, Vogel A M 1988 Monoclonal antibodies to cytokeratins in diagnostic immunocytochemistry. In: Wick M R, Siegal G P (eds) Monoclonal antibodies in diagnostic immunohistochemistry. Marcel Dekker, New York, p 51–70

Makin C A, Bobrow L G, Bodmer W F 1984 Monoclonal antibody to cytokeratin for use in routine histopathology. Journal of Clinical Pathology 37: 975–983

Manvel J 1988 Antibodies to human chorionic gonadotropin. In: Wick M R, Siegal G P (eds) Monoclonal antibodies in diagnostic immunohistochemistry. Marcel Dekker, New York, p 581

Manvel J C, Neihans G, Wick M R, Dehner L P 1987 Intermediate trophoblast in germ cell neoplasms. American Journal of Surgical Pathology 11: 693–701

Mazoujian G 1988 Gross cystic disease fluid protein-15. In: Wick M R, Siegal G P (eds) Monoclonal antibodies in diagnostic immunohistochemistry. Marcel Dekker, New York, p 505–519

Moll R, Franke W W, Schiller D L 1982 The catalog of human cytokeratins: patterns of expression in normal epithelia tumors and cultured cells. Cell 31: 11–24

Moll R, Lowe A, Laufer J et al 1992 Cytokeratin 20 in human carcinomas: a new histodiagnostic marker detected by monoclonal antibodies. American Journal of Pathology 140: 427–447

Nadji M, Tabei S Z, Castro A et al 1981 Prostate-specific antigen: an immunohistologic marker for prostatic neoplasms. Cancer 48: 1229–1232

Pfaltz M, Odermatt B, Christen B, Rüttner J R 1987 Immunohistochemistry in the diagnosis of malignant mesothelioma. Virchows Archiv A, Pathological Anatomy and Histopathology 411: 387–393

Stewart J F, Tattersall M H N, Woods R L, Fox R M 1979 Unknown primary adenocarcinoma: incidence of overinvestigation and natural history. British Medical Journal 1: 1530–1533

Swanson P E 1988 Monoclonal antibodies to human milk fat globule proteins. In: Wick M R, Siegal G P (eds) Monoclonal antibodies in diagnostic immunohistochemistry. Marcel Dekker, New York, p 227–283

Wang N S, Huang S N, Gold P 1979 Absence of carcino-embryonic antigen-like material in mesothelioma: an immunohistochemical differentiation from other lung cancers. Cancer 44: 937–943

Wick M R 1988 Monoclonal antibodies to carcino-embryonic antigen in diagnostic immunohistochemistry. In: Wick M R, Siegal G P (eds) Monoclonal antibodies in diagnostic immunohistochemistry. Marcel Dekker, New York, p 539–567

# 6. Soft-tissue tumours

## INTRODUCTION

Soft tissue is defined as non-epithelial extra-skeletal tissue with the exceptions of reticuloendothelial system, glia and supporting tissue of various parenchymal organs (Enzinger & Weiss 1988).

## EMBRYOLOGY

Embryologically, soft tissues are derived from mesoderm, with some contribution from neuroectoderm. Soft tissue is represented by connective tissue, adipose tissue, cartilage, muscle tissue, blood and lymph vessels, synovial tissue, and mesothelial tissue. It also includes by definition the peripheral nerves, the autonomic ganglia and paraganglionic structures.

## ANATOMY AND BIOCHEMISTRY

Anatomically, connective tissue, fat and vessels can be found throughout the body. Muscle tissue can be distinguished on the basis of morphological and functional criteria: skeleton muscles, smooth muscles (gastrointestinal tract, genitourinary tract, skin), and heart muscle. Synovial tissue can be found as the lining of joints, tendons and bursae. Cartilage is a specialized form of connective tissue. Its main functions are to support soft tissues, to provide sliding areas for joints, and it is essential for the development and growth of long bones before and after birth. The paraganglia can be found throughout the body as a widely dispersed system of neural crest cells arising in association with the segmental or collateral anatomic ganglia.

## IMMUNOCYTOCHEMICAL MARKERS IN SOFT-TISSUE STUDIES

The main tasks for immunocytochemistry in diseases involving soft tissues are:

1. as a tool for a more accurate identification of tumours and tumour-like lesions arising from soft tissues having an important impact on treatment and therapy
2. to distinguish soft-tissue tumours and tumour-like lesions from (undifferentiated) carcinoma, lymphoma and melanoma.

As stated above, immunocytochemistry in this area deals to a great extent with tumours arising from soft tissues. Soft-tissue tumours are masses occurring in soft tissues excluding lymphomas and tumours of the skin. Important information in regard to the differential diagnosis of soft-tissue tumours includes the age of the respective patient and the tumour location (for detailed explanations see textbooks on soft-tissue tumours).

With the advent of excellent and commercially available antibodies against structures of the cyto-skeleton and other markers, immunocytochemistry has become a recognized and important field for differential diagnosis of soft-tissue tumours. The most important antibodies and their main antigen distributions in soft-tissue tumours are:

- *Cytokeratin:* synovial sarcoma, epithelioid sarcoma, mesothelioma; aberrant expression in other sarcomas may occur
- *Vimentin:* almost all sarcomas; may be expressed by carcinomas
- *Desmin:* skeletal and smooth-muscle tumours
- *Myoglobin:* differentiated skeletal-muscle tumours

- *Factor VIII-related antigen (F-VIII-RAG):* angiomas and angiosarcomas, lymphangiomas
- *S-100 protein:* melanoma, granular-cell tumours, clear-cell sarcoma, histiocytosis X, benign nerve sheath tumours, benign chondroid tumours, sustentacular cells of paragangliomas, malignant schwannomas
- *Epithelial membrane antigen (EMA)/human milk fat globulin (HMFGII):* synovial sarcoma, epithelioid sarcoma, some mesotheliomas.

Additional use of other antibodies is suggested depending mainly on morphological criteria found in routine stains and/or clinical information.

**Histochemical stains**

Histochemical stains are of limited importance in the diagnosis of soft-tissue tumours. They are mainly performed to demonstrate fat, glycogen, mucopolysaccharides or enzymes. (For a more detailed description, see Mackenzie & Filipe 1983.)

**Immunocytochemistry of soft-tissue tumours**

For each tumour type only the most important markers which are detectable in formalin-fixed, paraffin-embedded tissues are listed in the form of diagnostic algorithms in Tables 6.1–6.12. Differential diagnostic comments are included in these wherever appropriate.

**Table 6.1** Tumours of fibrous tissue

| Fibrosarcoma | Differential diagnostic comments |
|---|---|
| – cytokeratin | + monophasic synovial sarcoma |
| | + mesothelioma |
| – S-100 protein | + melanoma |
| | +/– malignant schwannoma |
| – MAC387 | + malignant fibrous histiocytoma |
| – KP1 (CD68) | + |

**Table 6.2** Fibrohistiocytic tumours

| Tumour type | Differential diagnostic comments |
|---|---|
| *Juvenile xanthogranuloma* | |
| – S-100 protein | + neurofibroma |
| | +/– (myxoid) liposarcoma |
| *Atypical fibroxanthoma* | |
| – S-100 protein | + melanoma |
| – cytokeratin | – |
| | For the differential diagnosis of a melanoma both antibodies should be used! |
| *Malignant fibrous histiocytoma (MFH)* | |
| + MAC387; KP1 (CD68) | – fibrosarcoma |
| | – lymphomas |
| – LeuMI (CD15) | + Hodgkin's disease |
| – Ki-1 (CD30) | |
| – cytokeratin | + anaplastic carcinoma |
| +/– alpha-1-antitrypsin | |
| +/– lysozyme | both markers are rather unspecific (Soini & Miettinen 1989) |
| – myoglobin | +/– } rhabdomyosarcoma |
| – desmin | + } |
| + laminin | Few neoplastic cells in some cases are positive (Soini et al 1989) |
| –/+ Type IV collagen | |
| – S-100 protein | +/– liposarcoma |

**Table 6.3** Tumours of adipose tissue

| Tumour type | Differential diagnostic comment |
|---|---|
| Lipoma | |
| – MAC387 | Beham et al (1989) found a weak to |
| – laminin | moderate intracytoplasmatic S-100 protein |
| – Type IV collagen | staining in pleiomorphic, but not in spindle-cell lipomas |
| *Liposarcoma* | |
| +/– S-100 protein | – } Malignant fibrous |
| – MAC387 | + } histiocytoma (Hashimoto et al 1984) |

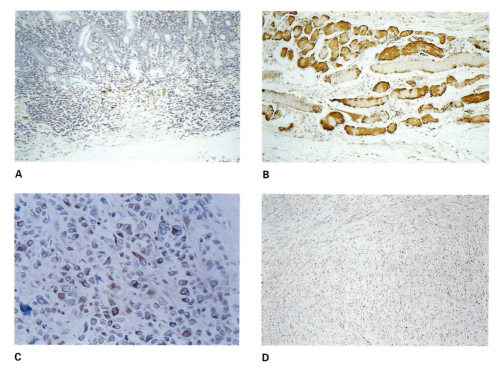

**Fig. 6.1**   Illustration of markers of value in the diagnosis of rhabdomyosarcoma. (**A**) Use of small intestinal biopsy as a convenient positive control tissue. (**B**) Strong staining of background skeletal muscle cells with myoglobin antibody. (**C**) Desmin staining of an embryonal rhabdomyosarcoma helping to identify the so-called tandem cells and racket-shaped cells considered to be characteristic of rhabdomyosarcomas. (**D**) Myoglobin staining in another case of embryonal rhabdomyosarcoma proving as a definitive diagnostic test (simple two-step indirect immunoperoxidase method).

**Table 6.4**   Tumours of muscle tissue

| Tumour type | Differential diagnostic comment |
| --- | --- |
| *Leiomyosarcoma* | |
| +/– desmin | See Enzinger & Weiss 1988, Hashimoto et al 1986 |
| + actin | See Tsukada et al 1987, Jones et al 1990 |
| – S-100 protein | +/– malignant schwannoma |
| | + neurolemmoma |
| *Epithelioid smooth-muscle tumours* | Desmin is very rarely expressed by these tumours (Enzinger & Weiss 1988, Appelman 1986) |
| *Rhabdomyoma* | |
| + desmin | – ⎫ |
| – S-100 protein | + ⎬ granular-cell tumour |
| + actin | ⎭ |
| *Rhabdomyosarcoma* | |
| +/– myoglobin (expressed by approximately 60% of rhabdomyosarcomas. Myoglobin is very rarely found in leiomyosarcomas; Leader et al 1989) | |
| + desmin | – malignant fibrous histiocytoma |
| – S-100 protein | + Triton tumours (Denk et al 1983) |
| + myosin | |
| + vimentin | |
| – NSE, chromogranin A | + primitive neuroectodermal tumour (PNET) |

Cytokeratin and neurofilament expression was found in some cases of rhabdomyosarcoma by Miettinen & Rapola (1989). Dodd et al (1989) described a positive staining with antibodies against troponin T in 'favourable' tumours. So far, however, this marker is not commercially available. Immunocytochemical application of vimentin, desmin and myoglobin in diagnosis of rhabdomyosarcoma is photomicrographically illustrated in Figure 6.1.

**Table 6.5**  Heterologous tumours with rhabdomyoblastic differentiation

In the following tumours, rhabdomyoblastic differentiation can be demonstrated immunohistochemically using antibodies to myoglobin, desmin and myosin:
1. Malignant mixed mesodermal tumours of uterus, ovary, and retroperitoneum (mixed Müllerian tumours)
2. Carcinosarcoma of breast and urinary bladder
3. Nephroblastoma
4. Mixed-type hepatoblastoma
5. Wilms' tumours
6. Malignant teratomas
7. Various neuroectodermal tumours: ganglioneuroma, medulloepithelioma, malignant schwannoma (malignant Triton tumour)
8. Pulmonary blastoma

**Table 6.6**  Tumours of blood and lymph vessels (see Figure 6.2 for photomicrographic illustration of the pattern of staining obtained with F-VIII-RAG, BMA 120 and JC/70)

| Tumour type | Differential diagnostic comments |
| --- | --- |
| *Haemangioma* | |
| + F-VIII-RAG (von Willebrand factor) | |
| + BMA 120 | See Alles & Bosslet 1988 |
| + JC/70 (CD31) | See Parums et al 1990 |
| + QBEND/10 (CD34) | See Ramani et al 1990 |
| *Angiosarcoma* | |
| + F-VIII-RAG | Abberrant F-VIII-RAG expression has been found in some anaplastic carcinomas! |
| + BMA 120 | |
| + JC/70 (CD31) | |
| + QBEND/10 (CD34) | |
| − cytokeratin | + carcinomas |
| + vimentin | +/− some carcinomas may express vimentin! |
| *Kaposi's sarcoma* | |
| + JC/70 (CD31) | |
| + QBEND/10 (CD34) | |
| − F-VIII-RAG | usually only expressed in occasionally spindled tumour cells (Millard & Heryet 1985, Parums et al 1990) |
| − HLA-DR Ia | + normal capillaries |
| *Glomus tumours* | |
| + JC/70 | See Parums et al 1990 |
| − F-VIII-RAG | + vascular tumours |
| − desmin | + myogenic tumours |
| *Haemangiopericytoma* | |
| + JC/70 | See Parums et al 1990 |
| − F-VIII-RAG | |
| − Ulex europaeus I agglutinin | |
| − BMA 120 | Tumour cells of haemangiopericytomas are negative for endothelial markers, whereas normal endothelial cells within the tumour show a positive staining |
| − actin | |
| − vimentin | |
| − desmin | |
| +/− S-100 protein | See Enzinger & Weiss 1988 |
| − MAC387 | + malignant fibrous histiocytoma |
| − cytokeratin and EMA | + synovial sarcoma |
| − renin | + renin-producing juxtaglomerular tumour (Gherardi et al 1974) |

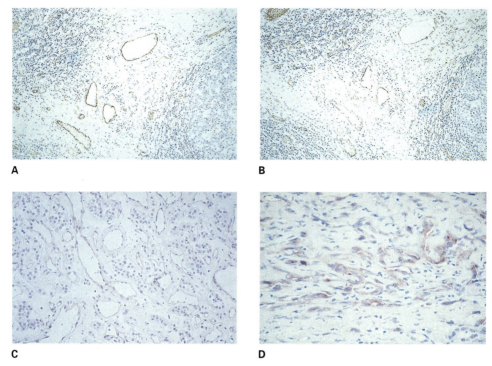

**Fig. 6.2**   Illustration of markers of importance in the diagnosis of blood and lymph vessel tumours. (**A**) and (**B**) Use of human tonsil as a convenient positive tissue for demonstration of Factor VIII-related antigen (von Willebrand factor) and JC/70 (CD31) respectively. (**C**) Staining of the endothelial cell lining in a case of glomangioma with the BMA 120 marker. (**D**) Staining of the neoplastic blood vessels with von Willebrand factor-specific antibody in a case of an angiosarcoma (simple two-step indirect immunoperoxidase method).

**Table 6.7**    Tumours of synovial tissue

| Tumour type | Differential diagnostic comments |
| --- | --- |
| *Synovial sarcoma* | |
| + cytokeratin | (spindle and epithelial cells) – fibrosarcoma – haemangiopericytoma |
| + EMA | (less intensive than cytokeratin in spindle and epithelial cells) |
| + vimentin | Cytokeratin and EMA are negative in tenosynovial giant-cell tumours (nodular tenosynovitis) |
| +/– CEA | (Corson et al 1984) |
| S-100 | Protein can be found very rarely in a few neoplastic spindle cells (Enzinger & Weiss 1988) |
| | +/– malignant schwannoma |
| | + melanoma |

**Table 6.8a**    Mesothelial tumours

| Tumour type | Differential diagnostic comments |
| --- | --- |
| *Benign mesothelioma of the genital tract (adenomatoid tumour)* | |
| – F-VIII-RAG | + vascular tumours |
| + EMA | |
| + cytokeratin | |
| *Localized fibrous mesothelioma (subserosal fibroma)* | |
| + vimentin | |
| – EMA | |
| – low molecular weight | + reactive fibrous proliferation |
| cytokeratin (CAM5.2) | + mesothelioma of connective tissue type (Al-Izzi et al 1989) |

**Table 6.8a** (*contd.*)

| Tumour type | Differential diagnostic comments |
|---|---|
| *Multicystic peritoneal mesothelioma*<br>+ cytokeratin<br>+ EMA<br>– F-VIII-RAG | – lymphangioma |
| *Malignant mesothelioma*<br>+ cytokeratin<br>+ EMA<br>+ vimentin }<br>– CEA   } | – localized fibrous mesothelioma<br>These two antibodies are the most important markers to distinguish<br>malignant mesothelioma from lung adenocarcinoma, whereas vimentin is very<br>rarely found in these tumours (Jasani et al 1985; see also p. 63) |
| – LeuM1<br>– beta-1 pregnancy-specific protein<br>– Ca19.9 | |

**Table 6.8b**  Tumours of peripheral nerves

| Tumour type | Differential diagnostic comments |
|---|---|
| *Benign schwannoma (neurolemmoma)*<br>+ S-100 protein<br>*Neurofibroma*<br>Only occasionally S-100 cells can be found in<br>neurofibromas. See Enzinger & Weiss 1988 | |
| *Granular-cell tumour (benign and malignant)* (see Figure 6.3 for photomicrographic illustration of the staining pattern obtained with S-100 and NSE) | |
| + S-100 protein | congenital gingival granular-cell tumour |
| – laminin | |
| + NSE | |
| + myelin proteins | (interstitial cells, Nathrath & Remberger 1986) |
| – GFAP | |
| – NF | |
| *Malignant schwannoma*<br>– cytokeratin<br>– EMA<br>+ S-100 protein (Weiss et al 1983)<br>+ myelin (Wick et al 1987)<br>+ NSE<br>+/– NF (occasionally; Matsunou et al 1985) | +<br>+ } synovial sarcoma<br>– |
| *Malignant Triton tumour (malignant schwannoma with rhabdomyoblastic differentiation)*<br>+ desmin<br>+ myoglobin<br>+ vimentin<br>+ S-100 protein | +<br>+ } rhabdomyosarcoma<br>+<br>– |
| *Glandular malignant schwannoma*<br>– cytokeratin<br>+ S-100 protein | +<br>– } synovial sarcoma (Enzinger & Weiss 1988) |
| *Malignant epithelioid schwannoma**<br>– cytokeratin<br>+ S-100 protein<br>– melanin stains | + carcinoma<br>+<br>+ } melanoma |
| *Neurotropic (desmoplastic) melanoma*<br>+ S-100 protein<br>– cytokeratin | – reactive fibroblastic proliferation of the skin<br>+ carcinoma |
| (See Figure 6.4 for photomicrographic illustration of the value of S-100 and a melanoma-specific marker, M3080, in the diagnosis of melanomas in general.) | |
| *Neuroepithelioma (peripheral neuroblastoma)*<br>– S-100 protein<br>– cytokeratin<br>– WBC<br>+ NSE and chromogranin A (Llombart-Bosch et al 1989) | + schwannoma<br>+ carcinoma<br>+ lymphoma |

*This tumour closely resembles melanoma or anaplastic carcinoma. It may be indistinguishable from non-pigmented melanoma.

**Table 6.9**   Paraganglioma

| Tumour type | Differential diagnostic comments |
|---|---|
| *Paragangliomas of various locations*<br>+ NSE<br>+ SF<br>+/- met-enkephalin<br>+ chromogranin A (Weiler et al 1988)<br><br>+ S-100 protein<br>+ GFAP (Schröder<br>  & Johannsen 1986) | The combined use of NSE, chromogranin A, and met-enkephalin shows a 100% positive staining of paragangliomas (Kliewer et al 1989)<br>- metastases of clear-cell carcinomas, e.g. renal-cell carcinomas) |
| *Gangliocytic paraganglioma*<br>+ NSE<br><br>+ NF<br>+ chromogranin A<br>+ S-100 protein<br>+ GFAP<br>+ various polypeptides (insulin, glucagon,<br>  leu-enkephalin, pancreatic polypeptide,<br>  somatostatin, vasoactive intestinal<br>  polypeptide, serotonin and others;<br>  Perrone et al 1985, Hamid et al<br>  1986, Scheithauer et al 1986) | Gangliocytic paraganglioma combines features of paragangliomas, carcinoids, and ganglioneuromas and is almost always found in the duodenum |

**Table 6.10**   Tumours of cartilage

| Tumour type | Differential diagnostic comment |
|---|---|
| + S-100 protein<br>+ vimentin | + } like<br>+ } normal chondrocytes |
| *Extraskeletal myxoid chondrosarcoma*<br>+ vimentin<br>+ S-100 protein<br>- GFAP<br>- EMA<br>- cytokeratin<br>- CEA | <br><br>+ } myxopapillary ependymoma (Specht et al 1986)<br>+ }<br>+ } pleiomorphic adenoma, chondroid syringioma, adenoidcystic carcinoma<br>+ } |

**Table 6.11**   Osseous tumours of soft tissue

| Tumour type | Differential diagnostic comment |
|---|---|
| + vimentin<br>- cytokeratin<br>- EMA<br>- MAC387<br>- S-100 protein<br>- cytokeratin<br>+/- NSE (Shimada et al 1988)<br>+ NF (Ushigome et al 1989) | + }<br>+ } synovial sarcoma<br>+ }<br>+ malignant fibrous histiocytoma<br>+/- liposarcoma<br>+ carcinoma |

**Table 6.12** Soft-tissue tumours of uncertain histogenesis

| Tumour type | Differential diagnostic comment |
|---|---|
| *Alveolar soft-part sarcoma* | |
| +/– desmin (Denk et al 1983, Lieberman et al 1989) | |
| +/– actin (Mukai et al 1986, Ordonez et al 1989) | |
| +/– vimentin (Denk et al 1983, Lieberman et al 1989) | |
| +/– NSE (Ordonez et al 1989) | |
| + S-100 protein (Lieberman et al 1989) | |
| – cytokeratin | + renal-cell carcinoma |
| | |
| *Epithelioid sarcoma* | |
| + cytokeratin | – ⎫ |
| + EMA (Miettinen et al 1982, | – ⎬ (malignant) fibrous histiocytoma, fibrosarcoma |
| Fisher 1988); | – ⎭ |
| + vimentin | |
| – S-100 protein | + melanoma |
| – F-VIII-RAG | + angiosarcoma |
| | |
| Alpha-1-antitrypsin, alpha-1-antichymotrypsin | |
| and CEA were demonstrated in some cases | |
| (Chase et al 1984) | |
| | |
| *Clear-cell sarcoma* | |
| + S-100 protein | – fibrosarcoma |
| | |
| *Extraskeletal Ewing's sarcoma* | |
| + vimentin | |
| +/– NSE | + ⎫ Merkel cell carcinoma |
| – chromogranin A | + ⎭ neuroblastoma PNET |
| +/– S-100 protein (Shimada et al 1988) | |
| – NF | |
| – GFAP | |
| – F-VIII-RAG | |
| – Ulex europaeus I agglutinin | |
| – desmin | + alveolar rhabdomyosarcoma |
| – cytokeratin | + small-cell carcinoma |
| – WBC | + lymphoma |

## REFERENCES AND FURTHER READING

Al-Izzi M, Thurlow N P, Corrin B 1989 Pleural mesothelioma of connective tissue type, localized fibrous tumour of the pleura, and reactive submesothelial hyperplasia. An immunohistochemical comparison. Journal of Pathology 158: 41–44

Alles J U, Bosslet K 1988 Immunocytochemistry of angiosarcomas. A study of 19 cases with special emphasis on the applicability of endothelial cell specific markers to routinely prepared tissues. American Journal of Clinical Pathology 89: 463–471

Appelman H D 1986 Smooth muscle tumours of the gastrointestinal tract: what we know that Stout didn't know. American Journal of Surgical Pathology 10: 83–85 (Suppl)

Beckstead J H, Wood G S, Fletcher V 1985 Evidence for the origin of Kaposi's Sarcoma from lymphatic endothelium. American Journal of Pathology 119: 294–300

Beham A, Schmid C, Hödl S, Fletcher C D M 1989 Spindle cell and pleomorphic lipoma: an immunohistochemical study and histogenetic analysis. Journal of Pathology 158: 219–222

Chase D R, Weiss S W, Enzinger F M, Longloss J M 1984 Keratin in epithelioid sarcoma. An immunohistochemical study. American Journal of Surgical Pathology 8: 435–441

Corson J M, Weiss L M, Banks-Schlegel S P, Pinkus G S 1984 Keratin proteins and carcinoembryonic antigen in synovial sarcomas: an immunohistochemical study of 24 cases. Human Pathology 15: 615–621

Denk H, Krepler R, Artlieb U, Gabbiani G, Rungger-Brändle E, Leoncini P, Franke W W 1983 Proteins of intermediate filament. An immunohistochemical and biochemical approach to the classification of soft tissue tumors. American Journal of Pathology 110: 193–208

Dodd S, Malone M, McCulloch W 1989 Rhabdomyosarcoma in children: a histological and immunohistochemical study of 59 cases. Journal of Pathology 158: 13–18

Enzinger F M, Weiss S W 1988 Soft tissue tumours, 2nd edn. C V Mosby, St Louis

Fisher C 1988 Epithelioid sarcoma: the spectrum of ultrastructural differentiation in seven immunohistochemically defined cases. Human Pathology 19: 265–275

Gherardi G, Arya S, Hickler R B 1974 Juxtaglomerular body tumor: a rare occult, but curable cause of lethal hypertension. Human Pathology 5: 236–239

Hamid Q A, Bishop A E, Rode J et al 1986 Duodenal gangliocytic paragangliomas: a study of 10 cases with

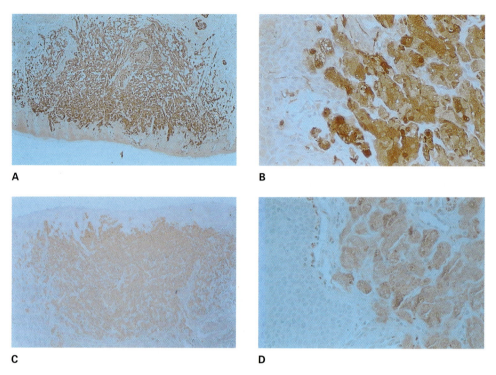

**A**

**B**

**C**

**D**

**Fig. 6.3** Illustration of the pattern of staining with S-100 and NSE in a case of a granular-cell tumour. (**A**) and (**B**) Low- and high-power views of S-100 staining. (**C**) and (**D**) Low- and high-power views of NSE staining in semi-adjacent sections (simple two-step indirect immunoperoxidase method).

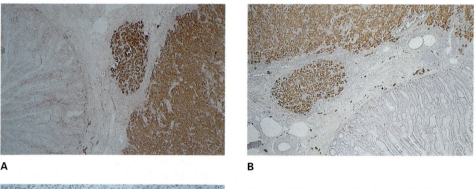

**A**

**B**

**C**

**Fig. 6.4** Illustration of the value of S-100 and a melanoma-specific marker, M3080, in the diagnosis of melanomas in general: (**A**) S-100 and (**B**) M3080 staining of a clinically occult amelanotic melanoma metastasis to the small intestine. The patient subsequently remembered the removal of a nodular skin lesion six years previously, the histology of which was not apparently investigated! (**C**) shows the typical S-100 positivity in a malignant melanoma. The S-100 is found in the cytoplasm and/or the nucleus. It should be noted that not all melanomas are S-100 positive (sensitivity approximately 90%) and that the additional use of the 'melanoma-specific antibodies' such as the M3080 may be helpful in the S-100-negative cases (simple two-step indirect immunoperoxidase).

immunohistochemical neuroendocrine markers. Human Pathology 17: 1151–1157

Hashimoto H, Daimaru Y, Enjoji M 1984 S-100 protein distribution in liposarcoma. An immunoperoxidase study with special reference to the distinction of liposarcoma from myxoid malignant fibrous histiocytoma. Virchows Archiv. A 405:1–10

Hashimoto H, Daimaru Y, Tsuneyoshi M, Enjoji M 1986 Leiomyosarcoma of external soft tissues. A clinicopathologic, immunohistochemical, and electron microscopic study. Cancer 57: 2077–2088

Jasani B, Edwards R E, Thomas N D, Gibbs A R 1985 The use of vimentin antibodies in the diagnosis of malignant mesothelioma. Virchows Archiv. A 406: 441–448

Jones H, Steart P V, Du Boulay C E H, Roche W R 1990 Alpha-smooth muscle actin as a marker for soft tissue tumours: a comparison with desmin. Journal of Pathology 162: 29

Kliewer K E, Wen D-R, Cancilla P A, Cochran A J 1989 Paragangliomas: assessment of prognosis by histologic, immunohistochemical, and ultrastructural techniques. Human Pathology 20: 29–39

Leader M, Patel J, Collins M, Henry K 1989 Myoglobin: an evaluation of its role as a marker of rhabdomyosarcomas. British Journal of Cancer 59: 106–109

Lieberman P H, Brennan M F, Kimmel M, Erlandson R A, Garin-Chesa P, Flehinger B 1989 Alveolar soft part sarcoma. A clinico-pathologic study on half a century. Cancer 63: 1–13

Llombart-Bosch A, Terrier-Lacombe MJ, Peydro-Olaya A, Contesso G 1989 Peripheral neuroectodermal sarcoma of soft tissue (peripheral neuroepithelioma): a pathologic study of ten cases with differential diagnosis regarding other small, round-cell sarcomas. Human Pathology 20: 273–280

Mackenzie D H, Filipe M I 1983 Soft tissue tumours. In: Filipe M I, Lake B D (eds) Histochemistry in pathology. Churchill Livingstone, Edinburgh, p 245–251

Matsunou H, Shimoda T, Kakimoto S, Yamashita H, Ishikawa E, Mukai M 1985 Histopathologic and immunohistochemical study of malignant tumours of peripheral nerve sheath (malignant schwannoma). Cancer 56: 2269–2279

Miettinen M, Lehto V-P, Vartio T, Virtanen I 1982 Epithelioid sarcoma. Ultrastructural and immunohistologic features suggesting a synovial origin. Archives of Pathology and Laboratory Medicine 10: 620–623

Miettinen M, Rapola J 1989 Immunohistochemical spectrum of rhabdomyosarcoma and rhabdomyosarcoma-like tumours. Expression of cytokeratin and the 68-kD neurofilament protein. American Journal of Surgical Pathology 13: 120–132

Millard P R, Heryet A R 1985 An immunohistological study of Factor VIII related antigen and Kaposi's sarcoma using polyclonal and monoclonal antibodies. Journal of Pathology 146: 31–38

Mukai M, Torikata C, Iri H, Mikata A, Hanaoka H, Kato K, Kageyama K 1986 Histogenesis of alveolar soft part sarcoma. An immunohistochemical and biochemical study. American Journal of Surgical Pathology 10: 212–218

Nathrath W B J, Remberger K 1986 Immunohistochemical study of granular cell tumours. Demonstration of neurone specific enolase, S 100 protein, laminin and alpha-1-antichymotrypsin. Virchows Archiv. (Pathological Anatomy) 408: 421–434

Ordonez N G 1989 The immunohistochemical diagnosis of mesothelioma. Differentiation of mesothelioma and lung adenocarcinoma. American Journal of Surgical Pathology 13: 276–291

Ordonez N G, Ro J Y, Mackay B 1989 Alveolar soft part sarcoma. An ultrastructural and immunocytochemical investigation of its histogenesis. Cancer 63: 1721–1736

Parums D V, Cordell J L, Micklem K, Heryet A R, Gatter K C, Mason D Y 1990 JC70: a new monoclonal antibody that detects vascular endothelium associated antigen on routinely processed tissue sections. Journal of Clinical Pathology 43: 752

Perrone T, Sibley R K, Rosai J 1985 Duodenal gangliocytic paraganglioma. An immunohistochemical and ultrastructural study and a hypothesis concerning its origin. American Journal of Surgical Pathology 9: 31–41

Ramani P, Bradley N J, Fletcher C D M 1990 QBEND/10, a new monoclonal antibody to endothelium: assessment of its diagnostic utility in paraffin sections. Histopathology 17: 237

Scheithauer B W, Nora F E, LeChango J, Wick M R, Crawford B G, Weiland L H, Carney J A 1986 Duodenal gangliocytic paraganglioma. Clinicopathologic and immunocytochemical study of 11 cases. American Journal of Clinical Pathology 86: 559–565

Schröder H D, Johannsen L 1986 Demonstration of S-100 protein in sustentacular cells of pheochromocytomas and paragangliomas. Histochemistry 10: 1023–1027

Shimada H, Newton W A, Soule E, Qualman S J, Aoyama C, Maurer H M 1988 Pathologic features of extraosseus Ewing's sarcoma: a report from the Intergroup Rhabdomyosarcoma Study. Human Pathology 19: 442–453

Soini Y, Miettinen M 1989 Alpha-1-antitrypsin and lysozyme. Their limited significance in fibrohistiocytic tumors. American Journal of Clinical Pathology 91: 515–521

Soini Y, Autio-Harmainen H, Miettinen M 1989 Immunoreactivity for laminin and type IV collagen in malignant and benign fibrous histiocytoma. Journal of Pathology 158: 223–228

Specht C S, Smith T W, DeGirolami U, Price J M 1986 Myxopapillary ependymoma of the filum terminale. A light and electron microscopic study. Cancer 58: 310–317

Tsukada T, Tippens D, Gordon D, Ross R, Gown A M 1987 HHF35, a muscle-actin-specific monoclonal antibody. I. Immunocytochemical and biochemical characterization. American Journal of Pathology 126: 51–60

Ushigome S, Shimoda T, Takaki K, Nikaido T, Takakuwa T, Ishikawa E, Spjut H J 1989 Immunocytochemical and ultrastructural studies of the histogenesis of Ewing's sarcoma and putatively related tumors. Cancer 64: 52–62

Weiler R, Fischer-Colbrie R, Schmid K W et al 1988 Immunological studies on the occurrence and properties of chromogranin A and B secretogranin II in endocrine tumors. American Journal of Surgical Pathology 12: 877–884

Weiss S W, Langloss J M, Enzinger F M 1983 The role of S-100 protein in the diagnosis of soft tissue tumors with particular reference to benign and malignant Schwann cell tumors. Laboratory Investigation 49: 229–306

Wick M R, Swanson P E, Scheithauer B W, Manivel J C 1987 Malignant peripheral nerve sheath tumor. An immunohistochemical study of 62 cases. American Journal of Clinical Pathology 87: 425–433

# 7. Neuroendocrine tumours

## INTRODUCTION

The cells of the endocrine system synthesize and release chemical messengers, the hormones, which control the interactions and coordination of the activities of various target tissues and cells. Most biological phenomena, however, are under the overlapping control of the endocrine and the nervous system. This interlocking communication network of endocrine and neural cells is regarded as constituting a single neuroendocrine system.

Disorders of the following components of this system are described below with respect to their immunocytochemical analysis and evaluation: pituitary, adrenals, thyroid gland, parathyroid, islets of Langerhans and the diffuse endocrine system.

## PITUITARY

### Embryology

The pituitary develops partly from oral ectoderm and partly from nerve tissue. The oral component, forming the adenohypophysis, arises as an out-pocketing (Rathke's pouch) from the roof of the primitive mouth of the embryo. The part of the pituitary that develops from nerve tissue is the neurohypophysis arising from the neural ectoderm of the floor of the forebrain.

### Anatomy and biochemistry

#### Adenohypophysis

The adenohypophysis consists of a pars distalis, which contains the secretory cells of the pituitary, the pars tuberalis (surrounding the pars infundibularis of the neurohypophysis) and the pars intermedia, which, in humans, is a rudimentary region made up of cords of weakly basophilic cells with small secretory granules.

#### Secretory cells of the adenohypophysis

1. Corticotrophic cells represent the weakly basophilic and PAS-positive cells and produce adenocorticotrophic hormone (ACTH).
2. Mammotrophic cells form part of the acidophilic cell population, produce prolactin, and constitute up to 20% of all cells.
3. Somatotrophic cells form the bulk of the acidophilic cell population, produce growth hormone (somatotropin, GH), and make up to 50% of all cells in the normal pituitary.
4. Thyrotrophic cells form part of the basophilic and PAS-positive cell population, and produce thyroid-stimulating hormone (TSH).
5. Gonadotrophic cells constitute the basophilic, large-cell population, producing follicle-stimulating hormone (FSH) and luteinizing hormone (LH). The secretory granules of these cells contain both FSH and LH.

Multiple hormone storage in normal cells of the anterior pituitary has been shown by immuno-electron microscopy (Newman et al 1989).

#### Neurohypophysis

It consists of the pars nervosa and the infundibulum, which connects the neurohypophysis with the hypothalamus. The neurohypophysis contains unmyelinated axons of neurosecretory cells (situated in the supraoptic and paraventricular nuclei). The hormones vasopressin (antidiuretic hormone, ADH) and oxytocin are stored in the neurohypophysis.

## Immunocytochemistry

### Neoplasms of the anterior pituitary

Antisera against the six hormones of the adeno-hypophysis (GH, prolactin, ACTH, TSH, FSH, LH) are used to demonstrate the possible hormonal composition of neoplasms of the anterior pituitary. These tumours are almost exclusively adenomas, whereas true primary carcinomas of the anterior pituitary which give rise to distant metastases are rarely found. Additionally antibodies against α-HCG should be used in the diagnosis of pituitary tumours (Landolt & Heitz 1986). Table 7.1 shows the percentages of the various hormone types found in pituitary adenomas (adopted from Horvath & Kovacs 1988). Usually a panel of antisera against six hormones (GH, prolactin, LH, FSH, TSH and ACTH) and occasionally α-HCG are also used on pituitary adenomas to help distinguish tumour cells from the non-neoplastic background pituitary cells. Null-cell adenomas are either negative or show a few scattered cells positive for one or more pituitary hormones, mainly TSH, FSH, and LH. Staining due to the five main pituitary hormone markers in a normal pituitary is illustrated in Figure 7.1, together with prolactin staining associated with a prolactinoma.

In a recent study (Schmid et al 1991b) we have shown that all pituitary adenomas express chromogranin B. An additional chromogranin A positivity was found in FSH/LH, TSH and the majority of clinically non-functioning null-cell adenomas. Chromogranin A and B may therefore be an additional help in the immunohistochemical differential diagnosis of pituitary adenomas.

***Growth hormone (GH) adenoma.*** GH cell adenomas are clinically associated with acromegaly and correspond to acidophilic adenomas by light microscopy. GH immunoreactivity is less pronounced in chromophobic GH cell adenomas than that seen in acidophilic tumours (Horvath & Kovacs 1988). Sometimes the staining is focal. GH-producing adenomas express chromogranin B; in some cases a co-localization of GH and alpha-subunit has been found in GH-secreting adenomas (Osamura & Watanabe 1987).

Acromegaly may also be caused by gangliocytomas of the pituitary (Scheithauer et al 1986), the mechanism of which is not yet clearly understood (Horvath & Kovacs 1991).

***Prolactin cell adenoma.*** Prolactin cell adenomas are the most frequently found hormone-producing tumours of the pituitary. Positive immunocytochemical staining with prolactin depicts characteristically as juxtanuclear punctate deposits representing the Golgi apparatus (Horvath & Kovacs 1988). The immunocytochemical staining may vary quite substantially and can even be negative in the absence of granules. Apparently prolactin can be released by these cells immediately to the extracellular space without the formation of secretory granules and a storage phase. Prolactin-secreting adenomas are chromogranin B positive and chromogranin A negative (Lloyd et al 1989, Schmid et al 1991b).

***Mixed growth hormone and prolactin adenoma.*** GH-producing tumours may occur in a mixed form with an uneven admixture of GH- and prolactin-positive cells. The GH and prolactin positivity is found associated with different cell populations. These tumours are chromogranin B positive.

***Thyroid-stimulating hormone (TSH) adenoma.*** Thyrotroph (micro-) adenoma may occur in long-standing hypothyroidism or in a few cases with hyperthyroidism associated with pituitary tumours and elevated TSH levels. Mixed tumours consisting of thyrotrophs and at least one other pituitary cell type have been reported. Antisera against TSH may cross-react with FSH and LH cells if adequate care is not taken to eliminate cross-reactive antibodies to the shared alpha-subunit. TSH-secreting adenomas are chromogranin A and B positive.

***Follicle-stimulating hormone (FSH)/lutein-***

**Table 7.1**   Percentages of hormone types found in pituitary adenomas

| Hormone | % |
| --- | --- |
| Prolactin cell adenomas | 28 |
| Clinically non-functioning adenomas (null-cell adenomas) and oncocytomas | 25 |
| ACTH and 'silent corticotrope adenomas' | 14 |
| GH cell adenomas | 14 |
| Plurihormonal adenomas | 8 |
| Mixed GH and prolactin adenomas | 5 |
| FSH/LH cell adenomas | 5 |
| TSH cell adenomas | 0.8 |

Adapted from Horvath & Kovacs (1988).

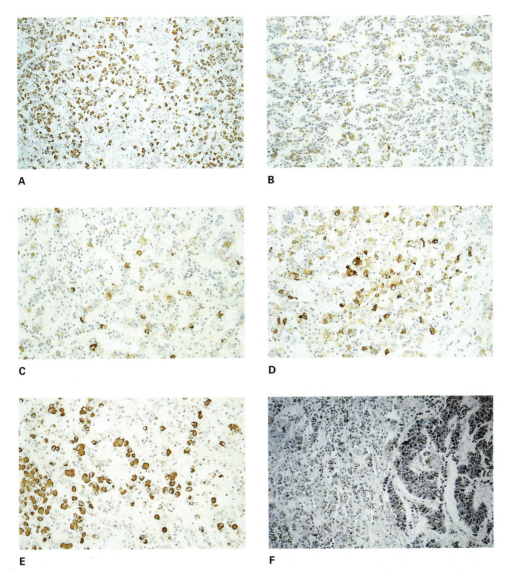

**Fig. 7.1** Illustration of staining of normal postmortem pituitary tissue with the five major pituitary hormone markers: (**A**) Growth hormone (GH); (**B**) prolactin (PRL); (**C**) luteinizing hormone (LH); (**D**) thyroid-stimulating hormone (TSH); and (**E**) adrenocorticotrophic hormone (ACTH). (**F**) shows staining of a prolactinoma and the background pituitary tissue obtained using antihuman PRL. (**A–E**) Simple two-step indirect immunoperoxidase technique; (**F**) DHSS immunoperoxidase procedure.

*izing hormone (LH) cell adenoma*. Gonadotrophs comprise up to 5% of all adenohypophyseal cell adenomas. The majority of gonadotroph adenomas are not associated with obvious clinical syndromes and the circulating levels of gonadotrophins are within normal range for the patient's age. Antisera against FSH and LH may cross-react with TSH-producing cells if the cross-reacting antibodies to the shared alpha-subunit are not adequately excluded. FSH/LH-producing adenomas express both chromogranin A and B.

*Corticotrophic cell adenoma*. ACTH-producing adenomas are either associated with Cushing's syndrome (hypercorticism) or with Nelson's syndrome (resulting in bilaterally adrenalectomized patients with Cushing's syndrome).

The most prominent immunocytochemical staining for ACTH is found in the periphery of the tumour cells.

ACTH and corticotrophin-releasing factor (CRF) may be produced in small-cell carcinomas of the lung (more than 50% of cases!), thymomas, pancreatic carcinomas and medullary thyroid carcinomas.

Clinically non-functioning adenoma (null-cell adenomas and pituitary oncocytomas). These tumours represent nearly 25% of surgically removed pituitary adenomas. They usually present by local symptoms. Histologically, two types can be distinguished by the mitochondrial content of the tumour cells, e.g. null-cell adenomas and pituitary oncocytomas. Null-cell adenomas are immunohistochemically negative or show various amounts of FSH, LH, TSH and α-HCG-positive cells, rarely other pituitary hormones. The majority of null-cell adenomas are positive for chromogranins A and B (Lloyd et al 1989, Schmid et al 1991b). Some cases, however, express only chromogranin B (Schmid et al 1991a).

**Silent adenoma**. There are three well-defined morphological entities, which are not related to any recognizable clinical syndromes:

1. Type I and II silent 'corticotrophic' adenomas. Both tumour types contain ACTH. Type I is additionally strongly PAS positive, whereas type II exhibits focally distributed PAS positivity in varying amounts. Electron microscopically the two types can be distinguished by the different size of their secretory granules.
2. Type III adenoma which mimics prolactin production. These tumours usually occur in young women. They are associated with oligomenorrhea or amenorrhea, galactorrhea, and slightly raised serum prolactin levels. Some cells may be immunocytochemically positive for any pituitary hormone and in some cases the tumours may be completely negative for all antisera used.

*Neoplasms of the posterior pituitary*

**Histiocytosis X involving the posterior pituitary**. The posterior pituitary may be completely destroyed by an accumulation of histiocytes, macrophages, lymphocytes, eosinophilic granulocytes and fibroblasts. The lesion may lead in severe cases to diabetes insipidus. The histiocytic accumulation is positive with antibodies against S-100 protein.

**Granular-cell tumours in the posterior pituitary**. Granular-cell tumours are the most frequently found tumours of the posterior pituitary (Scheithauer 1985). It is usual for these tumours to be positive for S-100 protein.

## ADRENAL GLANDS

### Embryology

The adrenal gland may be considered as two functionally and morphologically distinct organs (adrenal medulla and cortex). They are united during embryonic development. The adrenal medulla arises from neuroectoderm, whereas the cortex consists of cells originating from coelomic intermediate mesoderm.

### Anatomy and biochemistry

*Adrenal medulla*

The adrenal medulla is composed of chromaffin, polyhedral cells (phaeochromocytes) supported by a reticular fibre network. A few scattered parasympathetic ganglion cells can be found. Phaeochromocytes synthesize catecholamines and several other substances.

*Adrenal cortex*

In the adrenal cortex three layers can be distinguished, which, in humans, are not sharply defined:

1. The zona glomerulosa which produces mineralocorticoids (mainly aldosterone)
2. The zona fasciculata which produces and secretes glucocorticoids and small amounts of androgens and probably also oestrogens
3. The zona reticularis which produces androgens and probably also glucocorticoids and oestrogen.

### Immunocytochemistry

*Phaeochromocytoma*

The vast majority of phaeochromocytomas occur

as sporadic tumours. In a small group of patients, however, the tumour occurs as part of the multiple endocrine neoplasia type II syndromes (MEN IIA, Sipple's syndrome; MEN IIB, mucosal neuroma syndrome). Usually phaeochromocytomas are benign by morphological criteria, though approximately 4–7% are metastasizing tumours. Familial cases are bilateral in approximately 66% of cases, whereas sporadic cases are unilateral in more than 90% of cases. Phaeochromocytomas are chromaffin tumours which are positive for the Grimelius staining.

Phaeochromocytomas are immunocytochemically positive for the non-specific neuroendocrine markers NSE, chromogranins (A, B, and secretogranin II) and synaptophysin (Gould et al 1987, Schober et al 1987). In some cases, somatostatin, calcitonin and pituitary hormones can be found (O'Connor et al 1983, Tischler et al 1984, Roth et al 1986).

### Composite phaeochromocytoma

Mixed tumours with either phaeochromocytic and neuroblastomatous or phaeochromocytic and ganglioneuromatous components have been reported (Dawson & Tapp 1969, Mendelsohn et al 1979). VIP positivity (clinically associated with a Verner–Morrison syndrome) has been reported in the ganglioneuromatous component.

### Ganglioneuroma

Ganglioneuromas are benign tumours found in older children and young adults, arising in approximately 15–30% of cases in the adrenals. Ganglioneuromas are positive for S-100 protein and NSE. Ectopic hormone production may occur occasionally (Said & Faloona 1975, Mendelsohn et al 1979).

### Ganglioneuroblastoma

Ganglioneuroblastomas are composed of undifferentiated neuroblastic cells (positive for NSE and chromogranin A) and maturing ganglion cells (positive for NSE and S-100 protein). Some cases may show ectopic hormone production (ACTH, VIP) (Jansen-Goemans & Engelhardt

1977, Mendelsohn et al 1979, Mitchell et al 1976).

### Neuroblastomas

Neuroblastomas are the most common tumours in childhood and infancy; they are rarely found in adults. More than 50% of neuroblastomas arise within the adrenals. NSE and chromogranin A may be positive in neuroblastomas. Preservation of tissue may be crucial for the immunocytochemical staining (e.g. effects of preoperative treatment!). Neurofilament would be a highly specific marker for neuroblastomas. It is, however, undetectable in a high percentage of poorly differentiated tumours (Artlieb et al 1985).

Poorly differentiated neuroblastomas must be differentiated from other small, round-cell tumours of childhood such as Ewing's sarcoma, lymphomas, and soft-tissue sarcomas (Triche et al 1986).

### Adrenal cortex

Immunocytochemistry does not currently play any useful role in routine diagnosis of disorders of the adrenal cortex.

## THYROID GLAND

### Embryology

The thyroid is composed of two different cell types, the follicular cells and the C cells (parafollicular cells). The follicular cells are derived from the cephalic portion of the alimentary canal endoderm in the region of the developing tongue. The C cells are believed to be of neuroectodermal origin (neural crest). They develop in the ventral portion of each fourth pouch forming the ultimobranchial body, which fuses with the thyroid gland.

### Anatomy and biochemistry

The follicular cells synthesize the hormones thyroxine ($T_4$) and triiodothyronine ($T_3$) and store them in large quantities in the extracellular colloid. Thyroid colloid consists of thyroglobulin (a high molecular weight glycoprotein; mol. wt.

660 000). The activity of the follicle cells is controlled by the circulating levels of thyroid-stimulating hormone (TSH).

The C cells produce and secrete calcitonin (32 amino acids; mol. wt. 3500), which lowers the blood calcium levels by inhibiting bone reabsorption. The secretion of calcitonin is under the control of the blood calcium concentration.

Anatomically, the thyroid gland consists of two lobes, which are situated just below the cricoid cartilage. They are usually connected by the isthmus. Sometimes a so-called pyramidal lobe can be found. The C cells are confined normally to the middle of the upper third of the lateral lobes.

Abnormalities of the thyroid descent may result in the 'lingual thyroid' or the occurrence of heterotrophic thyroid tissue (larynx, trachea, etc.). Thyroidal tissue can develop in benign tumours of the ovary ('struma ovarii'). Occasionally, intra-thyroidal thymic tissue or parathyroid glands are found.

## Immunocytochemistry

(See Williams (1986) and Jasani & Newman (1989) for general reviews.)

*Tumours arising from thyroid follicular cells*

**Follicular adenoma.** One of the major problems in thyroid pathology is to distinguish follicular adenoma, in particular the so-called 'atypical' follicular adenoma (cf. Katoh et al 1989), from highly differentiated follicular carcinoma. Both tumour types are positive for thyroglobulin. In a recently published paper, Tuccari & Barresi (1990) claim that tissue polypeptide antigen (TPA) may be a useful tool to discriminate such difficult tumour types by means of immunocytochemistry. Also, Ca19-9 and Ca50 have been demonstrated in a majority of papillary and follicular thyroid carcinomas, whereas follicular adenomas were usually negative for these antibodies (Vierbuchen et al 1989). Several studies have stressed the value of the identification of extra-capsular vascular invasion in the diagnosis of a follicular carcinoma. Factor VIII-RAG immuno-localization, a reliable endothelial marker in normal and neoplastic vascular tissue, has been applied to the study of vascular invasion in follicular carcinoma with limited success (Harach et al 1983).

**Follicular thyroid carcinoma.** Follicular thyroid carcinomas are positive with antibodies against thyroglobulin. According to Harach & Fransilla (1988) highly and moderately differentiated follicular carcinomas show a high immunoreactivity with thyroglobulin (moderately differentiated tumours even more than highly differentiated ones). In a few cases follicular thyroid carcinomas show a weak keratin positivity (Permanetter et al 1982). Poorly differentiated follicular carcinomas are usually only weakly positive for thyroglobulin or even negative in some cases. In general, the immunoreactivity for thyroglobulin is found within the neoplastic cells rather than within the lumina (Williams 1986).

Oxyphilic and clear-cell variants of follicular thyroid carcinoma are (weakly to moderately) positive for thyroglobulin in approximately 80% of all cases (Harach & Franssila 1988). Therefore the differential diagnosis between a clear-cell follicular carcinoma and metastatic renal-cell carcinoma may be difficult or even impossible using thyroglobulin antibodies.

**Papillary thyroid carcinoma.** Papillary thyroid carcinoma is usually positive for thyroglobulin but less strong than follicular carcinoma. In most cases the staining pattern is a focal one. Using an antiserum to human epidermal keratin, Permanetter et al (1982) demonstrated that almost all papillary carcinomas stain positively in areas with papillary differentiation.

The thyroglobulin staining intensity decreases as the degree of de-differentiation increases, as in follicular thyroid carcinoma.

**Anaplastic thyroid carcinoma.** Anaplastic thyroid carcinomas show no immunoreactivity for thyroglobulin according to most authors. Positive staining may indicate remnants of differentiation in these tumours. Although positive staining in spindle- or giant-cell carcinomas has been reported (Burt & Goudie 1979, Böcker et al 1980, Albores-Saavedra et al 1983), these findings have to be interpreted with caution. The so-called small-cell type of anaplastic carcinoma almost certainly mimics other types of thyroid tumours such as malignant lymphoma (WBC positive)

(Burt et al 1985, Cameron et al 1975, Williams 1981), undifferentiated medullary carcinoma (positive for calcitonin, chromogranin A and CEA) (Mendelsohn et al 1980, Myskow et al 1986), or the so-called poorly differentiated 'insular' carcinoma (positive for thyroglobulin and, in some cases, calcitonin) (Carcangiu et al 1984).

Approximately 50% of anaplastic thyroid carcinomas are strongly positive for cytokeratins. Thyroid anaplastic carcinomas may also show co-expression of vimentin and cytokeratin (Mietinnen et al 1983).

*Tumours of thyroid C cells*

Although calcitonin production has been described in a variety of normal tissues, it is a standard marker for medullary thyroid carcinoma (MTC). Two other markers, calcitonin gene-related peptide (CGRP) and katacalcin, appear to be useful additional markers (Ali-Rachedi et al 1983, Sabate et al 1985, Williams et al 1987). Both are rarely used, however, in routine diagnostic practice.

Amyloid, found in a majority of cases of MTC, is positive for calcitonin, but not for CGRP (Williams et al 1987).

General neuroendocrine markers are positive in MTC, e.g. NSE (Tapia et al 1981), chromogranin A and B, secretogranin II (Schmid et al 1987b, 1992) and synaptophysin (Gould et al 1987).

CEA is present in the vast majority of MTC cases. It is of particular diagnostic value in undifferentiated MTC, where calcitonin expression is almost completely lost (Mendelsohn et al 1984). The occurrence of calcitonin-positive cells in anaplastic carcinomas (Nieuwenhuijzen Kruseman et al 1982) should be regarded with care, as long as no strong CEA immunoreactivity can be demonstrated in these cells.

Approximately 20% of MTC cases are part of the inherited MEN II syndromes (IIa: MTC, pheochromocytoma, hyperparathyroidism; IIb: MTC, pheochromocytoma, mucosal neuromata, marfanoid habitus). In the majority of MEN IIa cases, MTC represents the initial symptom of the disease. The prognosis of MEN IIb cases is significantly worse when compared to sporadic MTC and MTC associated with MEN IIa.

Familial MTC is preceded by C cell hyperplasia. The thyroid tissue bordering MEN II-associated MTC regularly contains residues of not yet neoplastically transformed diffuse or nodular C cell hyperplasia, whereas this finding is absent in sporadic MTC. It has been stressed by the WHO (Hedinger et al 1988) that identification of normal and hyperplasic C cells on H & E sections is not reliable. Thus immunolocalization of calcitonin is mandatory for the recognition or exclusion of hyperplastic C cells (Fig. 7.2b). 50 C cells per low-power field (x 10) have been taken to indicate hyperplasia.

*Mixed follicular/medullary thyroid carcinoma*

Mixed follicular/medullary carcinomas of the thyroid are rare tumours (Holm et al 1987). By definition, these tumours show thyroglobulin and calcitonin positivity within the same tumour. Thyroglobulin may be present in medullary carcinomas by entrapment or phagocytosis. Relatively often, non-neoplastic follicles can be found in MTC. However, since coproduction of thyroglobulin and calcitonin has been demonstrated in the primary tumour and its metastases (Pfaltz et al 1983), mixed follicular/medullary carcinoma has been accepted as a distinct pathological entity.

Figure 7.2 shows a photomicrograhic illustration of the use of thyroglobulin and calcitonin as markers in the diagnosis of thyroid follicular cell and C cell lesions.

*Malignant lymphomas*

Malignant lymphomas make up to 10% of all thyroid malignancies. The majority of thyroid lymphomas, as one might expect, do not express immunoglobulins. Approximately 80% of primary thyroid lymphomas are associated with thyroiditis in the non-neoplastic thyroid parenchyma (predominantly with Hashimoto's thyroiditis) (Williams 1981). The immunocytochemical typing of malignant thyroid lymphomas is the same as in systemic malignant lymphomas (see Chapter 4).

*Miscellaneous tumours*

**Primary thymoma of the thyroid.** There

are only a few reports dealing with this extremely rare tumour of the thyroid (Harach et al 1985, Miyauchi et al 1985, Asa et al 1988). The tumour may have a spindle-cell (Harach et al 1985) or squamous-cell appearance (Miyauchi et al 1985). Immunocytochemically the tumours were positive for low molecular cytokeratin and focally for high molecular epithelial keratins (Harach et al 1985, Asa et al 1988). NSE and CEA may be positive (Asa et al 1988).

*Sarcomas*. A variety of sarcomas have been described in the thyroid gland, the most important being fibrosarcoma and malignant haemangio-endothelioma (MHE).

MHE is a highly malignant tumour rarely found outside endemic goitre areas, which develops in most cases in a long-standing nodular goitre. Some authors regard MHE as a variant of anaplastic carcinoma. Its vascular origin has been confirmed, however, using antibodies against endothelial cell-specific markers (F-VIII-RAG, BMA 120). Furthermore, MHEs are positive for vimentin and negative for cytokeratin, whereas the majority of anaplastic thyroid carcinomas are negative for endothelial cell-specific markers (Tötsch et al 1990). However, other investigators found a higher percentage of both MHE and anaplastic carcinomas with a coexpression of endothelial and epithelial markers (Vollenweider et al 1989). According to the WHO classification (Hedinger et al 1988), tumours which express cytokeratins should be regarded as anaplastic carcinomas.

*Metastases to the thyroid*

The primary tumours commonly causing metastases to the thyroid are carcinomas of the breast, kidney, and lung and malignant melanomas (Shimaoka et al 1962, Czech et al 1982). The use of immunocytochemistry in differential diagnosis of metastatic tumours involving the thyroid is summarized in Table 7.2.

## PARATHYROID GLANDS

### Embryology

The parathyroid glands are derived from pharyngeal pouches. The inferior glands derive from the third pouch, the superior from the fourth. Parathyroid tissue may be found within the thyroid, the wall of the pharynx, and in the mediastinum beside and within the thymus.

### Anatomy and biochemistry

Usually there are four parathyroid glands situated behind the thyroid, one at each end of the upper and lower poles. The four glands have a total weight of about 400 mg. In 6–10%, more than four glands can be found (maximum up to 10). Rarely there are fewer than four glands. Heterotrophic parathyroid tissue can be found in the thymus, the thyroid, or within the wall of the pharynx.

Histologically, the parenchyma of the parathyroid is composed of two cell types. The majority of cells are the so-called 'chief cells'. The 'oxyphilic cells' appear at the age of seven and increase in number with age. In hyperplasia, a third cell type, the 'water clear cells', can be seen. The stroma of the parathyroid glands consists of various amounts of fat cells (approximately 40–70%). The fat content has been used in the past as an indicator of whether a gland is normal or hyperplastic.

### Immunocytochemistry

Parathyroid tissue is immunocytochemically positive with antibodies against parathyroid hormone (PTH) and chromogranin A (Weiler et al 1987, Schmid et al 1991a). PTH antibodies may be directed against the C-terminal fragment (hormonally inactive) or the N-fragment (hormonally active) of the PTH molecule. Because of its higher immunogenicity, most antibodies available are directed against the C-fragment. However, biologically active PTH can only be demonstrated using antibodies against the N-terminal fragment. The comparative immunocytochemical reactions

**Table 7.2** Immunocytochemistry in differential diagnosis of metastatic tumour in thyroid

| Metastatic tumour | Marker status | Differential diagnosis |
|---|---|---|
| Renal-cell carcinoma | thyroglobulin –ve | Clear-cell carcinoma of thyroid, usually thyroglobulin +ve |
| Melanoma | S-100 +ve | Medullary carcinoma of thyroid –ve |

**Table 7.3** Comparative immunocytochemical reactions of parathyroid and thyroid tissues

| Markers | Tumour type | |
| --- | --- | --- |
| | Parathyroid | Thyroid/C cell tissue |
| PTH | + | – |
| Thyroglobulin | – | + (thyroid follicular cells) |
| Chromogranin A | + | + (C cell) |
| Calcitonin | – | + (C cells) |

of parathyroid and thyroid tumours are summarized in Table 7.3.

## Parathyroid hyperplasia and adenoma

The diagnosis of a parathyroid adenoma is based on the finding of a single gland enlargement (Mendelsohn 1988a). In former years, up to 80% of cases of primary hyperparathyroidism have been considered to be caused by adenomas. In the last few years, however, studies have shown that the majority of cases of primary hyperparathyroidism are due to parathyroid hyperplasia (Ghandur-Mnaymneh & Kimura 1984). Immunocytochemical stains with PTH antibodies may help to distinguish suppressed parathyroid tissue situated adjacent to adenomas from adenomatous tissue by means of their different staining intensity. The suppressed tissue secretes almost no PTH which results in (increased) storage of the hormone and strong PTH-specific immunostaining. On the other hand, hyperplastic and adenomatous tissue shows a rather weak or sometimes focally moderate staining intensity with antibodies against PTH (Harach & Jasani 1992).

The oxiphilic cell adenomas of the parathyroid have been regarded as functionally inactive and therefore negative for PTH antibodies. Ordonez et al (1982), however, found a functional activity in some of these cases.

### Histochemistry

An important tool in distinguishing normal or suppressed chief cells from hyperplastic or adenomatous ones is the use of fat stains. On frozen sections, Oil-red O and Sudan IV stains demonstrate intracytoplasmic lipid droplets which apparently reflect the cell activity. In normal and suppressed tissue, chief cells contain, in almost every cell, intracytoplasmic lipid droplets, whereas

there is a greatly decreased number (less than 20%), and virtually no such cells in hyperplastic and adenomatous parathyroid tissue, respectively.

## Differential diagnosis of parathyroid neoplasms

In differentiating follicular thyroid adenoma from parathyroid adenoma with follicular (acinar) structures, immunocytochemical staining with thyroglobulin and PTH should be performed. Negativity for thyroglobulin virtually excludes thyroid adenoma. Intrathyroidal parathyroid carcinomas may mimic medullary thyroid carcinoma (Ordonez et al 1983, Mendelsohn 1988a) or follicular carcinoma. Immunocytochemistry with thyroglobulin, calcitonin and PTH will be helpful to obtain a diagnosis.

## ISLETS OF LANGERHANS

### Embryology

In early pancreatic development endocrine cells cannot be distinguished from exocrine cells. Apparently both pancreatic components arise from the pancreatic buds of the gut tube. The first clusters of primitive islets cells can be found in the 12th week of gestation. The first electron microscopically identifiable cells are the A cells, followed by the D and B cells, and finally the PP cells.

### Anatomy and biochemistry

The various cell types are not irregularly situated within the islets. The insulin-producing B cells are found in the centre of the islets, surrounded by a peripheral ring of glucagon-producing A cells. D and PP cells are found in smaller numbers between the A cells. The human pancreas additionally contains a network of VIP (vasoactive intestinal polypeptide)-containing fibres arising from local ganglia of the autonomic nervous system. This fibre network enmeshes and occasionally penetrates the islets (Bishop et al 1980).

### A cells

A cells produce glucagon and contain numerous granules (about 300 nm in diameter). A cells make up approximately 20% of the islet cell mass. They are rarely found in the so-called PP islets of the dorsal region of the pancreatic head. Characteristically, they form a mantle surrounding the centrally located B cells.

A cells are immunocytochemically positive for glucagon, NSE and chromogranin A and B (Schmid et al 1989).

### B cells

B cells produce insulin. Their granules are also about 300 nm in diameter but show a typical clear halo between the centre of the granule and their surrounding membrane. B cells make up more than 70% of all islet cells.

The B cells are situated in the centre of the islets and they are immunocytochemically positive for insulin, NSE and chromogranin A.

### D cells

D cells contain membrane-bound granules with a size of 150–400 nm. D cells produce somatostatin and make up fewer than 5% of the islet cells. Usually they are found in the periphery of the islet situated between A cells.

Immunocytochemically D cells are positive for somatostatin and NSE. They are most likely to be negative for chromogranins.

### PP cells (F cells)

PP cells are the rarest cell type found in the pancreatic islets of the anterior part of the pancreatic head as well as the remaining portions of the pancreas. PP cells contain granules with a size of 90–200 nm. The highest density of PP cells is found in the posterior part of the pancreatic head ('PP-rich islets'). PP cells are situated usually in the periphery of the islets. In PP-rich islets the PP cells are scantily distributed and the number of neighbouring B cells is substantially decreased.

Within the islet, the PP cells are usually situated in the periphery. PP cells are positive for PP, NSE and occasionally for chromogranin A and B (Schmid et al 1989).

### Other cell types

Other endocrine cells can be found within the islets and terminal ductules of the pancreas. Various substances have been reported to be produced by these cells (VIP, GIP, serotonin and others). However, it is now generally agreed that VIP is only present in nerve fibres and ganglion cells. Furthermore, gastrin, once claimed to be present in islet cells (Greider & McGuigan 1971), is not produced normally in the pancreatic islets. This, however, does not preclude expression of ectopic gastrin in neoplastic conditions of the pancreatic islets (see below).

## Nesidioblastosis (islet-cell hyperplasia)

Nesidioblastosis is a proliferation of islet cells within pancreatic ducts and ductules and the formation of new islets (Laidlaw 1938). These changes lead characteristically to an increase in the number of islets as well as an increase in their average size.

In some cases this hypertrophy of islet cells is difficult to judge. Therefore morphometric studies may be the only way to come to a definitive diagnosis (Klöppel et al 1974). Clinically, nesidioblastosis is found in most cases in young children presenting as hyperinsulinaemic hypoglycaemia with an increased number not only of B, but also of A, PP and D cells. This disease usually occurs sporadically. Familial cases, however, have been reported (Vance et al 1969, Woo et al 1976). Furthermore, nesidioblastosis may be the cause, in the absence of an islet-cell tumour, of such pancreatic endocrine syndromes as the Zollinger–Ellison and watery diarrhoea syndromes (Mendelsohn 1981, Nishiyama et al 1984, Mendelsohn 1988b). Immunohistochemically, all islet cells in nesidioblastosis can be demonstrated with NSE. Chromogranin A is also positive in the vast majority of islet cells, but questionably in D cells. The cells of the hyperplastic nodules have been shown to have polycrine potential in terms of their capacity to store/synthesize insulin and glucagon granules in the same cell (Newman et al 1986).

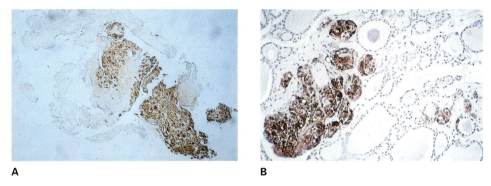

**Fig. 7.2** Illustration of the usefulness of thyroglobulin and calcitonin in diagnosis of thyroid tumours. (**A**) Thyroglobulin positivity of a lung metastasis identifying its thyroid follicular cell origin, and (**B**) calcitonin staining helping to identify the presence of nodular form C cell hyperplasia associated with the familial variety of medullary thyroid cancer (simple two-step indirect immunoperoxidase method).

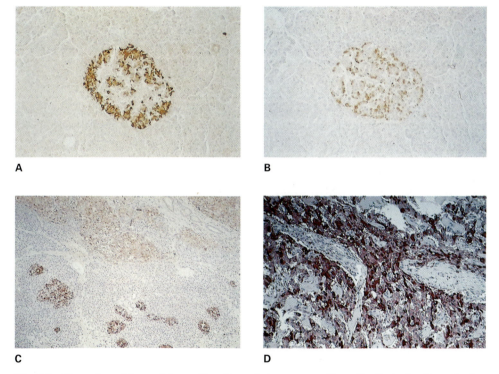

**Fig. 7.3** Illustration of the usefulness of insulin- and glucagon-specific antibodies in the diagnosis of pancreatic endocrine tumours. (**A**) and (**B**) Insulin- and glucagon-specific pattern of staining in a normal islet seen in a surgically removed pancreatic positive control tissue (simple two-step immunoperoxidase method). (**C**) Insulin staining of an insulinoma and a series of background islets. (**D**) Intense uniform staining of glucagon in a glucagonoma (APAAP technique).

## Tumours of endocrine pancreas (Schmid & Höfler 1991)

*Islet-cell tumours with production of orthotopic hormones*

**Insulinoma**. Insulinomas are the most common islet-cell tumours (approximately 75%). A rather low percentage of these tumours become malignant (4–16%). More than 50% of all insulinomas show multihormonal expression as evinced by immunocytochemistry (glucagon, PP and gastrin; a high proportion of gastrin-producing cells has been considered as an indicator of poor prognosis). A decrease in the insulin immunoreactivity may also indicate a poor prognosis. Insulinomas are rarely (less than 4%) part of an MEN I syndrome.

NSE and chromogranin are positive in insulinomas. A strong chromogranin A immunoreactivity has been observed in malignant insulinomas (Schmid et al 1987b).

**Glucagonoma**. Glucagonomas make up 1% of all pancreatic endocrine tumours. More than 60%, however, are malignant. A considerable number of PP cells can be demonstrated in most glucagonomas (Heitz et al 1982).

The value of insulin and glucagon in the diagnosis of insulinoma and glucagonoma is illustrated photomicrographically in Figure 7.3.

**Somatostatinoma**. Somatostatinomas are rare tumours and almost always malignant. Other hormones (mainly PP) may be associated with somatostatinomas.

**PP-oma**. These rare tumours are seldom found in a 'pure' form. PP cells can frequently be demonstrated in other pancreatic endocrine tumours (mainly in glucagonomas, but also in insulinomas, somatostatinomas, etc.). 'Pure' PP-producing tumours are usually benign and monohormonal by definition. Symptoms of inappropriate PP secretion are so far not known.

*Islet-cell tumours with production of ectopic hormones*

**Gastrinoma**. Gastrinomas can be found in the pancreas (20–25% amongst all pancreatic endocrine tumours), the duodenum, the stomach, and in the wall of the bile duct. More than 70% of gastrinomas are malignant and gastrinomas almost always occur as multiple tumours. Gastrinomas are the usual cause of the Zollinger–Ellison syndrome. In more than 50% of all gastrinomas, cells other than gastrin-producing cells can be found (somatostatin, VIP, PP).

**Serotoninoma**. Only rarely, islet-cell tumours are associated with a carcinoid syndrome. Immunohistochemically these tumours express serotonin. The term 'pancreatic carcinoid' should be avoided.

**VIP-oma**. These tumours account for fewer than 5% of pancreatic endocrine tumours and they are associated with the WHDA syndrome (Verner–Morrison syndrome). VIP-omas are malignant in 50–70% of cases. Immunocytochemically, VIP unfortunately cannot be demonstrated in all cases of clinically unambiguous VIP-omas. Probably the WHDA syndrome is not exclusively related to VIP. For instance, GIP, a secretin-like substance, and other peptides have been reported to cause WHDA syndrome.

**Other hormones**. Other hormones, such as ACTH, α-HCG, calcitonin, parathyroid hormone and neurotensin may be found in pancreatic islet tumours. Alpha-HCG expression may indicate malignancy; it is, however, not a proof for malignancy (Klöppel et al 1991).

*Mixed endoexocrine tumours of the pancreas*

The diagnosis of these rare tumours, which may be benign or malignant, can be exclusively made by means of immunocytochemistry and/or electron microscopy (Ulich et al 1982).

## DIFFUSE (NEURO-)ENDOCRINE SYSTEM

### Introduction

Feyrter introduced in 1938 the term 'diffuse endocrine system'. With the aid of a light microscope he detected and described 'clear' cells to which he attributed an endocrine function. These cells were subsequently found in various organs (gut, lung, pituitary, pancreas, thyroid, genitourinary system, skin). This 'diffuse endocrine system' is under the control of numerous regulatory peptides and a massive number of studies have been performed to elucidate the distribution of these peptides.

Despite the effectiveness of some histochemical stains (e.g. silver impregnation), immunocytochemistry has become the most popular tool for the demonstration of these regulatory peptides.

## General markers for the diffuse neuroendocrine system

### Neurone-specific enolase (NSE)

NSE was first thought to be present exclusively in neurones. Subsequently, however, NSE was demonstrated in endocrine cells and central and peripheral nerves. NSE is therefore a rather 'non-specific' neuroendocrine marker, being apparently present in a higher number of cells than can be demonstrated in comparative studies with a variety of peptides, amines, and enzymes using the most up-to-date methods. Problems concerning the specificity of NSE in immunocytochemical tumour diagnosis are mainly attributable to the polyclonal nature of the most frequently used antibodies against NSE. The recent introduction of monoclonal antibodies has helped to improve the specificity of this marker.

### Chromogranins and secretogranins

Chromogranin A and B and secretogranin II (for nomenclature see Eiden et al 1987) are soluble acidic glycoproteins of chromaffin granules. So far, only chromogranin A has been used broadly as an immunocytochemical marker. Chromogranin A has a widespread distribution in human endocrine tissues and tumours. However, there is still some controversy about its occurrence in the nervous system.

Chromogranin A has proved to be an extremely useful and reliable marker for a variety of (neuro-)-endocrine tumours containing granules. Monoclonal antibodies are available and excellent staining results can be obtained on conventionally fixed and processed tissues, although Rindi et al (1986) have pointed out that overfixation of tissues may cause false-negative immunocytochemical results. The use of antibodies against chromogranin B and secretogranin II has so far been restricted to re-

search. Reviews on chromogranins have recently been given by Wiedenmann & Huttner (1989) and Winkler & Fischer-Colbrie (1992).

### Synaptophysin

This relatively recently recognized marker (Gould et al 1987) seems to react specifically with pre-synaptic vesicles of cerebral and spinal neurones, of neuromuscular endplates and the retina. It also reacts with a variety of normal and tumorous neuroendocrine cells (e.g. adrenal medulla, islet cells). The usefulness of this integral, transmembrane protein as a routine marker in ICC has been reviewed by Wiedenmann & Huttner (1989).

### Leu7

Leu7 was initially found to react with natural killer cells of the lymphoid cell series. It has subsequently been shown to be a useful marker for endocrine cells (Bunn et al 1985, Michels et al 1987).

## Carcinoid tumours

In 1907 Oberndorfer introduced the term 'carcinoid tumour' for a group of epithelial neoplasms reminiscent of a carcinoma but with a favourable clinical outcome. Later these tumours were suspected to be endocrine in nature (Gosset & Masson 1914, Masson 1914).

### Carcinoids of the digestive tract

**Oesophagus**. True carcinoids of the oesophagus might not be as rare as reported in the literature (Ibrahim et al 1984). The majority of these neoplasms are poorly differentiated carcinoids with a poor clinical prognosis. Amongst other hormones, calcitonin and ACTH have been reported to be produced by these tumours.

**Stomach**. As stated for oesophageal carcinoids, carcinoid tumours of the stomach may be found more often than commonly suggested. This might be due to the fact that carcinoids of the stomach exhibit a variety of histological patterns sometimes almost indistinguishable from adenocarcinomas. Carcinoids of the stomach can be multiple. Some cases are associated with diffuse hyperplasia of neuroendocrine cells (argyrophilic cells) (Goldman

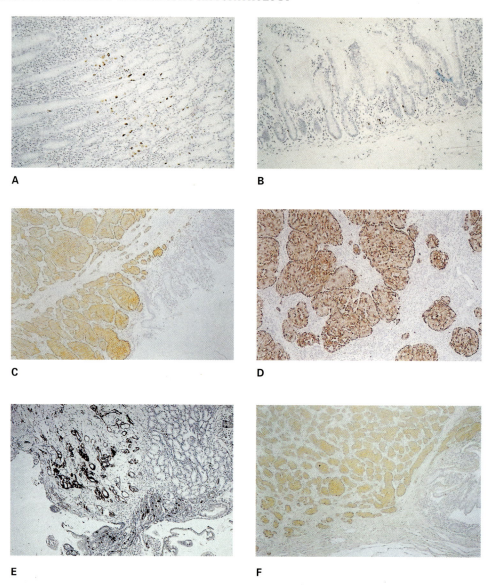

**Fig. 7.4** Illustration of the use of chromogranin A and serotonin in the diagnosis of carcinoid tumours. (**A**) and (**B**) Use of gut mucosa as a convenient positive control tissue for chromogranin A- and serotonin-based immunocytochemical analysis respectively. (**C**) and (**D**) Typically dual chromogranin A and serotonin staining of a small-bowel (midgut) carcinoid (simple two-step indirect immunoperoxidase method).

et al 1981). Carcinoids of the stomach may synthesize various products including serotonin, beta-MSH, ACTH and gastrin (the latter associated with the Zollinger–Ellison syndrome).

*Duodenum*. Usually, duodenal carcinoids histologically show an admixture of solid and trabecular patterns. In some cases, duodenal carcinoids cannot be distinguished from the islet-cell tumours of the pancreas by means of morphological criteria. In the majority of cases, duodenal carcinoids are clinically silent with the exception of gastrin production (Zollinger–Ellison syndrome). In a recently published study (Burke et al 1989) of 65 duodenal carcinoids, production of gastrin (65%), somatostatin (47%), serotonin (39%), calcitonin (19%), insulin (5%) and PP

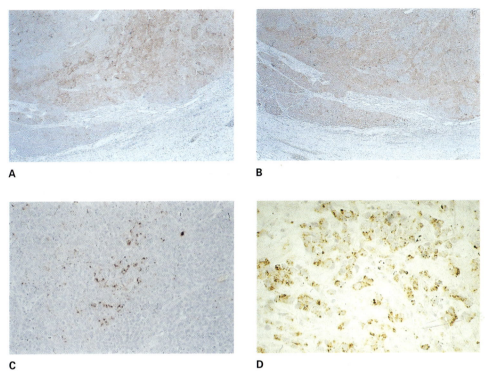

A    B

C    D

**Fig. 7.5**  Illustration of the typical staining pattern of a moderately differentiated neuroendocrine carcinoma of the colon with (**A**) CEA, (**B**) NSE and (**C**) chromogranin A. (**D**) illustrates the usefulness of secretogranin II in the diagnosis of neuroendocrine differentiation in an anaplastic lung carcinoma in which NSE, chromogranin A and chromogranin B were all negative. The demonstration of neuroendocrine differentiation has been shown to be of therapeutical and prognostic importance in lung cancer (simple two-step indirect immunoperoxidase method).

(3%) was described. Duodenal carcinoids may be associated with von Recklinghausen's neurofibromatosis (Griffiths et al 1984, Stephens et al 1987). Somatostatin-producing tumours may contain psammoma bodies (Dayal et al 1983, 1986).

The usefulness of chromogranin A and serotonin in the diagnosis of carcinoid tumours is photomicrographically illustrated in Figure 7.4.

*Jejunum and ileum*. Carcinoids of these sites are more often associated with carcinoid syndrome than carcinoids of all other sites. Midgut carcinoids may occur simultaneously with adenocarcinomas of the bowel. Immunocytochemical production of bombesin (or gastrin-releasing peptide) (Bostwick et al 1984), substance P, insulin, catecholamines, serotonin, and others have been reported.

*Appendix*. The appendix is the most common site for carcinoid tumours. They occur at any age and are usually found incidentally in routine appendectomies. Appendiceal carcinoids grow in various patterns:

1. Solid nests of isomorph cells with an excellent prognosis
2. The tubular appearance is associated with a slightly worse prognosis
3. The third type, the so-called adenocarcinoid or goblet cell carcinoid, however, has been shown to metastasize in approximately 15% of cases (Warkel et al 1978).

*Large bowel*. Carcinoids of the large bowel are not rare tumours and often present clinically, especially well-differentiated ones, as 'ordinary' polyps. The most common location is the caecum. Large-bowel carcinoids have been reported to synthesize and secrete substance P, neuropeptide Y (NPY), glucagon, somatostatin and catecholamines. Some cases may occur as adenocarcinoids with an admixture of an adenocarcinoma pattern without neuroendocrine differentiation and a more isomorphic carcinoid pattern, the latter being positive in immunocytochemistry for non-specific neuroendocrine markers.

**Gallbladder and extrahepatic biliary tree.** Somatostatin-producing tumours of the ampulla have been reported in patients with von Recklinghausen's neurofibromatosis (Hough et al 1983, Dayal et al 1986, Griffiths et al 1984). Carcinoid tumours of the gallbladder of all grades of differentiation may occur, but they are rare. An ACTH-producing carcinoid tumour of the gallbladder has been reported (Spence & Burns-Cox 1975).

**Meckel's diverticulum.** A few cases of carcinoids found in a Meckel's diverticulum have been reported (Wilson et al 1970).

*Bronchopulmonary neuroendocrine tumours*

Immunocytochemistry plays an important role in distinguishing neuroendocrine tumours of the lung from other lung carcinomas. NSE-specific antibodies and those against the chromogranin/ secretogranin group, and synaptophysin are useful as general markers to demonstrate the neuroendocrine nature of these tumours. However, it might be difficult to confirm the diagnosis immunocytochemically of less differentiated neuroendocrine tumours in small bronchial biopsies. A comparison of the WHO classification and the classification suggested by Gould et al (1984) is given in Table 7.4. We have decided to use the classification suggested by Gould et al (1984) in this book because of its emphasis on the neuroendocrine origin of these tumours.

**Bronchopulmonary carcinoid.** According to Gould et al (1984) the term 'bronchopulmonary carcinoid' should be histologically restricted to a case of a very well-differentiated, demonstrably neuroendocrine neoplasm with local invasiveness.

**Table 7.4** Classification systems for neuroendocrine tumours of lung

| WHO | Gould et al (1984) |
| --- | --- |
| Carcinoid, typical | Bronchopulmonary carcinoid |
| Carcinoid, atypical | Well-differentiated neuroendocrine carcinoma |
| Small-cell intermediate carcinoma (transitional) | Neuroendocrine carcinoma of intermediate-cell type |
| Small-cell carcinoma (oat-cell type) | Neuroendocrine carcinoma of small-cell type |

Clinically, the tumour may recur locally and may develop true metastases, but only late in its course.

These so-called 'typical' carcinoids of bronchopulmonary origin are always found invading the bronchial wall and in some cases even the adjacent pulmonary parenchyma. The vast majority of bronchopulmonary carcinoids show immunocytochemical positivity for the broad-spectrum neuroendocrine markers such as NSE, chromogranin A and B (Weiler et al 1987, Tötsch et al 1992) and synaptophysin (Lee et al 1987, Gould et al 1988). The most frequently demonstrated hormone (Gould et al 1984) is serotonin, followed by bombesin, VIP, gastrin leu-enkephalin, melanocyte-stimulating hormone (MSH), somatostatin, substance P, and calcitonin. Usually, immunostaining of two or more was obtained in this study. ACTH could be demonstrated by Gould et al (1988) only in a single case, a finding which is in contrast to reports from other investigators (Tsutsumi et al 1983, Gould et al 1984). Care has to be taken with regard to the fact that some cases show only occasional foci with clear-cut positive staining. Some cases, which are convincingly positive for broad-spectrum neuroendocrine markers may nevertheless fail to stain against the antibody panel mentioned above.

Large-cell anaplastic carcinomas of the lung show a neuroendocrine differentiation (demonstrated by markers as chromogranins or synaptophysin, but not by NSE, and/or electron microscopy) in approximately 20% of cases.

Bronchopulmonary carcinoids express cytokeratin and coexpress in some cases cytokeratin and neurofilament proteins (Lehto et al 1986).

**Neuroendocrine bronchopulmonary carcinomas.** This group comprises all cases of malignant epithelial neoplasms with the exception of typical carcinoids. Recognition of the neuroendocrine differentiation component of these tumours is considered to be a critical diagnostic criterion (Gould et al 1984).

*Well-differentiated neuroendocrine carcinomas (WDNE).* This group includes most cases of the formerly so-called 'atypical' carcinoids. These tumours show basic features of a typical carcinoid but with moderate-to-pronounced cellular pleomorphism and increased mitotic activity (up to

30 per 10 HPF). Clinically they tend to be clearly more aggressive than typical carcinoids. Besides their usual positivity for general neuroendocrine markers, such as synaptophysin (Lee et al 1987) and chromogranins (Weiler et al 1987, Tötsch et al 1992), these tumours synthesize a variety of hormones including bombesin, ACTH, calcitonin, serotonin, somatostatin, VIP, leu-enkephalin, gastrin and others. As in typical carcinoids the extent and intensity of immunohistochemical stains may vary quite considerably.

WDNE are cytokeratin positive. In a few cases coexpression of cytokeratin and neurofilament protein has been reported (Blobel et al 1985, Lehto et al 1986).

*Neuroendocrine carcinoma of intermediate-cell type (ICNC).* This tumour group behaves clinically as unfavourably as the small-cell variant of neuroendocrine carcinomas. The cells of this tumour type are, however, at least twice the size of small-cell carcinomas. Glandular and/or squamous differentiation may be found occasionally in these tumours, a feature which can also occur in the small-cell type. These findings, however, do not have any influence on their generally poor clinical course. At this level of differentiation, even the broad-spectrum neuroendocrine markers may fail to demonstrate the neuroendocrine nature of these tumours. Chromogranins have been demonstrated in approximately 50% of ICNC (Tötsch et al 1992).

Cytokeratin is expressed by this tumour type; in a few cases coexpression of cytokeratin and neurofilament has been demonstrated (Gould et al 1988).

*Neuroendocrine carcinoma of small-cell type (SCNC).* This term describes a group of tumours with a pronounced structural and functional heterogeneity so far classified as classical small-cell carcinoma (oat-cell carcinoma). As in neuroendocrine carcinomas of the intermediate-cell type, immunocytochemistry may fail to demonstrate the neuroendocrine origin. In a study performed on 19 neuroendocrine bronchopulmonary carcinomas of small-cell type, 12 cases were positive for NSE and 16 for chromogranins (5 cases were positive both for chromogranin A and B; 5 cases were only positive for chromogranin A and 6 only for chromogranin B) (Tötsch et al 1992). Gould

et al (1984) demonstrated ACTH, bombesin, calcitonin, somatostatin, and leu-enkephalin positivity in small-cell neuroendocrine carcinomas.

Neuroendocrine carcinomas of the small-cell type are positive for cytokeratins. Gould et al (1988) were unable to demonstrate neurofilament proteins in these tumours, a finding which is in accordance with our own results (unpublished observations).

*Neuroendocrine carcinomas of various locations*

Neuroendocrine carcinomas of all grades of differentiation can be found in almost all sites of the body, the most important being the urinary bladder, the kidney, and the pancreas. Figure 7.5 is included to illustrate the typical staining pattern of a moderately differentiated neuroendocrine carcinoma of the colon with NSE and chromogranin A and the usefulness of secretogranin II in the diagnosis of an anaplastic lung carcinoma.

*Carcinoid tumours of the ovary*

Ovarian carcinoids are rare tumours. One-third of these cases are associated with a carcinoid syndrome which is relieved after the removal of the tumour. Ovarian carcinoids may develop from neuroendocrine cells in gastrointestinal or respiratory epithelium of ovarian teratomas. A further possibility concerns C cells in thyroid tissue. True ovarian carcinoids are usually unilateral, whereas metastases of carcinoids to the ovaries are almost always bilateral or multifocal.

*Thymic carcinoid*

In the thymus, occasional cells which contain numerous dense-core endosecretory granules can be found (so-called 'Kulchitsky cells'). These cells probably give rise to carcinoid tumours of the mediastinum. The carcinoids of this region show a different morphology and clinical behaviour from 'classical' thymoma. Some authors consider these carcinoids to be tumours of extrathymic origin (Arya et al 1982). Carcinoids of the thymic region are usually associated with the MEN I syndrome. Ectopic ACTH production may cause Cushing's syndrome.

*Neuroendocrine (Merkel-cell) carcinoma of the skin*

Merkel cells are of neural crest origin. They are present at the undersurface of the epidermis and the oral mucosa. Merkel-cell carcinomas are positive for NSE and at least weakly positive for cytokeratin (Sibley et al 1985). Chromogranin A and secretogranin II immunoreactivity has been described in a limited number of Merkel-cell carcinomas (Weiler et al 1988). Synaptophysin has also been found in some cases of Merkel-cell tumours (Gould et al 1987, Buffa et al 1988) and neurofilament has been demonstrated in approximately half the cases of Merkel-cell carcinomas (Sibley et al 1985).

It might be difficult to distinguish Merkel-cell carcinoma from malignant melanoma. ICC staining with antibodies against cytokeratin (positive in Merkel-cell carcinomas) and vimentin (positive in melanomas) may be helpful as well as neuroendocrine markers (positive in Merkel-cell carcinomas) and S-100 protein (positive in melanomas).

## REFERENCES AND FURTHER READING

Albores-Saavedra J, Nadji M, Civantos F, Morales A 1983 Thyroglobulin in carcinoma of the thyroid. Human Pathology 14: 62–66

Ali-Rachedi A, Varndell I M, Facer P, Hillyard C J, Craig R K, MacIntyre I, Polak J M 1983 Immunohistochemical localisation of katacalcin, a calcium-lowering hormone cleaved from the human calcitonin precursor. Journal of Clinical Endocrinology and Metabolism 57: 680–682

Artlieb U, Krepler R, Wiche G 1985 Expression of microtubule-associated proteins, MAP-1 and MAP-2, in human neuroblastomas and differential diagnosis of immature neuroblasts. Laboratory Investigation 53: 648–691

Arya S, Gilbert E F, Hong R, Bloodworth J M B Jr 1982 The thymus. In: Bloodworth J M B Jr (ed) Endocrine pathology, general and surgical, 2nd edn. Williams & Wilkins, Baltimore, p 767–832

Asa S L, Dardick I, Van Nostrand A W P, Bailey D J, Gullane P J 1988 Primary thyroid thymoma: a distinct clinicopathologic entity. Human Pathology 19: 1463–1467

Bishop A E, Polak J M, Green I C, Bryant M G, Bloom S R 1980 The location of VIP in the pancreas of man and rat. Diabetologia 18: 73–78

Blobel G A, Gould V E, Moll R et al 1985 Coexpression of neuroendocrine markers and epithelial cytoskeletal proteins in bronchopulmonary neuroendocrine neoplasms. Laboratory Investigation 52: 39–51

Böcker W, Dralle H, Husselmann H, Bay V, Brassow M 1980 Immunohistochemical analysis of thyroglobulin synthesis in thyroid carcinomas. Virchows Archiv. A 385: 187–200

Bostwick D G, Roth K A, Barchas J D, Bensch K G 1984 Gastrin-releasing peptide immunoreactivity in intestinal carcinoids. American Journal of Clinical Pathology 82: 428–431

Buffa R, Rindi G, Sessa F et al 1988 Synaptophysin immunoreactivity and small clear vesicles in neuroendocrine cells and related tumours. Molecular and Cellular Probes 1: 367–381

Bunn A P, Linnoila I, Minna J D, Carney D, Gazdar A F 1985 Small cell lung cancer, endocrine cells of the fetal bronchus, and other neuroendocrine cells express the leu-7 antigenic determinant present on natural killer cells. Blood 65: 764–768

Burke A P, Federspiel B H, Sobin L H, Shekitka K M, Helwig E B 1989 Carcinoids of the duodenum. A histologic and immunohistochemical study of 65 tumors. American Journal of Surgical Pathology 13: 828–837

Burt A, Goudie R B 1979 Diagnosis of primary thyroid carcinoma by immunohistochemical demonstration of thyroglobulin. Histopathology 3: 279–286

Burt A D, Kerr D J, Brown I L, Boyle P 1985 Lymphoid and epithelial markers in small cell anaplastic thyroid tumors. Journal of Clinical Pathology 38: 893–896

Cameron R G, Seemayer T A, Wang N S, Ahmed M N, Tabah E J 1975 Small cell malignant tumors of the thyroid. A light and electronmicroscopic study. Human Pathology 6: 731–740

Carcangiu M L, Zampi G, Rosai J 1984 Poorly differentiated ('insular') thyroid carcinoma. A reinterpretation of Langhans' 'wuchernde Struma'. American Journal of Surgical Pathology 8: 655–668

Czech J M, Lichtor T R, Carney J A, van Heerden J A 1982 Neoplasms metastatic to the thyroid gland. Surgery, Gynecology and Obstetrics 155: 503–505

Dawson D W, Tapp E 1969 A compound tumor of the adrenal medulla. Journal of Pathology 97: 231

Dayal J, Nunnemacher G, Doos W G, DeLellis R A, O'Brien M J, Wolfe H J 1983 Psammomatous somatostatinomas of the duodenum. American Journal of Surgical Pathology 7: 653–665

Dayal Y, Tallberg K, Nunnemacher G, DeLellis R, Wolfe H 1986 Duodenal carcinoids in patients with and without neurofibromatosis. A comparative study. American Journal of Surgical Pathology 10: 348–357

Eiden L E, Huttner W B, Mallet J, O'Connor D T, Winkler H, Zanini A 1987 A nomenclature proposal for the chromogranin/secretogranin proteins. Neuroscience 21: 1019–1021

Feyrter F 1938 Über diffuse endokrine epitheliale Organe. Barth Leipzig, p 5–17

Ghandur-Mnaymneh L, Kimura N 1984 The parathyroid adenoma: a histopathologic definition with a study of 172 cases of primary hyperparathyroidism. American Journal of Pathology 115: 70–83

Goldman H, French S, Burbige E 1981 Kulchitzky cell hyperplasia and multiple metastasizing carcinoids of the stomach. Cancer 47: 2620–2624

Gosset H, Masson P 1914 Tumeurs endocrines de l'appendice. Presse Medicale 25: 237–246

Gould V E, Warren W H, Memoli V A 1984 Neuroendocrine neoplasms of the lung. Light microscopic, immunohistochemical, and ultrastructural spectrum. In: Becker K L, Gazdar A F (eds) The endocrine lung in health and disease. W B Saunders, Philadelphia, p 406–445

Gould V E, Wiedenmann B, Lee I et al 1987 Synaptophysin expression in neuroendocrine neoplasms as determined by immunocytochemistry. American Journal of Pathology 126: 243–257

Gould V E, Warren W H, Lee I 1988 Neuroendocrine neoplasms and related lesions of the lung. In: Mendelsohn G (ed) Diagnosis and pathology of endocrine diseases. J B Lippincott, Philadelphia, p 451–475

Greider M H, McGuigan J E 1971 Cellular localisation of gastrin in the human pancreas. Diabetes 20: 389–396

Griffiths D F R, Jasani B, Newman G R, Williams E D, Williams G T 1984 Glandular duodenal carcinoid-somatostatin rich tumour with neuroendocrine associations. Journal of Clinical Pathology 37: 163–169

Hagn C, Schmid K W, Fischer-Colbrie R, Winkler H 1986 Chromogranin A, B and C in human adrenal medulla and endocrine tissues. Laboratory Investigation 55: 405–411

Harach H R, Jasani B, Williams E D 1983 Factor VIII as a marker of endothelial cells in follicular carcinoma of thyroid. Journal of Clinical Pathology 36: 1050–1054

Harach H R, Day E S, Franssila K O 1985 Thyroid spindle-cell tumor with mucous cysts. An intrathyroid thymoma? American Journal of Surgical Pathology 9: 525–530

Harach H R, Franssila K O 1988 Thyroglobulin immunostaining in follicular thyroid carcinoma: relationship to the degree of differentiation and cell type. Histopathology 13: 43–54

Harach H R, Jasani B 1992 Parathyroid hyperplasia in tertiary hyperparathyroidism: a pathological and immunohistochemical reappraisal. Histopathology 20: 305–313

Hedinger C, Williams E D, Sobin L H 1988 Histological typing of thyroid tumours (International Histological Classification of Tumours; Vol 11) 2nd edn. Springer Verlag, Berlin

Heitz P U, Kasper M, Polak J M, Klöppel G 1982 Pancreatic endocrine tumors. Immunocytochemical analysis of 125 tumors. Human Pathology 13: 263–271

Holm R, Sobrinho-Simoes M, Nesland J M, Sambade C, Johannessen J V 1987 Medullary thyroid carcinoma with thyroglobulin immunoreactivity. A special entity? Laboratory Investigation 57: 258–264

Horvath E, Kovacs K 1988 Pathology of the hypothalamus and the pituitary gland. In: Mendelsohn G (ed) Diagnosis and pathology of endocrine diseases. J B Lippincott, Philadelphia. ch 11, p 379–412

Horvath E, Kovacs K 1991 The adenohypophysis. In: Kovacs K, Asa S L (eds) Functional endocrine pathology. Blackwell Scientific, Boston, Vol 1, p 240–281

Hough D R, Chan A, Davidson H 1983 Von Recklinghausen's disease associated with gastrointestinal carcinoid tumors. Cancer 51: 2206–2208

Ibrahim N B N, Briggs J C, Corbishley C M 1984 Extrapulmonary oat cell carcinoma. Cancer 54: 1645–1661

Jansen-Goemans A, Engelhardt J 1977 Intractable diarrhea in a boy with vasoactive intestinal polypeptide-producing ganglioneuroblastoma. Pediatrics 59: 710–712

Jasani B, Newman G R 1988 Applications of immunocytochemistry to thyroid tumours. In: Wynford-Thomas D, Williams E D (eds) Thyroid tumours: molecular basis of pathogenesis. Churchill Livingstone, Edinburgh, p 104–147

Katoh R, Jasani B, Williams E D 1989 Hyalinizing trabecular adenoma of the thyroid. A report of three cases with immunohistochemical and ultrastructural studies. Histopathology 15: 211–224

Klöppel G, Altenähr E, Reichel W et al 1974 Morphometric and ultrastructural studies in an infant with leucine-sensitive hypoglycemia, hyperinsulinism, and islet hyperplasia. Diabetologia 10: 245–257

Klöppel G, Höfler H, Heitz P U 1993 Pancreatic endocrine tumors in man. In: Polak J M (ed) Neuroendocrine tumors. Churchill Livingstone, Edinburgh (in press)

Laidlaw G F 1938 Nesidioblastoma, the islet tumor of the pancreas. American Journal of Pathology 14: 125–134

Landolt A M, Heitz P U 1986 Alpha-subunit-producing pituitary adenomas. Immunohistochemical and ultrastructural studies. Vichows Archiv. A 409: 417–431

Lee I, Gould V E, Moll R, Wiedenmann B, Franke W W 1987 Synaptophysin expressed in the bronchial tract: neuroendocrine cells, neuroepithelial bodies, and neuroendocrine neoplasms. Differentiation 34: 115–125

Lehto V P, Bergh J, Virtanen I 1986 Immunohistology in the classification of lung cancer. In: Hansen H H (ed) Lung cancer: basic and clinical aspects. Martinus Nijhoff, Boston, p 1–30

Lloyd R V, Iacangelo A, Eiden L E, Cano M, Jin L, Grimes M 1989 Chromogranin A and B messenger ribonucleic acids in pituitary and other normal and neoplastic human endocrine tissues. Laboratory Investigation 60: 538–556

Masson P 1914 La glande endocrine de l'intestine chez l'homme. Comptes Rendus de L'Academie des Sciences (Paris) 158: 59–76

Mendelsohn G, Egglestone J C, Olson J L et al 1979 Vasoactive intestinal peptide and its relationship to ganglion cell differentiation in neuroblastic tumors. Laboratory Investigation 41: 144–149

Mendelsohn G, Bigner S H, Egglestone J C, Baylin S B, Wells S A Jr 1980 Anaplastic variants of medullary carcinoma. A lightmicroscopic and immunohistochemical study. American Journal of Surgical Pathology 4: 333–341

Mendelsohn G 1981 Vasoactive intestinal polypeptide (VIP) and the spectrum of tumors producing the watery diarrhea syndrome. In: Fenoglio C M, Wolff M (eds) Progress in surgical pathology, Vol II, Masson, New York, p 199

Mendelsohn G, Wells S A, Baylin S B 1984 Relationship of tissue carcinoembryonic antigen and calcitonin to tumor virulence in medullary thyroid carcinoma. Cancer 54: 657–662

Mendelsohn G 1988a Pathology of parathyroid glands. In: Mendelsohn G (ed) Diagnosis and pathology of endocrine diseases. J B Lippincott, Philadelphia, p 139–177

Mendelsohn G 1988b The endocrine pancreas and diabetes mellitus: diagnosis and pathology. In: Mendelsohn G (ed) Diagnosis and pathology of endocrine diseases. J B Lippincott, Philadelphia, p 273–349

Michels S, Swanson P E, Robb J A, Wick M R 1987 Leu-7 in small cell neoplasms. An immunohistochemical study with ultrastructural correlations. Cancer 60: 2958–2964

Mietinnen M, Franssila K O, Lehto V-P et al 1984 Expression of intermediate filament proteins in thyroid gland and in thyroid tumors. Laboratory Investigation 50: 262–270

Mitchell C H, Sinatra F R, Crast F W et al 1976 Intractable watery diarrhea, ganglioneuroblastoma, and vasoactive intestinal peptide. Journal of Pediatrics 89: 593–596

Miyauchi A, Kuma K, Matsuzuka F et al 1985 Intrathyroidal

epithelial thymoma: an entity distinct from squamous cell carcinoma of the thyroid. World Journal of Surgery 9: 128–134

Molenaar W M, Baker D L, Pleasure D et al 1990 The neuroendocrine and neural profiles of neuroblastomas, ganglioneuroblastomas, and ganglioneuromas. American Journal of Pathology 136: 375–382

Myskow M W, Krajewsky A S, Dewar A E et al 1986 The role of immunoperoxidase techniques on paraffin embedded tissue in determining the histogenesis of undifferentiated thyroid neoplasms. Clinical Endocrinology 24: 335–341

Newman G R, Jasani B, Williams E D 1986 Multiple hormone storage by 'polycrine' cells in the pancreas (from case of nesidioblastosis). Histochemical Journal 18: 67–79

Newman G R, Jasani B, Williams E D 1989 Multiple hormone storage by cells of the human pituitary. Journal of Histochemistry and Cytochemistry 37: 1183–1192

Nieuwenhuijzen Kruseman A C, Bosman F T, van Bergen Henegouw J C, Cramer-Knijnenburg G, Brutel de la Riviere G 1982 Medullary differentiation of anaplastic thyroid carcinoma. American Journal of Clinical Pathology 77: 541–547

Nishiyama R H, Thompson N W, Lloyd R V et al 1984 Secretory diarrhea with islet cell hyperplasia and increased immunohistochemical reactivity to serotonin. Surgery 96: 1038–1044

Oberndorfer S 1907 Karzinoide Tumoren des Dünndarms. Frankfurter Zeitschrift für Pathologie 1: 426–

O'Connor D T, Frigon R P, Deftos L J 1983 Immunoreactive calcitonin in catecholamine storage vesicles of human phaeochromocytoma. Journal of Clinical Endocrinology and Metabolism 56: 582–585

Ordonez N G, Ibanez M L, Mackay B et al 1982 Functioning oxyphil cell adenomas of the parathyroid gland: immunoperoxidase evidence of hormonal activity in oxyphil cells. American Journal of Clinical Pathology 78: 681–688

Ordonez N G, Ibanez M L, Samaan N A et al 1983 Immunoperoxidase study of uncommon parathyroid tumors: report of two cases of nonfunctioning parathyroid carcinoma and one intrathyroid parathyroid tumor producing amyloid. American Journal of Surgical Pathology 7: 535–542

Osamura R Y, Watanabe K 1987 Immunohistochemical colocalisation of growth hormone (GH) and alpha-subunit in human GH secreting pituitary adenomas. Virchows Archiv. A 411: 323–330

Permanetter W, Nathrath W B, Löhrs U 1982 Immunohistochemical analysis of thyroglobulin and keratin in benign and malignant thyroid tumours. Virchows Archiv. A 398: 221–228

Pfaltz M, Hedinger C E, Mühlethaler J P 1983 Mixed medullary and follicular carcinoma of the thyroid. Virchows Archiv. A 400: 53–59

Rindi G, Buffa R, Sessa F, Tortora O, Solcia E 1986 Chromogranin A, B and C immunoreactivities of mammalian endocrine cells. Distribution, distinction from co-stored hormones/prohormones and relationship with the argyrophil component of secretory granules. Histochemistry 85: 19–28

Roth K A, Wilson D M, Eberwine J et al 1986 Acromegaly and phaeochromocytoma: a multiple endocrine syndrome caused by a plurihormonal adrenal medullary tumor. Journal of Clinical Endocrinology and Metabolism 63: 142–1426

Sabate M I, Stolarsky L S, Polak J M et al 1985 Regulation of neuroendocrine gene expression by alternative RNA processing. Journal of Biological Chemistry 260: 2589–2592

Said S I, Faloona G R 1975 Elevated plasma and tissue levels of vasoactive intestinal polypeptide in the watery diarrhea syndrome due to pancreatic, bronchogenic and other tumors. New England Journal of Medicine 293: 155–156

Scheithauer B W 1985 Pathology of the pituitary and sellar region: exclusive of pituitary adenoma. Pathology Annual 20: 67–155

Scheithauer B W, Kovacs K, Randall R V, Horvath E, Laws E R Jr 1986 Pathology of excessive production of growth hormone. Journal of Clinical Endocrinology and Metabolism 15: 655–681

Schmid K W, Fischer-Colbrie R, Hagn C, Jasani B, Williams E D, Winkler H 1987a Chromogranin A and B and secretogranin II in medullary thyroid carcinoma. American Journal of Surgical Pathology 11: 551–556

Schmid K W, Newman G R, Fischer-Colbrie R, Hagn C, Jasani B, Mikuz G, Winkler H 1987b Chromogranin A and B and secretogranin II in endocrine pancreatic tissue. Verhandlungen der Deutschen Gesellschaft für Pathologie 71: 311–313

Schmid K W, Weiler R, Xu R W, Hogue-Angeletti R, Fischer-Colbrie R, Winkler H 1989 An immunological study on chromogranin A and B in human endocrine and nervous tissues. Histochemical Journal 21: 365–373

Schmid K W, Hittmair A, Ladurner D, Sandbichler P, Gasser R, Tötsch M 1991a Chromogranin A and B in parathyroid tissue of primary hyperparathyroidism: an immunohistochemical study. Virchows Archiv. A 418: 295–299

Schmid K W, Kröll M, Hittmair A et al 1991b Chromogranin A and B in adenomas of the pituitary. An immunohistochemical study of 42 cases. American Journal of Surgical Pathology 15: 1072–1077

Schmid K W, Kirchmair R, Ladurner D, Fischer-Colbrie R, Böcker W 1992 Immunohistochemical comparison of chromogranins A and B and secretogranin II with calcitonin gene-related peptide expression in normal, hyperplastic and neoplastic C-cells of the human thyroid. Histopathology 21: 225–232

Schober M, Fischer-Colbrie R, Schmid K W, Bussolati G, O'Connor D T, Winkler H 1987 Comparison of chromogranins A, B, and secretogranin II in human adrenal medulla and phaeochromocytoma. Laboratory Investigation 57: 385–391

Shimaoka K, Sokal J E, Pickren J 1962 Metastatic neoplasms in the thyroid gland; pathological and clinical findings. Cancer 15: 557–565

Sibley R K, Dehner L P, Rosai J 1985 Primary neuroendocrine (Merkel cell) carcinoma of the skin. A clinicopathologic study of 43 cases. American Journal of Surgical Pathology 9: 95–108

Spence R W, Burns-Cox C J 1975 ACTH-secreting 'apudoma' of gallbladder. Gut 16: 473–475

Stephens M, Williams G T, Jasani B, Williams E D 1987 Synchronous duodenal neuroendocrine tumours in von Recklinghausen's disease – a case report of co-existing gangliocytic paraganglioma and somatostatin-rich glandular carcinoid. Histopathology 11: 1331–1340

Tapia F J, Barbosa A J A, Marangos P J, Polak J M, Bloom S R, Dermody C, Pearse A G E 1981 Neuron-specific enolase is produced by neuroendocrine tumours. Lancet 1: 808–811

Tischler A S, Lee Y C, Perlman R L et al 1984 Production of 'ectopic' vasoactive intestinal peptide-like and neurotensin-like immunoreactivity in human phaeochromocytoma cell cultures. Journal of Neuroscience 4: 1398–1404

Tötsch M, Dobler G, Feichtinger H, Sandbichler P, Ladurner D, Schmid K W 1990 Malignant hemangioendothelioma of the thyroid. American Journal of Surgical Pathology 14: 69–74

Tötsch M, Müller L C, Hittmair A, Öfner D, Gibbs A R, Schmid K W 1992 Immunohistochemical demonstration of chromogranins A and B in neuroendocrine tumors of the lung. Human Pathology 23: 312–316

Triche T J, Askin F, Kissane J M 1986 Neuroblastoma, Ewing's sarcoma and the differential diagnosis of small, round-blue-cell tumors. In: Finegold M, Bennington J L (eds) Pathology of neoplasia in children and adolescents. W B Saunders, Philadelphia, p 145–195

Tsutsumi Y, Osamura R Y, Watanabe K et al 1983 Immunohistochemical studies on gastrin-releasing peptide and adrenocorticotropic hormone-containing cells in the human lung. Laboratory Investigation 48: 623–632

Tuccari G, Barresi G 1990 Tissue polypeptide antigen in thyroid tumours of follicular origin: an immunohistochemical re-evaluation for diagnostic purposes. Histopathology 16: 377–381

Ulich T, Cheng L, Lewin K J 1982 Acinar-endocrine cell tumor of the pancreas. Report of a pancreatic tumor containing both zymogen and neuroendocrine granules. Cancer 50: 2099–2105

Vance J, Stoll R W, Kitabchi A E et al 1969 Nesidioblastosis in familial endocrine adenomatosis. Journal of the American Medical Association 207: 1679–1685

Vierbuchen M, Schröder S, Uhlenbruck G, Ortmann M, Fischer R 1989 CA 50 and CA 19-9 antigen expression in normal, hyperplastic, and neoplastic thyroid tissue. Laboratory Investigation 60: 726–732

Vollenweider I, Hedinger C, Saremanslani P, Pfaltz M 1989 Malignant haemangioendothelioma of the thyroid, immunohistochemical evidence of heterogeneity. Pathology, Research and Practice 184: 376–381

Warkel R L, Cooper P H, Helwig E B 1978 Adenocarcinoid, a mucin-producing carcinoid tumor of the appendix. A study of 39 cases. Cancer 42: 2781–2783

Weiler R, Feichtinger H, Schmid K W et al 1987 Chromogranin A and B and secretogranin II in bronchial and intestinal carcinoids. Virchows Archiv. A 412: 103–109

Weiler R, Fischer-Colbrie R, Schmid K W et al 1988 Immunological studies on the occurrence and properties of chromogranin A and B and secretogranin II in endocrine tumors. American Journal of Surgical Pathology 12: 877–884

Wiedenmann B, Huttner W B 1989 Synaptophysis and chromogranins/secretogranins – widespread constituents of distinct types of neuroendocrine vesicles and new tools in tumor diagnosis. Vichows Archiv. B 58: 95–121

Williams E D 1981 Malignant lymphoma of the thyroid. Journal of Clinical Endocrinology and Metabolism 10: 379–389

Williams E D 1986 Immunocytochemistry in the diagnosis of thyroid diseases. In: Polak M, Van Noordins (eds) Immunocytochemistry: modern methods and applications, 2nd edn. Wright, Bristol, p 533–546

Williams E D, Ponder B J, Craig R K 1987 CGRP in C cells and medullary carcinoma. Clinical Endocrinology 27: 104–107

Wilson G, Cheek R C, Sherman R T et al 1970 Carcinoid tumors. Current Problems in Surgery 1: 51–86

Winkler H, Fischer-Colbrie R 1992 The chromogranins A and B: the first 25 years and future perspectives. Neuroscience 49: 497–528

Woo D, Scopes J W, Polak J M 1976 Idiopathic hypoglycemia in sibs with morphological evidence of nesidioblastosis of the pancreas. Archives of Disease in Childhood 51: 528–536

# 8. Central nervous system tumours

## INTRODUCTION

The central nervous system (CNS) consists of the cerebral hemispheres, the cerebellum, the brain stem and the specialized tissues such as the retina, the pineal gland, the neurohypophysis and the choroid plexus.

## EMBRYOLOGY

The parenchymatous cells of the central nervous system tissues are all derived from the primitive neuroectoderm and consist of the various basic and specialized forms of neuronal and neuroglial cells.

In brief, at the time of the lateral flexion of the embryonic plate, the ectoderm lying over the notochord differentiates into the neural plate which gives rise to neural folds and ultimately to the neural tube. The wall of the neural tube, which is only one cell layer thick, is composed of the primitive medullary epithelial cells, from which almost all cells of the future central nervous system are developed. The lumen of the neural tube becomes the central canal of the spinal cord and ventricles of the brain.

The primitive medullary epithelial cells first undergo transformation into the spongioblasts which in turn are transformed into the astroblasts and thence to the astrocytes which constitute a particular type of neuroglial cell population. The residual primitive medulla epithelial cells become the cells lining the cavities, the ependymal cells, or transform into germinal cells to give rise to either the medulloblast or the neuroblast. The medulloblast is a bipotential cell in that it can give rise to either an astrocyte or an oligodendrocyte. The neuroblast ultimately differentiates into the adult neuronal cells.

The final type of central nervous system cell to develop is the microglial cell which develops from the adventitia of the blood vessels and is therefore mesodermal in origin, in contradistinction to all the other types of neuroglial cells which, as already discussed, are all neuroectodermal in origin.

## MORPHOLOGICAL AND FUNCTIONAL ANATOMY

### Astrocytes

Astrocytes form the support matrix of the CNS in which the nerve cells and cerebral capillaries are embedded. Fibrous astrocytes are responsible for scavenging debris and repairing central nervous tissue following injury, and are found primarily in the white matter. Protoplasmic astrocytes are found chiefly in the grey matter. The astrocytic neuroglial cells are distinguishable on the basis of their fairly consistent expression of glial fibrillary acidic protein (GFAP; 49 kDa) and because their cytology comprises a three-dimensional network of cell bodies and radiating processes.

### Ependymal cells

These line the luminal surfaces of the spinal canal and the brain ventricles. This type of neuroglial cell exhibits less strong and less consistent GFAP immunostaining compared to the astrocyte and gives rise to the choroid plexus responsible for the production of cerebrospinal fluid. The choroid plexus cells in addition express monoamine oxidase (MAO), Leu7 (CD57) and vimentin (VIM).

They also have a tendency to coexpress cyto-keratin (CK) in keeping with their morphological and functional epithelial cell-like character.

There are two types of these cells: the perineuronal oligodendrocytes surrounding the cell bodies of neurones known as the satellite cells, and the perivascular oligodendrocytes found in the vicinity of blood vessels. Both these types of neuroglial cells are important in the nutrition of neuronal tissue, and exhibit less strong and less consistent GFAP expression compared to the astrocyte. Mature oligodendrocytes have a tendency to express VIM.

## Neurones

These form cells which have a single process on one side of the cell body and several processes pushed out as dendrites at the opposite pole. The single process grows very considerably and forms the axon of the adult neurone. The neuronal cells have a fairly consistent tendency to express neurone-specific enolase (NSE) and may in addition exhibit neurofilament (NF; 68, 160 or 200 kDa proteins) and synaptophysin (SYNP; 38 kDa protein).

## Specialized cells

### Retinal cells

These are mainly neuronal cells in origin, comprising the photosensory receptors which are immunoreactive for S-antigen (48 kDa protein) capable of interacting with rhodopsin. These cells are associated with a specialized subset of neuroglial cells referred to as the Miller cells and the stellate astrocytes. The former are usually negative or very slightly positive for GFAP, but exhibit carbonic anhydrase isoenzyme and a myelin-associated glycoprotein suggesting their closer relationship to oligodendrocytes. However, these are VIM negative unlike the mature oligodendrocytes.

### Pineal cells

The pineal parenchymal cells, or pinealocytes, constituting the chief cells in the pineal gland, are specialized neuronal cells which are antigenically related to the photoreceptor cells of the retina in

that they exhibit the S-protein. The neuronal origin makes them exhibit NF and SYNP. The pineal gland also contains a moderate density of fibrillary astrocytes which are mainly concentrated at the periphery of the lobules and around the blood vessels, and specialize in modulation of the blood–pineal gland barrier function.

### Neurohypophysis

This forms the posterior wall of the pituitary, the stalk and the median eminence of the cinereum. The specialized neuroglial cells which form the bulk of the neurohypophysis, are referred to as pituicytes. These appear to be of astrocytic origin and have a strong tendency to express GFAP.

## ROLE OF IMMUNOCYTOCHEMISTRY

The vast majority of the CNS tumours in children as well as in adults are derived from neuroglial cell elements. This is because the capacity to undergo reactive hyperplasia is apparently restricted to these cells, in particular the astrocytes. The remarkable proliferative capacity of this type of cell probably accounts for the fact that astrocytic tumours constitute the highest proportion of CNS tumours in children (70–85%) and in adults (up to 45%, despite the inclusion of the relatively common meningiomas, acoustic schwannomas and pituitary adenomas). It also appears to be the case that the vast majority of oligodendroglial, ependymal and neuronal tumours are actually derived from glial/neuronal precursor cells.

This points to the possibility that these tumours are more likely to exhibit a variably mixed immunophenotype compared to their consistently pure normal counterpart making immunocytochemistry an essential tool for differentiating between neoplastic and hyperplastic or normal CNS cells. (See Figure 8.1 for a photomicrographic illustration.)

According to the expectations based on the mixed neuronal/neuroglial cell origins of the majority of the CNS tumours it is best to consider the division of these tumours into three categories:

1. predominantly neuronal
2. predominantly neuroglial
3. mixed neuroglial/neuronal.

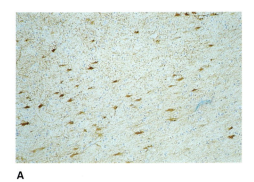 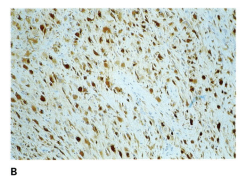

A B

**Fig. 8.1** Illustration of the value of immunocytochemistry in differentiation of neoplastic from normal/hyperplastic CNS cells. (**A**) and (**B**) GFAP staining of reactive and neoplastic astrocytes in a case of astrocytoma (DHSS immunoperoxidase procedure).

The role of immunocytochemistry in the diagnostic typing of the three categories of tumours is considered under these headings.

1. Predominantly neuronal cell-type tumours

a. *Medulloblastoma.* This tumour type is restricted to the cerebellum and takes its origin most probably from the fetal granular cell layer and its remnants. The majority of the medulloblastomas are positive for neurone-specific enolase (NSE) in addition to NF, SYNP and calcineurin (CALC). Only a small minority have been described to have in addition neoplastic cells of neuroglial origin exhibiting GFAP and S-100 immunostaining.

b. *Neuroblastomas.* These are very rare tumours taking their origin either from the granular layer of the cerebral hemispheres or the dentate fascia of the hippocampus. The tumours are consistently positive for NF (68 kDa, 160 kDa subunits) and NSE. They are generally negative for the GFAP.

2. Predominantly neuroglial cell-type tumours

These tumours are fairly consistently positive for the GFAP and show variable expression of Leu7 (CD57), S-100 and/or VIM. They are usually negative for NF, SYNP and CALC.

The three major types of tumour include astrocytomas, oligodendrogliomas and ependymomas, with their individual subtypes having the following immunocytochemical states (+ uniformly positive; +/– predominantly positive; –/+ predominantly negative; ? immunocytochemistry indeterminate.

a. *Astrocytomas:*

| Subtype | GFAP | Leu7 | S-100 | VIM |
|---|---|---|---|---|
| Protoplasmic | –/+ | ? | ? | ? |
| Fibrillary | + | +/– | +/– | +/– |
| Pilocytic | + | ? | ? | ? |
| Germistocytic | + | ? | ? | ? |
| Subependymal | + | ? | +/– | ? |
| Pleomorphic | + | ? | ? | ? |
| Desmoplastic | + | ? | ? | ? |

b. *Oligodendrogliomas:*

| Subtype | GFAP | Leu7 | S-100 | VIM |
|---|---|---|---|---|
| Pure oligodendroglial | + | + | + | ? |
| Mixed oligodendroglial/astrocytic | +/– | + | + | ? |

c. *Ependymomas:*

| Subtype | GFAP | Leu7 | S-100 | VIM |
|---|---|---|---|---|
| Epithelial | +/– | –/+ | +/– | ? |
| Papillary | +/– | –/+ | +/– | ? |
| Myxopapillary | +/– | –/+ | +/– | ? |
| Subependymal | +/– | –/+ | +/– | ? |

3. *Mixed neuronal/neuroglial cell-type tumours*

This type of tumour is in general characterized by NF, SYNP and/or CALC immunopositivity with variable expression of either GFAP, Leu7, S-100 and/or VIM

| Subtype | NF | SYNP | CALC | GFAP | Leu7 | S-100 | VIM |
|---|---|---|---|---|---|---|---|
| Medullo-epithelioma | +/– | +/– | +/– | –/+ | –/+ | –/+ | –/+ |
| Ganglioneuromas ganglion component | +/– | +/– | +/– | – | – | – | ? |
| Gangliogliomas glial component | – | – | – | +/– | +/– | +/– | ? |

4. *Spinalized cell tumours*

| (a) *Retinoblastoma* | NSE | NF | S-antigen | GFAP | Leu7 | S-100 |
|---|---|---|---|---|---|---|
| Neuronal component | + | + | + | – | – | – |
| Glial component | + | – | – | + | + | + |

(b) *Neurohypophysis*

| | NSE | NF 68 kDa | S-antigen | GFAP | Leu7 | S-100 |
|---|---|---|---|---|---|---|
| Pituicyte subtype | − | − | − | + | ? | ? |
| Granular cell subtype | − | − | − | −/+ | ? | ? |

(c) *Pineal*

| | NF | SYNP | S-antigen | GFAP |
|---|---|---|---|---|
| Parenchymal cells | + | + | + | − |
| Glial cells | − | − | − | + |

(d) *Choroid plexus*

| | GFAP | Leu7 | S-100 | VIM | CK | EMA | CEA |
|---|---|---|---|---|---|---|---|
| Papilloma/carcinoma | + | −/+ | −/+ | −/+ | −/+ | −/+ | −/+ |

5. *Miscellaneous intracranial tumours*

(a) *Meningiomas.* These may arise from the dura and/or the leptomeninges (arachnoid and pia mater). The tumour subtypes include meningiomatous, fibrous (fibroblastic), transitional (mixed), psammomatous, angiomatoid, haemangiomatous and papillary meningiomas respectively. All of these have the following immunocytochemical status:

| VIM | CK | EMA |
|---|---|---|
| +/− | −/+ | −/+ |

The various subtypes may be distinguished from their morphologically similar non-meningial tumorous counterparts as follows:

| Subtype | VIM | CK | EMA | GFAP | S-100 | Leu7 | F8R | ULEX |
|---|---|---|---|---|---|---|---|---|
| i) Meningiotheliomatous meningioma | +/− | −/+ | −/+ | − | −/+ | − | − | − |
| *vs* | | | | | | | | |
| protoplasmic astrocytoma | − | − | − | −/+ | ? | ? | − | − |
| oligodendroglioma | + | − | − | −/+ | + | + | − | − |
| ii) Fibrous meningioma | | | | | | | | |
| *vs* | | | | | | | | |
| neurofibroma | +/− | −/+ | −/+ | − | −/+ | − | − | − |
| schwannoma | −/+ | − | − | − | + | −/+ | − | − |
| xanthofibroma | +/− | − | − | −/+ | + | + | − | − |
| chordoma | +/− | −/+ | −/+ | − | −/+ | − | − | − |
| iii) Angiomatoid meningioma | | | | | | | | |
| *vs* | | | | | | | | |
| haemangiopericytoma | +/− | − | − | − | +/− | − | +/− | +/− |
| haemangioglioblastoma | +/− | − | − | − | − | − | − | +/− |

(b) *Peripheral nerve tumours*

| | VIM | S-100 | Leu7 | CFAP | Type I collagen | CD68 | Actin |
|---|---|---|---|---|---|---|---|
| i) Malignant schwannomas | +/− | + | + | −/+ | − | − | − |
| *vs* | | | | | | | |
| fibrosarcomas / malignant fibrous | +/− | − | − | − | + | − | − |
| histiocytomas | +/− | −/+ | −/+ | − | − | + | − |
| leiomyosarcomas | +/− | −/+ | −/+ | − | − | − | + |

| ii) Neurofibromas | S-100 | Leu7 | Type I collagen | Type II collagen | Types IV and V collagen |
|---|---|---|---|---|---|
| *vs* | + | + | − | − | + |
| fibromas | − | − | + | − | − |
| schwannomas | + | + | − | + | − |

(c) *Granular-cell tumours*

These are Schwann cell derived and are therefore uniformly positive for S-100(+) and Leu7(+), variably for VIM (+/−) and GFAP (−/+) and negative for Type I collagen (−), CD68(−) and actin(−).

(d) *Perineural tumours*

These are derived from perineural sheath cells and are S-100(−), Leu7(−) and EMA(+).

(e) *Neurothecomas*

These are questionably derived from either perineural or Schwann cells, and are liable to be variably positive for S-100, Leu7, VIM, GFAP and EMA.

(f) *Cavernous haemangiomas/haemangioblastomas/angiomas (von Hippel–Lindau syndrome)*

The association of retinal, cerebellar and spinal hepatic cysts, pancreatic islet tumours, renal-cell carcinomas and testicular cystadenomas is recognized as von Hippel–Lindau syndrome. Immunohistochemically, these have been shown to be positive for neurone-specific enolase (NSE) and polypeptide hormone, suggestive of their neuroectodermal origin.

(g) *Primary CNS lymphomas*

These are predominantly B cell in origin with the majority exhibiting monoclonal immunoglobulin immunophenotype. Only a very few cases of T cell lymphomas have been recorded.

   The differential diagnoses include transplantation, x-linked lymphoproliferative ten-

| | Subtype | PLAP | AFP | HCG | CEA | VIM | CYTK | EMA | NF | DES | GFAP |
|---|---|---|---|---|---|---|---|---|---|---|---|
| I | Germinoma | + | – | + | – | –/+ | –/+ | –/+ | – | – | – |
| II | Choriocarcinoma | – | – | + | – | – | + | + | – | – | – |
| IIIa | Yolk-sac carcinoma | – | + | + | – | – | –/+ | –/+ | – | – | – |
| IIIb | Endodermal sinus tumour | – | + | + | – | – | –/+ | –/+ | – | – | – |
| IIIc | Embryonal carcinoma | – | + | + | – | –/+ | –/+ | –/+ | – | – | – |
| IVa | Immature teratoma | – | – | – | – | –/+ | –/+ | –/+ | –/+ | –/+ | –/+ |
| IVb | Mature tertoma | – | – | – | – | +/– | +/– | +/– | +/– | +/– | +/– |
| V | Mixed germ-cell tumour | –/+ | –/+ | –/+ | –/+ | –/+ | –/+ | –/+ | –/+ | –/+ | –/+ |

dency, Epstein–Barr virus infection-related B cell lymphomas, all of which exhibit a tendency to be bi- or multiclonal with respect to the neoplastic B cells.

(h) *Histiocytosis X*
The malignant cells are uniformly S-100 positive and primary CNS involvement is seen in about 50% of the cases.

(i) *Germ-cell tumours*
These include germinomas and tumours devised from totipotential germ cells. These may be distinguished on the basis of the immunocytochemical profiles given above.

(j) *Paragangliomas*
According to the WHO classification scheme, these are divisible into four categories:
- (a) Phaechromocytomas (arising within adrenal medulla)
- (b) Sympathetic paragangliomas
- (c) Parasympathetic paragangliomas
- (d) Paragangliomas from uncertain cell of origin.

The tumours of this type are uniformly positive(+) for NSE and PGP9.5 and predominantly positive (+/–) for NF, Leu7, SYNP and neuropeptides such as methionin–enkephalin, VIP and somatostatin. .
The tumours are predominantly negative(–/+) for calcitonin and ACTH and only very occasionally show positivity for GFAP and CYTK. All paragangliomas show uniform(+) S-100 positivity

in sustentacular cells usually found at the periphery of the tumour cell groups.

*Special notes on CNS-based immunocytochemical markers*

(a) *Neurone-specific enolase (NSE)*
This marker is based on the γγ isoenzyme expressed by both the normal and neoplastic neuronal and neuroglial cells as well as neoplastic meningeal, Schwann and choroid plexus cells. Neoplastic stromal cells, apart from the endotrichial cells in cerebellar haemangiomas, are also positive. At the ultrastructural level the NSE positivity is localizable in the cytoplasmic as well as in the membranous compartments.

(b) *Calcineurin (CALC)*
This represents a calcium-dependent calmodulin-stimulated phosphoprotein phosphatase.

(c) *S-100*
This is a 21 kDa dimeric calcium-binding protein involved in the regulation of microtubule assembly and stabilization. It is most useful in the immunocytochemical differentiation of Schwann cells from perineural cells.

(d) *Retinal S-antigen*
This is a 50 kDa protein produced by retinocytes and pineal parenchyma cells. It is a useful negative marker in the diagnosis of cerebral neuroblastomas and cerebral neurocytomas.

### FUTHER READING

Garson J A, Bourne S P, Allan et al 1988 Immunohistological diagnosis of primary brain lymphoma using monoclonal antibodies: confirmation of B-cell origin. Neuropathology and Applied Neurobiology 14: 19–37

Gould V E, Rorke L B, Jansson D S et al 1990 Primitive neuroectodermal tumors of the central nervous system express neuroendocrine markers and may express all classes of intermediate filaments. Human Pathology 21: 245–252

Heitz P U, Roth J, Zuber C et al 1991 Markers for neural and endocrine cell in pathology. In: Gratzl M, Langley K (eds) Markers for neural and endocrine cells: molecular and cell biology, diagnostic applications. VCH Publishers, New York, p 203–216

Ismail S M, Jasani B, Cole G 1985 Histogenesis of haemangioblastomas: an immunocytochemical and ultrastructural study in a case of von Hippel – Lindau syndrome. Journal of Clinical Pathology 38: 417–421

Jasani B, Thomas N D, Wilkins P R, Cole G 1986 Retrospective immunohistochemical phenotyping of primitive neuroectodermal tumours. Journal of Pathology 148: 104A

Rubinstein L J 1986 Inaugural Dorothy S Russell Memorial Lecture: Immunohistochemical signposts—not markers—in neural tumour differentiation. Neuropathology and Applied Neurobiology 12: 523–537

Russell D S, Rubinstein L J 1989 Pathology of tumours of the nervous system, 5th edn. Edward Arnold, London

# 9. Reproductive organ tumours

## INTRODUCTION

Amongst the reproductive organs, the majority of the immunocytochemical applications have been confined to the study of neoplastic diseases arising from the testis, ovary, prostate and breast.

The aim of this chapter is to review these in relation to the principle tumour types of these organs.

## TESTIS

### Embryology

The testes develop retroperitoneally from the genital ridge in the dorsal wall of the abdominal cavity. Subsequently, they are suspended within the scrotum at the ends of the spermatic cord. Malpositioned testes (cryptorchidism) may be found at any point in the pathway of descent. The undescended testis bears both the risk of sterility and/or tumour development.

## Anatomy and biochemistry

The testis has two functions—reproductive and hormonal. The normal testis consists of approximately 250 testicular lobules. Each lobule contains several seminiferous tubules which are surrounded by intertubular connective tissue. The testicular lobules are united with straight tubules which communicate with the rete testis and the epididymis.

Microscopically, the seminiferous tubules consist of three components: a tunic of fibrous connective tissue, a basal lamina and the germinal epithelium. The germinal epithelium consists of cells that constitute the spermatogenic lineage and supporting (Sertoli) cells. The spaces between the seminiferous tubules are filled with connective tissue, nerves, blood and lymphatic vessels, and the interstitial (Leydig) cells. Leydig cells produce testosterone.

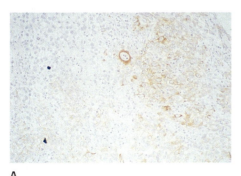
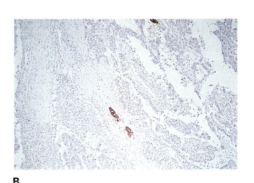

A B

**Fig. 9.1** Illustration of the value of cytokeratin and β-HCG in the diagnosis of testicular tumours. (**A**) Use of cytokeratin in recognition of therapeutically and prognostically important embryonal carcinomatous change in a testicular seminoma. (**B**) Demonstration of syncytiotrophoblastic giant cells with β-HCG staining in a testicular embryonal carcinoma. It is of interest to note that even a few syncytiotrophoblastic giant cells are sufficient to cause substantially raised serum β-HCG levels (simple two-step indirect immunoperoxidase method).

## Immunocytochemical markers

Immunocytochemical markers useful in the study of the testes and testicular tumours include the beta-subunit of human chorionic gonadotrophin (β-HCG), alpha-l-fetoprotein (AFP), cytokeratin, vimentin, alpha-l-antitrypsin (AAT), placental alkaline phosphatase (PLAP), S-100 protein, NSE and various other neuroendocrine markers, CEA, LCA (CD45), testosterone, and oestradiol.

## Immunocytochemistry of individual testicular tumours (classified according to Mikuz 1993)

### Germ-cell tumours of testis

**Seminoma**. Seminomas are the commonest type of germinal tumour (approximately 40%), hardly ever occurring in infants. Seminomas peak in the fourth decade. Pure seminomas do not stain immunocytochemically with HCG or AFP. HCG staining can be demonstrated, however, in syncytiotrophoblastic and intermediate trophoblastic cells (Niehans et al 1988, Karayannopoulou & Damjanov 1989). Rarely, clusters of cytokeratin-positive cells can be found in seminomas. The usual negativity for cytokeratin in seminomas may be helpful to distinguish them from embryonal carcinomas which are almost always cytokeratin positive. Approximately half of seminoma cases express vimentin. PLAP and NSE positivity can be found in the majority of cases.

Spermatocytic seminomas do not express HCG and cytokeratins. They are PLAP positive and in some cases vimentin can be demonstrated (Karayannopoulou & Damjanov 1989). Figure 9.1 illustrates the value of cytokeratin and β-HCG in the diagnosis of a seminoma/embryonal carcinoma.

**Embryonal carcinoma**. This category also includes yolk-sac tumours and polyembryomas.

*Embryonal carcinoma (malignant teratoma, undifferentiated)*. Embryonal carcinoma occurs mostly in patients aged between 20 and 40 years of age and constitutes approximately 20% of testicular tumours. Embryonal carcinomas are typically negative for HCG, with the exception of syncytiotrophoblastic elements, which show a strong immunoreactivity, whereas AFP is virtually never found within these cells. AFP positivity occurs, however, in approximately 30% of embryonal carcinomas. Embryonal carcinomas express cytokeratin. Some cases may coexpress cytokeratin and vimentin. Like seminomas, a high proportion of embryonal carcinomas show PLAP- and NSE-positive tumours.

*Yolk-sac tumour*. Yolk-sac tumours are cytokeratin positive and show a positive staining reaction for AFP either throughout the tumour or in a focal distribution. Approximately half the cases in the study of Niehans et al (1988) showed positivity for PLAP, NSE and AAT. CEA-positive cells are found only occasionally.

*Polyembryoma*. This is an extremely rare tumour in its pure form. More often, it forms a component of embryonal carcinomas or teratomas. Polyembryoma consists of the so-called 'embryoid body' resembling the embryonic disc. This disc is made up of undifferentiated large cells which are surrounded by loose mesenchyme with trophoblastic elements. HCG-, cytokeratin- and vimentin-positive cells have been described in these tumours.

*Combined tumours*. Embryonal carcinoma may be combined with a malignant teratoma, intermediate differentiation (= teratocarcinoma), or a yolk-sac tumour and/or polyembryoma.

**Teratoma**. Teratomas make up about 10% of testicular neoplasms. They may occur at any age. Teratomas are a complex group of tumours depicting various cellular and organoid components of more than one germ-cell layer. Histologically, two variants can be distinguished: mature teratoma (malignant teratoma, differentiated) and teratoma with malignant transformation of epithelial and/or mesenchymal components (malignant teratoma, intermediate differentiation). Immunocytochemically, the different components of teratomas show the same set of staining reactions as the respective tissues of the various germ layers which they represent. Cells with endocrine differentiation may give rise to tumour components resembling testicular carcinoids.

*Testicular carcinoid*. Testicular carcinoids are rare tumours. There are two theoretical pathways concerning their origin. They may either originate as 'pure' primary carcinoids or as part of a teratoma (Talerman 1986, Wheeler 1989). Whereas their histogenesis within a teratoma is readily apparent, the origin of pure carcinoids is uncertain. The high proportion of teratomas with neuroendocrine differentiation makes it much more likely that testicular carcinoids originate as a predominantly unicomponent development of a teratoma rather than from any neuroendocrine cells. In this context, it is noteworthy that neuroendocrine cells have not been found to date in the normal testis. Immunohistochemically, neuroendocrine differentiation has been demonstrated in differentiated components of testicular teratomas (Brodner et al 1980, Bosman & Louwerens 1981, Niehans et al 1988, Pichmann et al 1993).

*Choriocarcinoma*. Choriocarcinomas are highly malignant tumours composed, by definition, of both cytotrophoblast and syncytiotrophoblast. Choriocarcinomas are virtually always positive for HCG and cytokeratin. Some cases may contain AAT- and/or CEA-positive cells. NSE and PLAP can be demonstrated in approximately 50% of cases.

*Seminoma combined with other germ-cell tumours*. All germ-cell tumours of the testis may be found in an admixed form. For prognostical and therapeutic reasons the occurrence of embryonal carcinoma, polyembryoma, teratoma, or choriocarcinoma in a seminoma has to be excluded.

*Sex-cord tumours*

*Leydig-cell tumour and Sertoli-cell tumours*. These tumours may occur in a pure form or in a mixed Leydig-/Sertoli-cell form. The Leydig-cell elements show a strong positivity for testosterone. Occasionally Sertoli cells also stain for testosterone. Recently, McLaren & Thomson (1989) described S-100 protein expression in a Leydig-/Sertoli-cell tumour as well as in normal Leydig cells and Sertoli cells. Sertoli cells and Sertoli-cell tumours are usually vimentin positive.

*Sertoli-cell/mesenchyme tumours*. These tumours are composed of various amounts of stromal and Sertoli-cell-like elements. The tumour may even resemble rhabdomyosarcoma. Immunocytochemically, the tumour expresses vimentin,

in some cases testosterone and/or oestradiol. Desmin and myoglobin negativity may help to distinguish it from rhabdomyosarcoma.

*Granulosa-cell tumour*. Granulosa-cell tumours are usually associated with clinical manifestations of hormone production. Immunocytochemically, granulosa-cell tumours stain for oestradiol, progesterone and even testosterone (Taylor and Warner 1983).

*Tumours of gonadal stroma*

*Gonadoblastoma*. Gonadoblastomas consist of highly undifferentiated cells which may stain immunocytochemically for testosterone and/or oestradiol. The differential diagnosis of a malignant lymphoma may be difficult without the intervention of the appropriate set of immunocytochemical markers.

*Mixed germ-cell/gonadal stroma tumours*
*Paratesticular tumours*
*Adenomatoid tumour*
*Mesothelioma of the tunica vaginalis testis*
*Rhabdomyosarcoma*

See *Miscellaneous mesenchymal tumours* (p. 111).

OVARY

Like the testes, the ovaries arise as a thickened multilayered epithelium from the medial side of the mesonephric ridge in the fifth week of gestation. This epithelium extends along the ridge and thickens through further proliferation to form the genital ridge. The proliferating epithelium at this stage in the male begins to be organized into cellular cords referred to as testis cords, whilst in the female large numbers of cells simply remain below the surface coelomic epithelium or the germinal epithelium. The testis cords develop further to become the rete testis, whilst the female equivalent develops into the rete complex. The clusters of cells forming the rete complex are separated from each other by fine septae of undifferentiated mesenchyme which may or may not contain the primitive sex cells.

In the fifth month of gestation, the ovary becomes invaded by mesenchyme from the region of the mesovarium, which ultimately gives rise to the stroma of the gland. The cell clusters surrounding the primitive sex cells become flattened to form capsular cells which multiply to form the stratum granulosum. This in turn becomes surrounded by thecal cells derived from the stromal cells. These primordial follicles ultimately disappear and are replaced by second-generation sex cells derived from either the coelomic (germinal) epithelium or the primitive sex cells themselves.

## Development of ovarian follicles

Enmeshed within the stroma are the numerous ovarian follicles, in different states of development, the most mature being the vesicular or the Graafian follicles. These consist of an outer layer of the flattened thecal cells and an inner layer of the more exuberant cells forming the stratum granulosum. The innermost layer of the stratum granulosum, the cumulus ovaricus, surrounds the ovum.

As the follicle matures during the first half of the menstrual cycle under the stimulus of follicle-stimulating hormone, it approaches the surface of the ovary and ultimately bursts through the surface, releasing the ovum surrounded by the cells of the cumulus ovaricus, into the fimbriated end of the fallopian tube. The residual Graafian follicle undergoes changes to become the corpus luteum. In the absence of fertilization of the ovum, the latter degenerates within eight days or so into simple scar tissue. If, on the other hand, fertilization has taken place, the corpus luteum enlarges under the influence of the sex hormones to reach a size of approximately 2.5 cm in diameter by mid-pregnancy. After the pregnancy it degenerates to a size of about 1 cm in diameter.

## Anatomy and biochemistry

Three distinct types of tissue elements comprising the ovary give rise to the vast majority of the ovarian tumours. These include:

1. The epithelium associated with surface epithelial glands and cysts
2. The sex cord–stromal tissue with specialized forms of epithelium associated with granulosa and thecal cells

3. The germ cells consisting of ova present within the primary or developing follicles.

It is important to note that the outer aspect of the ovary is covered with the so-called surface, coelomic, or germinal epithelium which is histogenetically distinct from the epithelium associated with the superficial glands and cysts. For instance, it is consistently immunoreactive for both cytokeratin and vimentin, a finding which supports the view that it is derived as an extension of the neighbouring mesothelium.

The sex cord–stromal tissue is a specialized form of ovarian tissue derived from the mesenchyme. It consists of the epithelial components (theca and granulosa) of the various forms of ovarian follicles. The follicles are embedded within smooth muscle bundles separated by nests of cells resembling endometrial stromal cells, adipose cells, neuroendocrine cells and spindle-shaped fibroblastic-like cells.

The sex cord cells possess both steroidogenic potential and responsiveness to gonadotrophins derived either from the placenta (human chorionic gonadotrophin, HCG) or the anterior pituitary (follicle-stimulating hormone (FSH) and luteinizing hormone (LH)). The granulosa cells are responsive to both FSH and LH, whilst the thecal cells are primarily responsive to LH. Both these types of cells have the capacity to produce oestradiol and express oestradiol receptors, whilst the granulosa cells, under the effect of LH or HCG, also have the potential to produce progesterone and prostaglandins.

The neuroendocrine cells consist of the hilus cells, which are morphologically identical to the testicular Leydig cells. They are mostly present in the hilum in close association with nerves. Their number and location are, however, highly variable, being more readily found in postmenopausal women. They are responsive to chorionic gonadotrophin and undergo hyperplasia in response to iatrogenic influences or pregnancy, or choriocarcinoma-related high levels of chorionic gonadotrophin.

The germ cells in the adult ovary virtually all exist only as ova encapsulated within follicles in different stages of maturation. Any uncapsulated primordial germ cells usually fail to survive beyond the fifth month of gestation.

## Immunocytochemical markers of relevance in the study of ovarian tumours

Immunocytochemical markers have been used mainly for achieving a better understanding of the histogenesis and the nature of ovarian tumours rather than for purely diagnostic purposes.

For the study of the common epithelium-derived tumours, antibodies to cytokeratin, vimentin, carcinoembryonic antigen (CEA), epithelial membrane antigens (EMA and HMFGII), and two epithelial tumour antigens, CA19-9 and CA125, have been used widely. Amylase has also been used as a relatively specific marker of the serous and endometrioid variety of epithelial tumours.

As for the various sex cord–stromal and germ-cell tumours, the use of antibodies to neurone-specific enolase (NSE), serotonin, ACTH, gastrin, somatostatin and other peptide hormones in relation to neuroendocrine tumours, HCG and α-antitrypsin (α-AT), placental alkaline phosphatase (PLAP) and alpha-fetoprotein (AFP) for germ-cell tumours, and steroid hormones and steroid receptors vimentin and desmoplakin for sex cord–stromal tumours, have proved valuable.

## Immunocytochemistry of ovarian tumours

### General account

The bulk of the ovarian tumours seems to be derived from the common type of epithelium associated with the superficial glands and cysts. These are listed in Table 9.1 in the order of their incidence relative to the other types of ovarian tumours. Together they account for about 70% of all ovarian tumours. The germ-cell and sex cord–stromal tumours account for up to 25% of the other ovarian tumours, the rest (5–10%) being of metastatic origin. For further details the reader is referred to the accounts by Czernobilsk (1987), Talerman (1987), Young and Scully (1987), Saksela (1988) and Rosai 1989.

### Benign and malignant Brenner tumours

Brenner tumours are relatively rare (0.5–1.7% of all ovarian tumours). The majority of all types of Brenner tumours are positive with antibodies to CEA. In Brenner tumours the number of CEA-positive cases apparently does not reflect the degree of malignancy. Brenner tumours express cytokeratin, whereas no vimentin or desmin can be found. The cytokeratin subunit pattern of Brenner tumours resembles that of papillary cancer of the urothelial epithelium, supporting the theory that Brenner tumours exhibit a urothelial epithelium differentiation. About one-third of Brenner tumours contain a small amount of cells with neuroendocrine differentiation. Amongst the hormones demonstrated are serotonin, neurotensin and somatostatin.

Ovarian epithelial tumours are very prevalently positive for CA19-9, CA125, EMA and HMFGII. These markers, though not in any way specific for the ovarian carcinomas, have nevertheless proved useful in clinical follow-up studies as sensitive markers of residual tumour burden following surgery and chemotherapeutic measures (Maughan et al 1988, 1989).

Receptors for oestrogens, progesterone and androgens, though expressed in over 50% of ovarian tumours, are rarely applied as markers, as they do not seem to correlate well with histological grade, prognosis or antihormone responsiveness of the tumour.

### Common epithelial tumours

These include in the main the serous, mucinous, endometrioid and Brenner varieties.

Table 9.1 Main tumour types of the ovary and their relative incidence

| Tumour type | Relative incidence (compared to all ovarian tumours) (%) |
| --- | --- |
| *Common epithelial* | 65 overall |
| Serous | 25 |
| Mucinous | 20 |
| Endometrioid | 10–20 |
| Brenner | 1–2 |
| *Germ cell* | 20 overall |
| Teratoma | –20 |
| Dysgerminoma | –1 |
| Yolk sac (or endodermal sinus) | rare |
| Embryonal | rare |
| Choriocarcinoma | rare |
| *Sex cord–stromal* | 5 overall |
| Granulosa cell | |
| Thecal cell | |
| Leydig cell | |

*Serous and sero-papillary tumours.* Serous cystadenomas make up approximately 25% of all benign tumours, serous borderline tumours and serous cystadenocarcinomas about 50% of malignant tumours of the ovary. These tumours are only occasionally positive for CEA. Malignant serous tumours may coexpress cytokeratin and vimentin (Mietinnen et al 1983).

*Mucinous tumours.* Mucinous cystadenomas make up approximately 20% of benign tumours of the ovary. Mucinous cystadenomas rarely become malignant (approximately 10% of malignant ovarian tumours). CEA is found in approximately 15% of mucinous cystadenomas, approximately 80% of borderline tumours, and in all mucinous cystadenocarcinomas of the ovary. Thus there is an increasing number of CEA-positive cases with increasing degree of malignancy in these tumours. Both benign and malignant mucinous tumours express cytokeratin, but no vimentin.

As recently shown, a high proportion of argentaffin and argyrophil cells in mucinous tumours of the ovary produce polypeptide hormones, e.g. gastrin (in some cases clinically associated with the Zollinger–Ellison syndrome), somatostatin, ACTH, secretin, neurotensin, pancreatic polypeptide, enkephalin, glucagon and serotonin (reviewed by Scully et al 1984).

*Endometrioid carcinoma.* This almost certainly develops out of a pre-existing endometriosis. Endometrioid carcinomas express cytokeratin and CEA but not vimentin or desmin.

The serous and endometrioid tumour types are distinguishable from the mucinous variety by their expression of amylase. This enzyme-based antigen is expressed by 25% of serous and endometrioid tumours but virtually none of the mucinous type.

*Sex-cord and germinal tumours*

*Granulosa-cell tumour.* Granulosa-cell tumours are the most common malignant hormone-secreting ovarian neoplasm (6% amongst all malignant tumours of the ovary). They secrete oestrogens, causing clinical symptoms in 75% of patients. Immunocytochemically, granulosa-cell tumours express vimentin, but not cytokeratin. Their intermediate filament pattern allows their differentiation from poorly differentiated carcinomas which usually express cytokeratin and occasionally show cytokeratin/vimentin coexpression. A peripheral staining with desmoplakin can be found in granulosa-cell tumours, which may be helpful to distinguish them from stromal tumours.

*Thecoma.* Thecomas occur predominantly in women aged 50 to 60 years and these tumours are very rarely malignant. Like granulosa-cell tumours, thecomas are positive for vimentin and negative for cytokeratin. Since thecomas may secrete steroid hormones and promote endometrial hyperplasia or carcinoma, they should be distinguished from a related neoplasm, the fibroma. The distinction between these tumours, however, is not clear cut. Unfortunately, immunocytochemistry cannot contribute to the solution of this problem since both tumours express vimentin.

*Sertoli–Leydig-cell tumours (androblastoma).* Sertoli–Leydig-cell tumours are rare (fewer than 1% of all ovarian tumours). However, they are the most common virilizing tumours of the ovary. Sertoli–Leydig-cell tumours usually express both cytokeratin and vimentin. Approximately 20% of these tumours contain heterologous elements, which are composed in the majority of cases of glandular and cystic structures lined by gastrointestinal-type epithelium. Somatostatin, ACTH, gastrin, neurotensin and glucagon have been demonstrated in the gastrointestinal-type epithelium.

*Dysgerminoma.* Dysgerminomas are the most common malignant germ-cell tumour of the ovary. Dysgerminomas do not express cytokeratin. HCG can easily be demonstrated with immunocytochemistry in the cytoplasm of syncytiotrophoblastic giant cells, which are found in approximately 5% of dysgerminomas. However, dysgerminomas may be HCG positive even in the absence of these syncytiotroblastic giant cells. Serum HCG levels are used for monitoring the adequacy of treatment and for early detection of recurrence.

*Embryonal carcinoma.* This tumour is histologically similar to the much more common homologous neoplasm of the testis. Embryonal carcinomas almost always contain syncytiotrophoblastic giant cells which are HCG positive. AFP is also almost always positive. Both markers are clinically valuable markers for follow-up monitoring.

*Teratoma and teratocarcinoma.* The majority of ovarian teratomas are benign (so-called 'dermoid' cysts). Both benign and malignant teratomas generally express their differentiation-related intermediate filament pattern which may include GFAP, NF and myelin basic protein in elements of neural differentiation. Teratomas are almost always (at least focally) cytokeratin positive.

***Struma ovarii***. A teratoma which consists predominantly or exclusively of thyroid tissue is called 'struma ovarii'. In some cases, they may be found in the wall of dermoid cysts. Functionally, they are usually silent, rarely they may cause hyperthyroidism. Immunocytochemically, thyroglobulin can be demonstrated. Rare examples of a malignant struma ovarii have been reported.

***Carcinoid***. Primary ovarian carcinoids occur rarely. Most arise as metastases from neuroendocrine cells in respiratory or gastrointestinal epithelium. Another source might be the C cells in thyroid tissue. Ovarian carcinoids exhibit two distinct histological patterns, which may be admixed, but usually one pattern is predominant. The most common 'insular' pattern is associated in one-third of cases with a carcinoid syndrome. The 'trabecular' carcinoid is characterized by its columnar and ribbon-like growth pattern. The so-called 'strumal carcinoid' consists of trabeculae and glands lined by carcinoid cells and thyroid follicles.

Immunocytochemically, ovarian carcinoids are positive with NSE and chromogranin A.

It may be difficult to distinguish primary ovarian carcinoid from metastatic carcinoid to the ovary. Metastases, however, ofter occur bilaterally, whereas primary ovarian carcinoids almost always occur unilaterally.

***Endodermal sinus tumour***. This highly malignant tumour occurs mainly in children and young women. In the tumour tissue as well as in the patient's serum in a high proportion of cases of endodermal sinus tumours, alpha-l-fetoprotein (AFP) can be demonstrated. Since AFP may be focally distributed, several tumour blocks should be investigated immunocytochemically. In order to avoid false-negative results it may even be necessary to use frozen sections.

***Choriocarcinoma***. Choriocarcinomas may rarely occur in a pure, non-gestational primary germ-cell tumour (less than 0.6%) or often as a component in mixed germ-cell tumours. Human chorionic gonadotrophin (HCG) can be demonstrated in both types on formalin-fixed, paraffin-embedded tumour tissue.

*Miscellaneous mesenchymal tumours*

A variety of benign and malignant mesenchymal tumours may arise from the pluripotential Müllerian epithelium or from the non-specific ovarian stroma, as shown in Table 9.2.

Immunocytochemical markers used in the study of these tumours are essentially the same as those discussed for soft-tissue tumours and lymphocytic tumours in Chapters 4 and 6, respectively.

Two further tumour types under this category need mention.

***Mixed malignant mesodermal tumours (mixed Müllerian tumours; MMT)***. MMT is much rarer in the ovary than in the uterus. It has to be distinguished histologically from malignant ovarian teratoma. The carcinomatous component of MMT expresses cytokeratin, the sarcomatous stroma vimentin, and desmin can be demonstrated in areas with smooth muscle differentiation. In heterologous tumour elements other markers (e.g. myoglobin in striated muscle cell) can be found. Cytokeratin is also expressed in areas of epithelioid differentiation in the endometrial-type stromal sarcomas.

***Benign mesothelioma of the genital tract (adenomatoid tumour)***. Adenomatoid tumours

**Table 9.2** Miscellaneous mesenchymal tumours of the ovary

|  | Benign | Malignant |
|---|---|---|
| Arising from the pluripotential Müllerian epithelium | Chondroma Osteoma | Chondrosarcoma Osteosarcoma Rhabdomyosarcoma |
| Arising from the non-specific ovarian stroma | Fibroma Neurofibroma Ganglioneuroma Leiomyoma Myxoma Haemangioma and lymphangioma Lipoma | Fibrosarcoma Neurofibrosarcoma<br><br>Leiomyosarcoma Myxosarcoma Angiosarcoma<br>Liposarcoma Malignant lymphoma |

of the ovary are very rare tumours. They are positive for EMA and cytokeratin. The negative F-VIII-RAG staining may help to distinguish them from vascular tumours.

*Metastases to the ovary*

Approximately 10% of all tumours of the ovary are of metastatic origin. The main primary site is a carcinoma of the endometrium, followed by the gastrointestinal tract, namely the stomach (so-called 'Krukenberg tumour'), and the breast. Rarely, malignant tumours of the cervix, fallopian tube, pancreas, gallbladder, lung, kidney, thyroid or skin metastasize to the ovaries.

## PROSTATE

### Embryology and development

The prostate gland is the result of 14–20 out-growths from the proximal part of the urethra. These mainly arise from the lateral aspects of the urethral tube in the third month of gestation. The rest develop from its dorsal and ventral aspects. In relation to the orifices of the mesonephric ducts, about one-third of the outgrowths arise on the cephalic side and the rest on the caudal side. From their initial solid cord-like form they develop into tubular structures. These gradually invade the surrounding mesenchyme which is destined to become muscular tissue.

### Anatomy and biochemistry

The prostate is partly a glandular and partly a muscular organ. The muscular tissue constitutes the main stroma of the prostate, the fibrous con-nective tissue being very scanty and forming thin trabeculae between muscle bundles in which blood and lymphatic vessels and nerves are dis-tributed. The muscular tissue is at its most dense near the urethral opening where hardly any glands are present. Away from the bladder towards the apex of the gland the muscular meshwork be-comes looser and sponge-like as the prostatic glands increase in numbers. The glandular tissue consists of follicular lining with many papillary projections. The glandular acini open into elon-gated canals which link up to 12–20 small excre-tory ducts. The acinar and ductal lining is made up of a single layer of columnar cells.

The prostatic glands and the muscular stroma are under the influence of testosterone and un-dergo age-related hyperplasia/hypertrophy after puberty. Thus from a prepubertal weight of 8 g it rises to 20 g by the age of 21–30 years and remains steady until the 4th decade. Thereafter, there is a progressive increase in the incidence of nodular hyperplasia/hypertrophy experienced by the whole gland as a result of accumulation of dihydro-testosterone, mainly due to its decreased catabolism and enhanced intracellular binding. The weight of the gland may increase from anywhere between 20 and 100 g to over 800 g in exceptional cases.

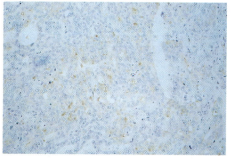
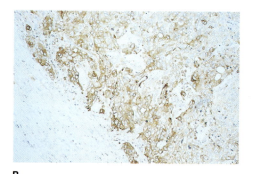

A  B

**Fig. 9.2** Illustration of the value of prostatic-specific antigen (PSA) and prostatic acid phosphatase (PAPh) in the diagnosis of a poorly differentiated prostatic adenocarcinoma. (**A**) PSA, and (**B**) PAPh. The positivity for these markers in a poorly differentiated tumour not only establishes that diagnosis but also provides optimism for treating definitively an otherwise highly malignant tumour. Note that the staining due to PAPh is usually more extensive than PSA in the same tumour (simple two-step indirect immunoperoxidase method).

The glandular cells of the prostate produce two varieties of proteins which are more or less specific for the tissue. Prostate-specific antigen, PSA, is a glycoprotein with a molecular weight of 33 kDa. The molecule has no enzymatic or any other types of known functions. The other molecule is referred to as prostatic acid phosphatase (PAPh). This is an acid phosphatase capable of hydrolysing phosphoric acid esters at acid pH. Several isoenzymes of PAPh are produced by the prostate and these are confined largely to lysosomes of the prostate epithelium. Only two of these isoenzymes are secreted into seminal fluid.

## Immunocytochemical markers

Antibodies to PSA and PAPh (directed against the seminal fluid isoenzymes) have proved extremely useful in the diagnosis of poorly differentiated metastatic prostatic cancers, or various unusual variants of prostatic adenocarcinomas mimicking or overlapping with other tumour types (see Figure 9.2 for a photomicrographic illustration). The small-cell carcinoma variant with its neuroendocrine features, in addition to being strongly positive for PSA and PAPh, may express serotonin, calcitonin, bombesin, ACTH, somatostatin activity, and/or antidiuretic hormone (i.e. vasopressin) activities. Prostatic carcinomas have also been shown to be positive for keratin, Leu7, epithelial membrane, CEA and gastrin to varying degrees.

### Immunocytochemistry of main prostatic tumours

Carcinoma of the prostate represents the most important tumour type from diagnostic and differential diagnostic viewpoints. Prostatic carcinomas are essentially all adenocarcinomas. These are divisible into two main categories: adenocarcinomas arising from the peripherally located acini or the small 'secondary' ducts; or the carcinoma arising from the centrally located large 'primary' ducts. The vast majority of the prostatic carcinomas belong to the former category.

Monoclonal antibodies to PSA and polyclonal antibodies to PAPh are both available commercially. These allow positive identification of prostatic carcinomas of all varieties except the least differentiated types, in routinely prepared formalin-fixed, paraffin-embedded tissue sections. The PSA and PAPh have therefore been most useful in the identification of the prostatic origin of metastatic tumours and the differential diagnosis between poorly differentiated prostatic and transitional-cell tumours.

In most people's experience, PSA is a more sensitive and specific marker compared to PAPh. The latter marker has been recorded as frequently staining breast carcinoma and occasionally renal-cell carcinoma (Yam et al 1983). In comparative studies by Nadji et al (1980) and Ellis et al (1984), overall, sensitivities of 99.1% (108 out of 109 cases) and 87.2% (95 out of 109 cases) were recorded for PSA and PAPh, respectively. In both the studies, PSA was found to be 100% specific, with none of the non-prostatic cancers, including 17 bladder cancers, giving any staining (Nadji et al 1980). Interestingly, only 4 out of a total of 95 cases (4.2%) of prostatic carcinomas were found to be CEA positive. These four cases were both PSA and PAPh positive (Ellis et al 1984). Thus a CEA+/PSA–/PAPh– tumour found in the prostate may be considered with confidence to be of a non-prostatic origin. This rule is particularly helpful in differentiation of primary transitional-cell carcinoma of the prostate from a bladder or urethral carcinoma extending into the prostate. Up to 35% (7 out of 20 cases) of bladder transitional-cell carcinomas have been noted by Heyderman et al (1984) to be positive for CEA. This group also observed all the bladder tumours to be negative for PAPh.

Finally, in relation to bone metastasis, Mansi et al (1988) have noted that immunocytochemical staining of bone marrow aspirate and trephine for PSA and PAPh is more sensitive than conventional staining. It is also more reliable than serum analysis of these markers and isotope scanning in identification of purely local disease—a point which is of vital importance when considering the cost-effectiveness of radical surgery for this condition (Moertel 1979).

## Neuroendocrine features associated with prostatic tumours

Neuroendocrine differentiation in prostatic carcinomas has been described as occurring in one of four different forms. Resolution of its diagnostic or prognostic significance usually requires a combined use of histological, histochemical and immunohistochemical techniques.

The commonest variety relates to histochemically (i.e. Grimelius's argyrophilia) and/or immunohistochemically (chromogranin A immunoreactivity) detectable neuroendocrine differentiation seen in up to two-thirds of an unselected series of prostatic adenocarcinomas (Abrahamsson et al 1989). The extent of such differentiation in the tumour cell population seems to correlate directly with the degree of tumour progression.

The next most common type is seen in approximately 10% of the cases defined histologically as mixed prostatic adenocarcinoma—small-cell carcinoma or carcinoid tumours (Turbat-Herrera et al 1988). The neuroendocrine component typically shows a positivity for neurone-specific enolase and chromogranin A and a negativity for prostate-specific antigen. In approximately 50% of cases it is liable to show a staining for calcitonin or synaptophysin and, in occasional cases, evidence of ectopic expression of corticotrophin or para-thyroid hormone immunoreactivity. Again, with these tumours, the extent of neuroendocrine differentiation seems to correlate with a poorer prognosis.

The third variety relates to pure small-cell carcinomas or carcinoid tumours of the prostate gland origin. Because of the rarity of this type of tumour, it is important to exclude a metastatic deposit from a lung small-cell carcinoma (Turbat-Herrera et al 1988) or the possibility of an extensive neuroendocrine differentiation in a terminally aggressive prostatic carcinoma (Schron et al 1984). The combined and judicious use of prostate-specific antigen and neuroendocrine markers is likely to help in the differential diagnostic analysis of this type of tumour.

Finally, in transurethral prostatic resection biopsies, cellular foci composed of paraganglion cells may occasionally be found to resemble an invasive carcinoma. Again, the use of neuroendocrine markers in conjunction with prostatic markers is likely to prove helpful in avoidance of the potential diagnostic pitfall (Rode et al 1990).

# BREAST

## Embryology and development

The glandular tissue of the breast is derived from the ectoderm and represents a modified sweat gland covered by a large amount of fatty subcutaneous tissue in the adult female. The embryonic mammary gland arises as a mammary bud extending out of the mammary streak occurring symmetrically on either side of the body. At birth the gland consists of branching cords of epithelial cells which constitute several secondary ducts connected to the nipple by a single primary milk duct. The peripheral regions of the ducts end in swollen structures known as terminal end buds (TEBs) which represent the main growth regions of the glands and are sensitive to maternal hormones. Following the withdrawal of these hormones after birth, the growth activity with the TEBs diminishes leaving behind blunt-ended ducts.

At puberty, under the action of the ovarian hormones, the TEBs begin to undergo growth once again. The growth is associated with both an increase in ductal length and extensive branching. After a while the density of TEBs begins to diminish as they become differentiated into smaller units, the alveolar buds (ABs). The ABs further differentiate into lobules. The mammary gland differentiation continues to increase with each successive menstrual cycle, reaching maximum maturity during pregnancy and lactation.

## Anatomy and biochemistry

The fully developed breast gland represents a complex branching structure composed of two main components: the terminal duct lobular unit (TDLU) and the large duct system. The TDLU consists of the terminal ductule and the lobule connected to it and represents the secretory unit of the gland. It connects up with the subsegmental duct. This in turn is linked to the segmental duct which joins up with the collecting (lactiferous) duct leading finally to the nipple.

The ductal–lobular epithelium is made up of two cell layers: the inner is represented by glandular cells with secretory and absorptive functions, whilst the outer layer is composed of the myoepithelial cells with a contractile function mediated via their actin filaments.

The growth and function of the ductal–lobular unit is oestrogen dependent with essential contributions from progesterone and pituitary hormones, in particular prolactin. The effect of the oestrogen is transmitted via oestrogen receptors located in the nuclear compartment.

In the absence of milk production, the major secretory product of the breast lobule consists of a carbohydrate- and lipid-rich protein complex referred to as human milk fat globulin, HMFG. The carbohydrate-rich fraction is referred to as HMFGI and corresponds to the epithelial membrane antigen, EMA, in terms of its immunoreactivity. On the other hand, the protein-rich component has a unique immunoreactivity and is termed HMFGII.

The ductal–lobular epithelium rests on a continuous basement membrane which is relatively specifically demonstrable with antibodies to laminin and Type IV collagen.

## Immunocytochemical markers

Antibodies to HMFGI, or EMA, and HMFGII have proved to be the most sensitive immunocytochemical markers of breast glandular epithelium. In addition, lactalbumin and CEA have also been used for the marking of the breast epithelium. On the other hand, antibodies to actin, and to a lesser extent S-100, have proved effective for delineating the myoepithelial cell component.

More recently, antibodies to protein extracted from fluid aspirates of gross cystic disease (GCD) of the breast in premenopausal women, have shown the gross cystic disease fluid protein-15 (GCDFP-15) to be a reliable marker of the apocrine glandular epithelium found in both benign and malignant conditions of the breast. Also, monoclonal antibodies against the oestrogen receptor protein have proved effective in lightly fixed frozen sections. These antibodies have recently been shown by some workers to be effective also in formalin-fixed, paraffin-embedded tissue sections provided protease pretreatment and a powerful secondary signal amplification system, e.g. silver intensification, are employed (Jackson et al 1989, Gee et al 1992).

Factor VIII-related antigen (F-VIII-RAG), laminin and collagen Type IV have been used in the detection of invasive breast tumours.

## Immunocytochemistry of breast tumours

Immunocytochemistry plays a rather limited role in relation to the diagnosis of breast tumours. Most of its use is directed at resolving diagnostic difficulties only occasionally encountered with invasive breast tumours.

Invasive ductal and invasive lobular carcinomas represent the two main types of invasive tumours of the breast. These may be further ramified into apocrine, mucinous, papillary or inflammatory types according to the cell type, the type and amount of secretion, architectural features, and the pattern of spread involved, respectively.

Immunocytochemistry plays two quite distinct roles with respect to the diagnosis of primary and secondary breast tumours, as discussed below.

## Primary breast tumours

The principle function of immunocytochemistry is that of diagnosing minimal invasion around the lobule as well as excluding any lymphatic, vascular or perineural space invasion.

In relation to the minimum invasive disease, laminin and collagen Type IV have been found to show a discontinuous linear pattern or are completely absent, in contrast to the continuous pattern exhibited by them with wholly intraduct lesions. In addition, absence of myoepithelial cells around tumour foci, as evidenced by a negative staining reaction with actin or S-100, is further confirmation of minimal invasion.

Lymphatic vessel invasion may be at times quite difficult to distinguish from artifactual tissue retraction around small tumour nests. Although reliable histological criteria are available to overcome this form of diagnostic difficulty, it is sometimes necessary to use F-VIII-RAG or *Ulex europeaus* lectin positively to identify or exclude the presence of an endothelial lining around the specified tumour foci.

As for perineural sheath invasion, S-100 and Leu7, two markers relatively specific for Schwann cells, may be used to identify more precisely the position of the tumour in relation to a nerve bundle.

## Breast tumour metastases

With respect to metastatic breast cancer, immunocytochemistry has been employed mainly to improve the sensitivity of detection of breast tumour cells in axillary lymph nodes in order to assess the degree of invasion for a more accurate prognostic evaluation, and in order to identify breast as an occult source of metastatic disease.

Immunocytochemistry has been used only to a limited extent to distinguish invasive breast carcinoma from other epithelial malignancies. This is because the most sensitive breast epithelial markers, EMA and HMFGII, are expressed by virtually all other types of carcinoma. The recently introduced breast apocrine epithelial marker, GCDFP-15, though expressed by only approximately 50% of primary breast cancers (and approximately 30% of all breast cancers) is more specific. Apart from breast carcinomas it has been found to be positive only in extramammary Paget's disease and a number of sweat gland tumours (Mazouhian 1988).

## Detection of lymph node micrometastases

The lymph nodes metastases are present most frequently in the axillary nodes. These are found in 40–50% of cases. The yield increases by a further 20% if each node is serially sectioned and examined microscopically. The cost-effectiveness of this approach is, however, questionable. Nevertheless, immunocytochemical detection of micrometastases in lymph nodes has been considered to offer a more sensitive as well as worthwhile exercise (O'Dowd et al 1991). Thus, in 60 cases with 'node-negative' status and a 5-year follow-up available, 37% of the cases were found to be node positive on review with immunocytochemically stained serial sections prepared using CEA, EMA, HMFGII and cytokeratin antibodies. Of the 63% immunocytochemically 'node-negative' cases only one case was found to have died, the rest being alive and well without recurrent breast carcinoma 5 years after mastectomy. On the other hand, amongst the cases with immunocytochemical positivity, eight cases had succumbed to the carcinoma. This study clearly indicates the need for a large multicentre survey to evaluate more fully the prognostic significance of 'micrometastases' detected by the given set of immunocytochemical markers. Figure 9.3 illustrates the use of EMA and cytokeratin in the detection of lymph node metastasis in breast cancer.

## Identification of occult breast carcinoma

Occasionally the finding of a single enlarged axillary lymph node in an adult female may be involved with metastatic poorly differentiated tumour in the presence of a radiologically normal breast and an absence of tumour elsewhere. The diagno-

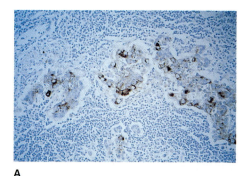
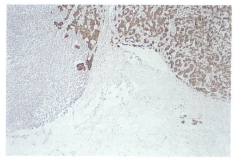

**A**  **B**

**Fig. 9.3** Illustration of the use of epithelial membrane antigen (EMA) and cytokeratin in the demonstration of lymph metastasis in breast cancer. (**A**) EMA, and (**B**) cytokeratin. These markers provide an excellent tool for the detection of micrometastases, the presence of which may be of both therapeutic and prognostic importance (simple two-step indirect immunoperoxidase method).

sis under these circumstances is most likely (>90%) to be either a metastatic breast carcinoma or a melanoma. Immunocytochemical markers such as cytokeratin, CEA and EMA or HMFGII are likely positively to identify a carcinomatous tumour, whilst S-100, melanoma marker (M3080 or HMB45) and vimentin are likely to be useful for identification of a melanoma. It should, however, be borne in mind that S-100 positivity has been recorded in 10–45% of unselected breast carcinomas.

## Oestrogen receptors

Immunocytochemistry of oestrogen receptors has largely been confined to study of lightly fixed frozen sections taken from freshly frozen breast tumour tissue, mainly for the purpose of assessing prognosis and the responsiveness of the tumour to hormonal manipulations and antioestrogen therapy (see Wold 1988 and Ch. 11 for further discussion).

REFERENCES AND FURTHER READING

**Testis**

Bosman F T, Louwerens J K 1981 APUD cells in teratomas. American Journal of Pathology 104: 174–180

Brodner O G, Grube D, Helmstaedter V, Kreienbrink M E, Wurster K, Forssmann W G 1980 Endocrine GEP-cells in primary testicular teratoma. Virchows Archiv. A 388: 251–262

Karayannopoulou G, Damjanov I 1989 Immunohistochemistry of testicular tumors. In: Damjanov I, Cohen A H, Mills S E, Young R H (eds) Progress in reproductive and urinary tract pathology, Vol 1. Field & Wood, New York, p 149–162

McLaren K, Thomson D 1989 Localization of S-100 protein in a Leydig and Sertoli cell tumour of testis. Histopathology 8: 649–652

Niehans G A, Manivel J C, Copland G T, Scheithauer B W, Wick M R 1988 Immunohistochemistry of germ cell and trophoblastic neoplasms. Cancer 62: 1113–1123

Mikuz G 1993 Tumoren des Hodens und der paratestikulären Strukturen. In: Histologische Tumorklassifikation. Histopathologische Nomenklatur und Klassifikation der Tumoren und tumorartigen Veränderungen. Springer Verlag, Vienna (in press)

Pichmann S, Mikuz G, Schmid K W 1993 Chromogranins A and B in nonseminomatous testicular tumors. An immunohistochemical study. Journal of Urogenital Pathology (in press)

Talerman A 1986 Germ cell tumors. In: Talerman A, Roth L M (eds) Pathology of the testis and its adnexa. Churchill Livingstone, Edinburgh, p 29–66

Taylor C R, Warner N E 1983 Immunohistological techniques for the diagnosis of ovarian and testicular neoplasms. In: Filipe M I, Lake B D (eds) Histochemistry in pathology. Churchill Livingstone, Edinburgh, p 252–262

Wheeler J E 1989 Testicular tumors. In: Hill G S (ed) Uropathology, Vol 2. Churchill Livingstone, New York, p 1047–1100

**Ovary**

Czernobilsky B 1987 Common epithelial tumours of the ovary. In: Kurman R J (ed) Blaustein's Pathology of the female genital tract. Springer-Verlag, New York, ch 18, p 560–606

Maughan T S, Fish R G, Shelly M, Jasani B, Williams G T, Adams M 1988 Antigen C A 125 in tumour tissue and serum from patients with adenocarcinoma of the ovary. Gynaecologic Oncology 30: 342–346

Maughan T S, Fish R G, Shelly M D, Jasani B, Williams G T, Adams M 1989 CA125 in ovarian tumour tissue at second laparotomy. British Journal of Cancer 5: 259

Mietinnen M, Lehto V P, Virtanen I 1983 Expression of intermediate filaments in normal ovaries and ovarian epithelial, sex cord–stromal, and germinal tumours. International Journal of Gynaecological Pathology 2: 64–71

Rosai J 1989 Female reproductive system. In: Rosai J (ed) Ackerman's Surgical pathology. C V Mosby, St Louis, ch 19, p 1120–1164

Saksela E 1988 Advances in immunohistochemistry of ovarian tumours. In: Nogales F (ed), Current topics in pathology, Vol 78: Ovarian Pathology. Springer-Verlag, Berlin, p 135–155

Scully R E, Aguirre P, DeLellis R A 1984 Argyrophilia, serotonin, and peptide hormones in the female genital tract and its tumours. A review. International Journal of Gynaecological Pathology 3: 51–70

Talerman A 1987 Germ cell tumours of the ovary. In: Kurman R J (ed) Blaustein's Pathology of the female genital tract. Springer-Verlag, New York, ch 20, p 660–721

Young R H, Scully R E 1987 Sex cord–stromal, steroid cell, and other ovarian tumours with endocrine, paraendocrine, and paraneoplastic manifestations. In: Kurman R J (ed) Blaustein's Pathology of the female genital tract. Springer-Verlag, New York, ch 19, p 607–658

**Prostate**

Abrahamsson P A, Falkner S, Fait K, Grimelius L 1989 The course of neuroendocrine differentiation in prostatic carcinomas. An immunohistochemical study testing chromogranin A as an 'endocrine marker'. Pathology Research and Practice 185: 373–380

Ellis D W, Brown B M E, Richardson T C 1984 Epithelial markers in prostatic, bladder, and colorectal cancer: an immunoperoxidase study of epithelial membrane antigen, carcino embryonic antigen, and prostatic acid phosphatase. Journal of Clinical Pathology 37: 1363

Heyderman E, Brown B M, Richardson T C 1984 Epithelial markers in prostate, bladder and colorectal cancer: an immunoperoxidase study of epithelial membrane antigens, carcinoembryonic antigen, and prostatic acid phosphatase. Journal of Clinical Pathology 37: 1363–1369

Limas C 1988 Monoclonal and polyclonal antibodies to prostatic acid phosphatase and prostate specific antigen. In: Wick M R, Siegal G P (eds) Monoclonal antibodes in diagnostic immunohistochemistry. Marcel Dekker, New York, ch 12, p 383–399

Mansi J L, Berger U, Wilson P, Shearer R et al 1988 Detection of tumour cells in bone marrow of patients with prostatic carcinoma by immunocytochemical techniques. Journal of Urology 139: 545–548

Moertel C D 1979 Adenocarcinoma of unknown origin. Annals of Internal Medicine 91: 646

Nadji M, Tabei S Z, Castro A et al 1980 Prostatic origin of tumors. An immunohistochemical study. American Journal of Clinical Pathology 73: 735–739

Nadji M, Tabei S Z, Castro A, Chu T M et al 1981 Prostatic-specific antigen: an immunohistologic marker for prostatic neoplasms. Cancer 48: 1229–1232

Rode J, Benley A, Parkinson 1990 Paraganglial cells of urinary bladder and prostate: potential diagnostic problem. Journal of Clinical Pathology 43: 13–16

Rosai J 1989 Male reproductive system. In: Rosai J Ackerman's Surgical pathology. C V Mosby, St Louis, Vol 2, ch 18, p 923–948

Schron D S, Gipson T, Mendelsohn G 1984 The histogenesis of small cell carcinoma of the prostate. An immunohistochemical study. Cancer 53: 2478–2480

Turbat-Herrera E A, Herrera G A, Lott R L, Grizzle W E, Bonnin J M 1988 Neuroendocrine differentiation in prostatic carcinomas. A retrospective autopsy study. Archives of Pathology and Laboratory Medicine 112: 1100–1105

Yam L T, Winkler C F, Janckila A T et al 1983 Prostatic cancer presenting as metastatic adenocarcinoma of undetermined origin. Cancer 51: 283–287

## Breast

Bettelheim R, Price K N, Gelber R D et al (International Ludwig Breast Cancer Study Group) 1990 Prognostic importance of occult axillary lymph node micrometastases from breast cancers. Lancet 335: 1565–1568

Gee J M W, Amselgruber W M, Jasani B, Nicholson R I 1992 Use of the dinitrophenyl hapten sandwich staining procedure (DHSS) to localise estrogen receptors in paraffin-embedded tissues. Journal of Histochemistry and Cytochemistry 39: 1659–1670

Jackson P, Teasdale J, Cowen P N 1989 Development and validation of a sensitive immunohistochemical oestrogen receptor assay for use on archival breast cancer tissue. Histochemistry 92: 149–152

Mazoujian G 1988 Gross cystic disease fluid protein-15. In: Wick M R, Siegal G P (eds) Monoclonal antibodies in diagnostic immunohistochemistry. Marcel Dekker, New York, p 505–519

O'Dowd G M, Kay E W, Hourihane D O'B 1991 Nodal micrometastases in breast carcinoma – occult malignancy or voodoo? Journal of Pathology 164: 365A

Rosai J 1989 Breast. In: Rosai J Ackerman's Surgical pathology. C V Mosby, St Louis, ch 20, p 1193–1267

Swanson P E 1988 Monoclonal antibodies to human milk fat globule proteins. In: Wick M R, Siegal G P (eds) Monoclonal antibodies in diagnostic immunohistochemistry. Marcel Dekker, New York, p 227–283

Wells C A, Heryet A, Brochier J et al 1984 The immunocytochemical detection of axillary micrometastases in breast cancer. British Journal of Cancer 50: 193–197

Wold L E 1988 Immunohistochemical localisation of oestrogen receptors with monoclonal antibodies. In: Wick M R, Siegal G P (eds) Monoclonal antibodies in diagnostic immunohistochemistry. Marcel Dekker, New York, p 367–382

# 10. Paediatric tumours

## INTRODUCTION

Childhood tumours are defined as neoplasms arising in children below the age of 15. About two-thirds of these tumours are accounted for by brain tumours and various forms of childhood leukaemias. Of the remainder, the majority are classifiable as the so-called 'small-round-cell tumours' of childhood. The main ones include lymphomas (13.2%), neuroblastoma (9.6%), rhabdomyosarcoma (5.3%) and Ewing's sarcoma (1.7%).

The role of immunocytochemistry in paediatric tumours is first and foremost related to resolution of differential diagnostic and prognostic problems posed by the small-round-cell tumours.

The main aim of this chapter is to highlight the use of immunocytochemistry in the typing and subtyping of the major variety of the small-round-cell tumours in a conventional histopathological setting. Emphasis is therefore given to immunocytochemical markers which are known to work well in formalin-fixed, paraffin-embedded tissue sections.

The use of immunocytochemistry in the diagnosis of other varieties of paediatric tumours is summarized in a section at the end of this chapter. For further details, the reader is referred to the excellent contributions included in Bennington (1986) and the articles by Mieran et al (1985) and Darbyshire et al (1986).

## IMMUNOCYTOCHEMISTRY OF SMALL-ROUND-CELL TUMOURS OF CHILDHOOD

As mentioned above, these include, in the main, lymphoma, neuroblastoma, rhabdomysarcoma and Ewing's sarcoma.

Below, brief summaries of immunocytochemical markers useful for diagnostic and prognostic typing of each variety of these tumours are given, followed by a discussion of the markers which have proved most useful in their differential diagnoses.

### Lymphoma

Lymphomas account for 10–15% of all childhood malignancies, of which approximately 40 and 60 per cent respectively are of the Hodgkin's and the non-Hodgkin's varieties.

#### Non-Hodgkin's lymphomas

The non-Hodgkin's childhood lymphomas, unlike the adult lymphomas, have a tendency to involve the extranodal tissue either as primary or secondary tumour presentation. The main types and subtypes and their respective immunophenotypes are listed in Table 10.1. The diagnostically useful markers for which antibodies which work well in formalin-fixed, paraffin-embedded tissues are available include CD45, CD3, CD20 and CD68.

**Table 10.1** Classification and immunophenotype of childhood non-Hodgkin's lymphomas

| Type/subtype | Immunophenotype |
|---|---|
| 1. Lymphoblastic lymphoma | T, pre-B or non-B/non-T |
| 2. T-cell leukaemia/lymphoma | T |
| 3. Undifferentiated (small, non-cleared cell) lymphomas | |
|    a. Burkitt's lymphoma | B |
|    b. Non-Burkitt's lymphoma | Usually B, may be non-B/non-T, rarely T |
| 4. Large-cell lymphoma | Usually B, may be non-B/non-T, rarely histiocytic |
| 5. Malignant histiocytosis | True histiocytes (rare) |

**Table 10.2**   Immunocytochemical markers useful in differential diagnosis of CD45-large-cell lymphomas

| Differential diagnosis | Marker status |
|---|---|
| 1. Undifferentiated carcinoma | Cytokeratin; CEA; EMA (HMFGII) |
| 2. Malignant histiocytosis | CD68 (KP1) |
| 3. Certain variants of Hodgkin's lymphomas | CD15 (LeuM1); CD30 (Ki-1, BerH2) |
| 4. Granulocytic sarcoma | |
| 5. Extraosseous Ewing's | |

It is important to note that whilst 80–100% of the undifferentiated (small, non-cleared cell) lymphomas (100%), T-cell leukaemias/lymphomas (100%) and lymphoblastic lymphomas (82%) have the tendency to exhibit CD45+ status, only 60% of the large-cell lymphomas are likely to express this marker.

Thus, as indicated in Table 10.2, additional markers are usually necessary in order to resolve any differential diagnostic problems posed by the CD45-large-cell non-Hodgkin's lymphoma variety.

*Hodgkin's lymphomas*

These are classifiable according to the Rye modification of the Lukes and Butler's classification into four main varieties as listed in Table 10.3.

The main difficulty encountered in the diagnosis of Hodgkin's lymphoma and its subtypes is the identification of the neoplastic cell component as being Reed–Sternberg cell and/or the so-called 'L and H' cell. Whilst morphological criteria are available to identify these cells, immunocytochemistry is likely to be more useful in particularly difficult cases and other diseases mimicking Hodgkin's disease (see Table 10.4). In this context it is noteworthy that the Hodgkin's cells are usually positive for CD15 (LeuMI) and CD30 (BerH2), two markers which are both effectively detectable in formalin-fixed, paraffin-embedded tissue sections.

**Table 10.3**   Classification of Hodgkin's lymphomas (Rye Modification Scheme)

1. Lymphocyte predominance
2. Nodular sclerosis
3. Mixed cellularity
4. Lymphocyte depletion

**Table 10.4**   Immunocytochemical markers useful in differential diagnosis of Hodgkin's disease

| Differential diagnosis | Useful markers |
|---|---|
| *Reactive conditions* | |
| 1. Non-specific lymphoid hyperplasia | |
| 2. Drug-induced hyperplasia | CD15 (LeuM1); |
| 3. Toxoplasmosis | CD30 (Ki-1, BerH2) |
| 4. Infectious mononucleosis | to exclude Hodgkin's |
| 5. Herpes zoster | cells |
| 6. Dermatopathic lymphadenitis | |
| *Neoplastic conditions* | |
| 1. Eosinophilic granuloma | CD68 (KP1) |
| 2. Metastatic carcinoma | Cytokeratin; CEA; EMA (HMFGII) |
| 3. Non-Hodgkin's lymphoma | CD45, CD3, CD20 |

**Neuroblastomas**

These are thought to arise from primitive cells of neural-crest origin. The putative stem cell, the 'sympathogon', is assumed to differentiate into sympathoblasts which are responsible for giving rise to the various types of neuroblastomas described. They also give rise to chromaffin or non-chromaffin paraganglionic cells responsible for the development of phaeochromocytoma and paraganglioma, tumours which are described in detail elsewhere in this book.

Neuroblastomas are divided into three main types according to their prognostic behaviour (see Table 10.5). Of these, the highly malignant variety which is the least differentiated is likely to pose the most difficult diagnostic problems.

Immunocytochemistry is useful for both diagnostic recognition and prognostic classification of such tumours. Thus, these tumours are invariably neurone-specific enolase (NSE) positive, and the positivity of certain tumour cell components, such as ganglion cells and the sustentacular cells, is indicative of a better prognosis compared to the tumours which are uniformly negative for S-100. Accordingly, only 40% of the Grade IV tumours are found to be positive for S-100 compared to

**Table 10.5**   Neuroblastoma—prognostic variants

| Prognostic category | Type |
|---|---|
| 1. Benign | Ganglioneuroma |
| 2. Intermediate malignancy | Ganglioneuroblastoma |
| 3. Highly malignant | Small-round-cell neuroblastoma |

100% of the Grades I to III neuroblastomas (see Shimada et al (1985) for a more detailed account).

## Rhabdomyosarcoma

The childhood rhabdomyosarcomas tend to be less differentiated (embryonal or botryoid types) compared to those encountered in adulthood (usually well differentiated) or adolescence (usually the alveolar type). The diagnostic problems usually arise with the least differentiated forms, referred to as either embryonic sarcoma, embryonal sarcoma with suspicion of rhabdomyosarcoma, undifferentiated sarcoma, or sarcoma of undetermined histogenesis.

In the light of the availability of effective chemotherapy for rhabdomyosarcoma it is important that every method capable of recognizing skeletal muscle cell origin of the tumour is vigorously pursued. Immunocytochemistry in conjunction with electron microscopy has proved quite valuable in achieving this goal.

Myoglobin has consistently proved to be the most specific marker of rhabdomyosarcoma with sensitivity ranging from 50 to 89%. Desmin, on the other hand, although more sensitive (80–100%) is reactive with tumours of smooth muscle origin and occasional fibrosarcoma and fibrous histiocytoma.

The recent introduction of a monoclonal antibody to a smooth muscle actin ($\alpha$-SMA) which is effective in formalin-fixed, paraffin-embedded tissue (Jones et al 1990) is likely to alleviate at least one of these problems.

## Ewing's sarcoma

This is a rare tumour which usually arises as a primary bone tumour in the childhood period with the peak incidence between 10 and 15 years of age.

Histologically, the tumour consists of small, round hyperchromatic cells which are otherwise devoid of any form of differentiation of organization. The lack of cellular differentiation is usually so complete that, apart from recognizing the tumour as being of mesenchymal origin, no further clues are revealed even by extensive ultrastructural or immunocytochemical studies. The histopathologist is usually therefore forced to rely upon clinicopathological information and report the morphological features as being consistent with those of a Ewing's sarcoma. His main problem is to ensure that other forms of undifferentiated small-round-cell tumours involving the bone are excluded before coming to this conclusion. Immunocytochemistry is able to play a prominent role in positive identification of such bone tumours as well as helping with diagnosis or exclusion of Ewing's sarcoma arising in an extraosseous location, as described next.

## DIFFERENTIAL DIAGNOSIS OF SMALL-ROUND-CELL TUMOURS OF CHILDHOOD

Although the small-round-cell tumours comprise only 20–30% of all tumours encountered in childhood, the diagnostic problems posed by the most difficult of these tumours seem to test and occupy the histopathologist's acumen out of all proportion to the frequency with which these tumours are encountered.

The most exacting of the difficulties faced relates to the differentiation of a neuroblastoma metastasizing to bone from a primary bone Ewing's sarcoma. This is especially important in the light of the fact that the two types of tumour in this situation have very different prognostic indices—75% long-term survival if it is Ewing's sarcoma and only 2.5% if it is a neuroblastoma. The other diagnostic difficulties relate to differentiation of a primary bone lymphoma from a primary bone Ewing's sarcoma, and embryonal rhabdomyosarcoma and an extranodal lymphoma from an extraosseous soft-tissue Ewing's sarcoma.

Three main immunocytochemical markers have proved useful in resolving these difficulties with specificity and sensitivity as indicated in Table 10.6.

It is evident from the table that differentiation of a neuroblastoma from a Ewing's sarcoma is not entirely satisfactorily achieved because of the unexpected variable reactivity for neurone-specific enolase (NSE) shown by the latter variety of tumour. In order to overcome this handicap of NSE, Triche et al (1986) have examined the value of

**Table 10.6**  Specificity and sensitivity of main markers in differential diagnosis of small-round-cell tumours of childhood

| Tumour type | Markers and reactivity (%) | | |
|---|---|---|---|
| | NSE | Myoglobin | CD45 |
| Neuroblastoma | 100 | 0 | 0 |
| Rhabdomyosarcoma | <25 | 50–90 | 0 |
| Lymphoma | 0 | 0 | 80–100 |
| Ewing's sarcoma | Variable | 0 | 0 |

matrix protein markers such as laminin, Type IV collagen and stromal collagen Types I, III and V, as well as fibronectin.

Their data indicate that whilst laminin, Type IV collagen and fibronectin are expressed by both neuroblastoma and Ewing's sarcoma, the expression of Type I and III collagen is restricted to Ewing's sarcoma.

It is to be noted that rhabdomyosarcoma is also capable of expressing Types I and III collagen. However, it also expresses Type V collagen which is unique to it and not expressed by either neuroblastoma, Ewing's sarcoma or lymphoma. A diagnostic algorithm of small-round-cell tumours which takes these points into account is given in Table 10.7.

## Nephroblastoma (Wilms' tumour)

Nephroblastoma is a malignant embryonal tumour of the kidney usually consisting of three components—blastemal cells, abortive tubules, and a spindle-cell stroma. Some nephroblastomas may only contain one component (monomorphic nephroblastoma). Nephroblastoma is one of the more common organ cancers in children under the age of 10.

**Table 10.7**  Diagnostic algorithm of small-round-cell tumours of childhood based on immunocytochemical marking

| Marker status Tumour type | NSE | Stromal collagen I | III | V | Myoglobin | CD45 |
|---|---|---|---|---|---|---|
| Neuroblastoma | + | – | – | – | – | – |
| Ewing's sarcoma | + | + | + | – | – | – |
| Rhabdomyosarcoma | + | + | + | + | + | – |
| Lymphoma | – | – | – | – | – | + |

## Typical nephroblastoma

'Typical nephroblastoma' can be divided into several subtypes: the epithelial-predominant type, the blastemal-predominant type, the stromal-predominant type and the mixed type. Immunocytochemical results (Schmidt 1989) with antibodies against cytokeratin, vimentin, NF and EMA are given in Table 10.8.

Occasionally other differentiations such as striated muscle, smooth muscle, cartilage, bone, collagenous fibrous tissue and fat cells can be found in typical nephroblastomas. Muscle differentiation can be confirmed with antibodies against desmin or myoglobin.

## Congenital mesoblastic nephroma (CMN)

This is a low-grade malignant nephroblastoma with an excellent prognosis. The tumour cells are vimentin positive. Enclosed pre-existent tubules express cytokeratin.

## Fetal rhabdomyomatous nephroblastoma (FRN)

The fetal rhabdomyomatous nephroblastoma is a subtype of the stromal-predominant type of nephroblastoma. Its prognosis is worse than previously suggested. Vimentin can be found in blastemal and stromal cells.

**Table 10.8**  Immunocytochemical subtyping of nephroblastic tumours

| Tumour type | Markers | | | |
|---|---|---|---|---|
| _Epithelial-predominant type_ | VIM | KER | NF | EMA |
| Blastemal component | +/– | – | – | – |
| Tubular component | – | +* | + | +* |
| Stromal component | + | – | – | – |
| _Blastemal-predominant type_ | | | | |
| Blastemal component | + | – | – | – |
| Tubular component | – | +* | – | +* |
| Stromal component | + | – | – | – |
| _Stromal-predominant type_ | | | | |
| Stromal component | + | – | – | – |
| Blastemal component | +/– | – | – | – |
| Tubular component | – | +* | – | +* |
| _Mixed type_ | | | | |
| Blastemal component | + | + | – | – |
| Tubular component | – | +* | – | +* |
| Stromal component | + | – | – | – |

\* Only higher differentiated tubular cells.

## Cystic partially differentiated nephroblastoma (CPDN)

This is a low-grade variant of nephroblastoma which contains striated muscle cells. These are desmin positive. A diagnostic algorithm of small-round-cell tumours of childhood based on the above discussion is summarized in Table 10.7.

## IMMUNOCYTOCHEMISTRY OF OTHER TYPES OF PAEDIATRIC TUMOURS

### Nephroblastoma with focal or diffuse anaplasia

All subtypes of typical nephroblastomas may focally or diffusely contain areas with anaplasia. The occurrence of anaplasia is associated with a poor prognosis.

### Clear-cell sarcoma of the kidney

This tumour has a strong preponderance among males and occurs almost without exception within the first 2 years of life. The tumour cells are vimentin positive and cytokeratin and EMA negative.

### Malignant rhabdoid tumour of the kidney (MRTK)

This usually occurs within the first 2 years of life and has a very poor prognosis. The tumour cells are strongly positive with vimentin antibodies. Some tumour cells may express EMA. Usually no cytokeratin and desmin expression can be demonstrated. Tamm–Horsfall protein (THP) expression has also been described in these and other childhood renal tumours (Kumar et al 1987, 1988).

### Rhabdomyomatous, focally rhabdomyosarcomatous nephroblastoma

Schmidt (1989) adds this tumour as a high-grade malignant variant of nephroblastoma to other nephroblastoma classifications. Three of the four cases of his series consisted mainly of striated muscle cells. Only small areas with blastemal and/or tubular differentiation were found.

REFERENCES AND FURTHER READING

**Introduction**

Bennington J L 1986 Pathology of neoplasia in children and adolescents. W B Saunders, Philadelphia, Vol 18, ch 5–10
Darbyshire P J, Bourne S P, Allan P M, Berry J, Oakhill A, Kemshead J T, Coakham H B 1987 The use of a panel of monoclonal antibodies in pediatric oncology. Cancer 59: 726–730
Mierau G W, Berry P J, Orsini E N 1985 Small round cell neoplasms: can electron microscopy and immunohistochemical studies accurately classify them? Ultrastructural Pathology 9: 99–111

**Lymphoma**

Kjeldsberg C R, Wilson J F 1986 Malignant lymphoma in children. In: Bennington J L (ed) Pathology of neoplasia in children and adolescents. W B Saunders, Philadelphia, Vol 18, ch 5, p 87–125

**Neuroblastoma**

Shimada H, Aoyama C, Chiba T, Newton W A Jr 1985 Prognostic subgroups for undifferentiated neuroblastoma: immunohistochemical study with anti-S100 protein antibody. Human Pathology 16: 471–476
Triche T J, Askin F B, Kissane J M 1986 Neuroblastoma, Ewing's sarcoma, and the differential diagnosis of small, round, blue-cell tumours. In: Bennington J L (ed) Pathology of neoplasia in children and adolescents. W B Saunders, Philadelphia, Vol 18, ch 7, p 145–159

**Rhabdomyosarcoma**

Bale P M, Parsons R E, Stevens M M 1986 Pathology and behaviour of juvenile rhabdomyosarcoma. In: Bennington J L (ed) Pathology of neoplasia in children and adolescents. W B Saunders, Philadelphia, Vol 18, ch 8, p 196–222
Jones H, Steart P V, Du Boulay C E H, Roche W R 1990 Alpha-smooth muscle actin as a marker for soft tissue tumours: a comparison with desmin. Journal of Pathology 162: 29–33

**Ewing's sarcoma**

Triche T J, Askin F B, Kissane J M 1986 Neuroblastoma, Ewing's sarcoma, and the differential diagnosis of small, round, blue-cell tumours. In: Bennington J L (ed) Pathology of neoplasia in children and adolescents. W B Saunders, Philadelphia, Vol 18, ch 7, p 145–195

**Small-round-cell tumours—differential diagnosis**

Beckwith J B 1986 Wilms' tumour and other renal tumours of childhood. In: Finegold M (ed) Pathology of neoplasia in children and adolescents. W B Saunders, Philadelphia, p 313–332
Kumar S, Marsden H B, Jasani B, Kumar P 1987 Study of

childhood renal tumours using a monoclonal antibody to Tamm–Horsfall protein. Journal of Clinical Pathology 40: 1456–1462

Kumar S, Jakate S M, Marsden H B, Kumar P, Jasani B 1988 Tamm–Horsfall protein is a marker of renal and extra-renal rhabdoid tumours. International Journal of Cancer 41: 386–389

Mierau G W, Berry P J, Orsini E N 1985 Small round cell neoplasms: can electron microscopy and immunohistochemical studies accurately classify them? Ultrastructural Pathology 9: 99–111

Schmidt D 1989 Nephroblastomas (Wilms' tumours) and special variants. Pathologic anatomy, classification, differential diagnosis. In: Seifert G (ed) Progress in Pathology, Vol 133. Gustav Fischer Verlag, Stuttgart

Triche T J, Askin F B, Kissane J M 1986 Neuroblastoma, Ewing's sarcoma, and the differential diagnosis of small, round, blue-cell tumours. In: Bennington J L (ed) Pathology of neoplasia in children and adolescents. W B Saunders, Philadelphia, Vol 18, ch 7, p 145–195

Wick M R 1988 Antibodies to desmin on diagnostic pathology. In: Wick M R, Siegal G P (eds) Monoclonal antibodies in diagnostic immunohistochemistry. Marcel Dekker, New York, ch 4, p 98–99

# 11. Prognostic typing of tumours

## INTRODUCTION

Prognostic analysis of neoplastic diseases similar to their diagnostic typing is based on well-established criteria of histopathological techniques (see Ch. 3).

The main aim of this type of analysis is to predict the deleterious effect of the tumour on the remaining lifespan of the patient bearing it. However, it also includes the subclassification of the tumour according to its expected responsiveness to an established treatment regimen.

To achieve these aims, a histopathologist attempts to identify the tumour initially as benign or malignant. The malignant tumour is further classified according to its grade of cytological differentiation and stage of its invasion.

In the vast majority of cases, the distinction between a benign and a malignant tumour is consistently well achieved on histological grounds alone in the hands of an expert, as is the designation of a malignant tumour to a low-, intermediate- or high-grade category. However, whilst there is virtually 100% correlation between the assigned benign or malignant histological character of a tumour and its clinical behaviour, the same is not always true of malignant tumours, given different prognoses on the basis of their differing histological gradings. This lack of correlation is naturally of great concern at the individual patient level of management since there is a real danger of either under- or overtreating a tumour on the basis of prognosis made on histological grounds.

This dilemma has led to the development of more specific tests of tumour behaviour and/or treatment responsiveness based on more dependable biochemical and cell biological principles and techniques. Whilst these have genuine contribu-

tions to make towards improving the accuracy of prognostic analysis, their full potential in diagnostic histopathology is hampered by their generally complex, time-consuming and expensive character. The tests are also destructive of the biopsy material and often fail to take any account of tumour heterogeneity and contribution of non-neoplastic elements. Immunocytochemistry, with its capacity to identify biochemically and cell biologically important molecules in an intimate relation to the cells producing or responsive to them, offers a powerful yet practical and economical alternative. This has been made possible largely by the advent of the monoclonal antibody technology capable of generating suitable primary probe reagent to a complex variety of biochemicals.

Three types of monoclonal antibodies have proved useful in prognostic analysis of malignant tumours: cell lineage specific, growth regulatory protein specific, and proliferating cell specific. The most lucrative applications to date of each of these types of antibody marker are reviewed below as a way of illustrating the powerful role played by immunocytochemistry in prognostic analysis of tumours in the context of diagnostic histopathology.

## CELL LINEAGE MARKERS

The most genuine advance so far made into cell lineage-specific antibodies relates to prognostic classification of lymphoreticular tumours.

Brown et al (1989) have analysed 51 cases of high-grade non-Hodgkin's lymphomas (NHL) for which long-term follow-up (14–28 years) was already available. Using a set of five antibody reagents to T and B cell-specific and effective on formalin-fixed, paraffin-embedded tissues, 43 of these were classified to be of B cell lineage and 8 to be of the T cell phenotype. The antibodies used included L26 (CD20 cytoplasmic domain) and 4KB5 for typing the B cell lineage, and UCHL-1 (CD45RO), polyclonal CD3 and DF-TI for typing the T cell phenotype.

The background information to these antibodies is summarized in Table 11.1.

In terms of survival, it seems according to this study, that high-grade B cell NHL cases have a much better survival rate beyond 5 years than their T cell NHL counterparts. It is nevertheless emphasized that the data are not entirely definitive because of the small numbers of T cell tumours included in the study and, in spite of their relatively mild therapy, the patients included in the study were not treated uniformly according to strict protocols. It is, however, noteworthy that previous studies by Brisbane et al (1983) and Grogan et al (1985) in a collective total of 20 cases of T cell lymphomas have recorded median survival of 9–11 months.

Thus, in conclusion, it appears that T cell lymphomas do have a more aggressive clinical course than the B cell NHL necessitating accurate subtyping of every NHL using immunocytochemical markers into their T cell and B cell variants to allow for their better management.

## GROWTH REGULATORY PROTEIN MARKERS

In the past 25 years, numerous series have confirmed that breast carcinomas which contain oestrogen receptors exhibit more favourable prognosis and predictable responsiveness to antioestrogen therapy (Singhakowinta et al 1980, Rubens & Hayward 1985, Horwitz 1988). Also, those with oestrogen-rich tumours have longer disease-free

and survival-to-term periods than those lacking these receptors (Allegra et al 1979). The latter finding in particular has led to the recommendation that all patients presenting with breast cancer should have their tumour oestrogen receptor status assessed prior to therapy (De Sombre et al 1979).

Oestrogen receptor status of a breast cancer lesion is biochemically definable on the basis of the dextran-coated charcoal assay. This method, although especially helpful in defining the concentration and the affinity of oestrogen receptors, is expensive, difficult to perform and demanding of fresh biopsy material. In addition, it fails to give sufficiently accurate assessment of the likelihood of responsiveness to hormonal therapy, or the duration of the disease-free interval following the initial treatment, or the overall length of survival. This is partly because the assay is unable to take account of tumour heterogeneity with respect to oestrogen receptor distribution and the relative contribution to oestrogen receptor content made by the included non-neoplastic elements (McClelland et al 1986). Furthermore, there are other factors, including breast cancer cellularity (Parham et al 1989) and the progesterone receptor status (Pertschuk et al 1988, Foekens et al 1989), important in accurate assessment of clinical response to endocrine therapy.

Immunocytochemical assay of oestrogen receptor status has helped to overcome some of these handicaps. The applicability of this approach on a worldwide basis has been made possible recently by the introduction of a commercially developed assay, oestrogen receptor immunocytochemical assay (ERICA) by Abbott. The assay is based on one (Mab H222) of several monoclonal antibodies to oestrogen receptors developed initially by Green et al (1980). It has been shown to be more efficient than the dextran-coated charcoal assay and equal in efficiency to a novel nuclear binding assay which currently represents the best method for assessing the functional status of steroid receptors (Reiner et al 1986, Kinsel et al 1989). It is the very first commercial immunocytochemical assay sold in the form of the Abbott kit to have received the approval of the Food and Drug Administration (FDA) of the USA, for diagnostic use.

ERICA's one handicap is that it relies on fresh frozen tissue sections for its success, which makes

**Table 11.1** Lineage-specific antibody markers useful in prognostic subclassification of non-Hodgkin's lymphomas

| Antibody | Antigen and cell lineage specificity | Source/reference |
|---|---|---|
| L26 | CD20 cytoplasmic domain; B cells | Ishii et al 1984; Mason et al 1988 |
| 4KB5 | CD45R; B cells | Pulford et al 1987 |
| UCHL-1 | CD45R; T cells | Smith et al 1986 |
| DF-TI | T cells | Stross et al 1989 |
| Polyclonal anti-T3 | CD3; T cells | Mason et al 1988 |

its routine applicability somewhat cumbersome, and the results lack morphological clarity and exact correlation with formalin-fixed, paraffin-embedded tissue sections used for diagnostic and histopathological assessment of the tumour. This difficulty, as well as the need to wholly preserve true cut and small tumour specimens (< 1 cm diameter) for histological studies (Eskelinin et al 1989), has prompted several workers to adapt ERICA to routinely processed specimens. Pioneering studies by Shimada et al (1985), Pousen et al (1985) and Shintaku & Said (1987) have recorded an overall concordance rate of 82–86% with respect to the corresponding results obtained with dextran-coated charcoal and frozen section-based assays, respectively. This initial success has encouraged Jackson et al (1989) to apply a modified ERICA to the study of oestrogen receptor status in archival material with the aim of assessing the prognostic value of this novel approach (Cowen et al 1990). According to the results of this study, patients with oestrogen receptor-rich tumours showing Grade I histology and associated with a node-negative and postmenopausal status, have significantly better prognosis than those with either Grade II or III histology and node-positive and premenopausal status, or with oestrogen receptor-negative, Grade I and/or postmenopausal status. The only parameter to have an overwhelming influence on the prognosis was found to be the node-negative status which indicated a favourable prognosis even in oestrogen-negative cases. The overall findings of the study performed by Cowen et al (1990) are summarized in Table 11.2 with the aim of providing a ready-reckoner chart for working out the prognosis, given the immunocytochemical-derived oestrogen receptor status and the various histological prognostic indices.

A commercial progesterone receptor immunocytochemical assay (PgR-ICA) similar to ERICA is now available for the study of progesterone receptor status in both frozen and routine paraffin-embedded sections (Perrot-Applanat et al 1989). However, it has limited sensitivity (< 70%) and is not yet approved by the FDA for diagnostic use. In Figure 11.1 the staining due to modified ERICA and PgR-ICA in a breast carcinoma obtained in formalin-fixed, paraffin-embedded tissue sections is photomicrographically illustrated.

## MARKERS OF CELL PROLIFERATIVE ACTIVITY

The proliferative activity of a tissue or a tumour is determined by its mean growth fraction (i.e. average numbers of cells in cell cycle phases G to M) and mean cell cycle time (i.e. average time taken by a dividing cell from one mitosis to the next). (See Wright (1984) for a review.)

In general, the higher the proliferative activity of a tumour, the greater is its malignant potential and the worse is the overall survival time from the time of diagnosis (Toubiana & Courdi 1989).

Accurate measurement of the growth rate of tumours is achieved by using either tritiated thymidine (Malaise et al 1973) or bromodeoxyuridine incorporation (Dean et al 1984), or flow cytometry (Quirke & Dyson 1986). However, all these methods are complex, expensive and labour intensive and therefore not suitable for the frequent demand arising from routine diagnostic histopathology. Hence, once again immunocytochemistry has been relied upon to provide a compromise alternative which is simple, more economical and yet relatively accurate.

Histopathologists are accustomed to counting mitotic figures to provide a crude index of the proliferative potential of a malignant tumour. This, however, relates to a very narrow part of the cell cycle and is therefore subject to unacceptable

**Table 11.2**  Breast tumour ER, grade, nodal and menopausal status and prognosis

| ER status | Grade I | Grade II/III | Node – | Node + | Premenopausal | Postmenopausal |
|-----------|---------|--------------|--------|--------|---------------|----------------|
| ER+       | F       | P            | F      | P      | P             | F              |
| ER–       | P       | P            | F      | P      | P             | P              |

F = favourable prognosis; P = poor prognosis (both in terms of disease-free interval following initial treatment, and survival to term as assessed over a 5-year follow-up period (Cowen et al 1990)).

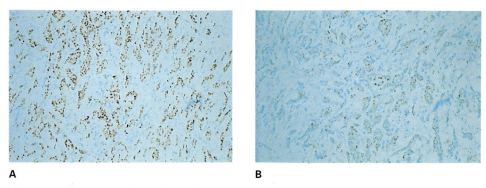

A                                                            B

**Fig. 11.1**    Illustration of the efficiency of the modified commercially available ERICA and PgR-ICA immunoperoxidase procedures in the demonstration of (**A**) oestrogen receptor (ER) and (**B**) progesterone (PR) in formalin-fixed, paraffin-embedded tissue sections taken from a breast carcinoma. (Courtesy of Dr Julia Gee, Tenovus Institute, University of Wales College of Medicine, Cardiff, Wales, UK.)

levels of error in tumours showing only a few mitotic figures.

Recently, a series of antibodies has been identified to nuclear proteins more or less specifically associated with cycling cells, which are expressed over a much wider span of the cell cycle including the late $G_1$, S, $G_S$ and M phases. So far, two such proteins have received the attention of specialist histopathologists interested in typing the proliferative activity of tumours as a means of assessing their prognosis. These include Ki-67 antigen and proliferating cell nuclear antigen (PCNA) or cyclin (Brown & Gatter 1990, Hall et al 1991).

Although the use of monoclonal antibodies to Ki-67, in combination with flow cytometry, has shown Ki-67 to be expressed in all phases of the cell cycle, except the $G_0$ phase, its distribution as elicited by immunocytochemistry is limited to its appearance in the late $G_1$ phase in the perinucleolar region rising to its peak karyoplasmic and perichromosomal expression in prophase and metaphase. Thereafter the Ki-67 immunocytochemical staining is seen to diminish rapidly during anaphase and telophase (Braun et al 1988, Guilland et al 1989) to apparently undetectable levels during most of the interphase.

Immunocytochemical identification of Ki-67 in a tumour cell population therefore allows many more cells to be taken into account for the estimate of the growth fraction based on mitotically active cells than that allowed by the mitotic figures count. Unfortunately, in solid tumours not all the cycling cells, and particularly the nutritionally de-

prived cells in and around the centre of a large tumour, obey a regular expression of Ki-67 during the late $G_1$ to M phases (Baisch & Gerdes 1987). Thus sometimes Ki-67 expression is found to persist beyond the mitotic phase well into the $G_1$ phase, and sometimes it seems to fail to appear at all in the S, $G_2$ and M phases (Verheijen et al 1989). The errors introduced by such variation in Ki-67 expression, taken together with the fact that immunocytochemical identification fails to provide any account of the mean cell cycle length, may be responsible for the failure of this marker to live up to its full promise as a superior prognostic indicator, especially in solid tumours (see the extensive data reviewed by Brown & Gatter 1990). Interestingly, in this study tumours presenting as bone marrow metastases from all varieties of non-Hodgkin's lymphomas as well as plasma cell malignancies gave the most dependable results with Ki-67 immunocytochemistry. Thus regardless of the histological type and grade of the tumour, all cases with more than 5% of Ki-67-positive tumour cells had an unfavourable clinical course (Thaler et al 1987). The only other example of superiority of Ki-67 antigen detection over that based on histologically determined mitotic index and cytological grade of the tumour was found in connection with soft-tissue sarcomas (Ueda et al 1989). The other major disadvantage of Ki-67 marker is its ineffectiveness on formalin-fixed, paraffin-embedded tissue sections. Its optimum detectability is limited to fresh frozen tissue sections fixed minimally with acetone (Ostmeiser &

Suter 1989). This particular handicap of Ki-67 had led to increasing focus on the use of PCNA as a more practical and suitable marker for use in diagnostic histopathology.

Recently a monoclonal antibody, PC10, specific to formalin fixation and paraffin-embedding-resistant epitope of PCNA, has been investigated by Hall et al (1990) on a wide variety of normal tissues and a limited range of lymphoma biopsies. Their preliminary observations confirm that the immunolocalization of this highly conserved 36 kDa acidic nuclear protein is intimately associated with the DNA synthesis phase of the cell cycle (Matthews et al 1984) and that its results are comparable to those yielded by Ki-67 immunocytochemistry. However, the PCNA expression varies from that of Ki-67 in certain types of tumours studied so far, e.g. breast and gastric carcinomas.

This seems to be due to some deregulation of PCNA synthesis in certain neoplastic cells adjacent to non-neoplastic stromal cells (Hall et al 1990).

In summary, immunocytochemical analysis of cell lineage-, growth regulatory- and proliferative activity-specific antigens in malignant tumours offers a limited but definite advantage over histological criteria applied alone for prognostic assessment of malignant conditions. Further work in this important field of inquiry is likely to extend the value of immunocytochemistry to a greater variety of tumours than that so far afforded by the limited number of follow-up studies performed with the current set of markers.

## CARCINOEMBRYONIC ANTIGEN (CEA) AS A PROGNOSTIC MARKER IN COLORECTAL CARCINOMA

### Introduction

CEA was originally described by Gold & Freedman in 1965. It was proposed as a useful prognostic marker for colorectal cancer (Minton & Martin 1978, Midiri et al 1985, Minton et al 1985). As a diagnostic marker, however, it has proved untenable because of its expression by various tumorous and non-tumorous conditions of many tissues.

### Immunocytochemical reactivity of CEA

However, different authors have reported different results in regard to the CEA content of colorectal carcinomas (Denk et al 1972, Bordes et al 1973, Wagener et al 1978, Phil et al 1980, Rognum et al 1980, 1982) and there is a well-known discrepancy between the serum CEA levels and the clinical course. Midiri et al (1985) stated that the number of immunocytochemically CEA-positive cases decreased with the grade of malignancy and tumour stage. We, however, found no CEA-negative colorectal carcinomas regardless of their differentiation grade (Schmid et al 1989). Hamada et al (1985) published an immunohistochemical grading of colorectal carcinomas by localizing the CEA in the tumour cells. They distinguished an 'apical' type from 'cytoplasmic' and 'stromal' ones and found a correlation of these types with elevated serum CEA levels.

Denk et al (1972) and Zamcheck & Kupchick (1979) found that a decrease in the immunocytochemical CEA content corresponds to the decrease in the grade of differentiation. Like other authors (Bordes et al 1973, Phil et al 1980, Wagener et al 1981), we found by measuring the immunoreactivity of CEA by a microdensitometric method (Schmid et al 1989) no unambiguous correlation between the grade of differentiation and the CEA content in colorectal carcinomas. We concluded that a low CEA immunoreactivity in the tumour and/or an increased preoperative serum CEA level may be considered as prognostically unfavourable. CEA determinations both in the serum and the tumour, however, seem to be of less clinical importance than generally assumed.

REFERENCES AND FURTHER READING

**Cell lineage markers in non-Hodgkin's lymphoma**

Brisbane J U, Berman L D, Neiman R S 1983 Peripheral T-cell lymphoma: a clinicopathologic study of nine cases. American Journal of Clinical Pathology 79: 285–293
Brown D C, Heryet A, Gatter K C, Mason D Y 1989 The prognostic significance of immunophenotype in high grade non-Hodgkin's lymphoma. Histopathology: 14: 621–627
Grogan T M, Fielder K, Rangel C, Jolley C J et al 1985 Peripheral T-cell lymphoma: aggressive disease with heterogeneous immunotypes. American Journal of Clinical Pathology 83: 279–288

Ishii Y, Takami T, Yuasa H et al 1984 Two distinct antigen systems in human B lymphocytes identification of cell surface and intracellular antigens using monoclonal antibodies. Clinical and Experimental Immunology 58: 183–192

Mason D Y, Krissansen G W, Davey F R et al 1988 Antisera against epitopes resistant to denaturation of T3 (CD3) antigen can detect reactive and neoplastic T cells in paraffin embedded tissue biopsy specimens. Journal of Clinical Pathology 41: 121–127

Pulford K A F, Falini B, Heryet A et al 1987 A new monoclonal anti-B cell antibody for routine diagnosis of lymphoid tissue biopsies. In: McMichael A et al (eds) Leucocyte typing III. Oxford University Press, Oxford, p 828

Smith S H, Brown M H, Rowe D et al 1986 Functional subsets of human helper–inducer cells defined by a new monoclonal antibody, UCHL-1. Immunology 58: 63–70

Stross W P, Warnke R A, Flavell D J et al 1989 Molecule detected in formalin fixed tissue by antibodies MT1, DF-T1 and L60 (Leu-22) corresponds to CD43 antigen. Journal of Clinical Pathology 42: 953–961

**Growth regulatory protein markers**

Allegra J C, Lippman M E, Simon R et al 1979 Association between steroid hormone receptor status and disease-free interval in breast cancer. Cancer Treatment Reports 63: 1271–1277

Cowen P N, Teasdale J, Jackson P, Reid B J 1990 Oestrogen receptor in breast cancer: prognostic studies using a new immunohistochemical assay. Histopathology 17: 319–325

De Sombre E R, Carbone P P, Jensen E V et al 1979 Special report: steroid receptors in breast cancer. New England Journal of Medicine 301: 1011–1012

Eskelinin M, Collan Y, Puttinen J, Valkamo E 1989 Frozen section diagnosis of breast cancer. Acta Oncologica 28: 183

Foekens J A, Portengen H, van Putton W L T et al 1989 Prognostic value of oestrogen and progesterone receptors measured by enzyme immunoassays in human breast cytosols. Cancer Research 49: 5823–5828

Green G L, Fitch F W, Jensen E V 1980 Monoclonal antibodies to estrophilin: probe for the study of oestrogen receptors. Proceedings of National Academy of Sciences USA 77: 157–161

Horwitz K B 1988 The central role of progesterone receptors and progestational agents in the management and treatment of breast cancer. Seminars in Oncology 15: 14–19

Jackson P, Teasdale J, Cowen P N 1989 Development and validation of a sensitive immunohistochemical oestrogen receptor assay for use on archival breast cancer tissue. Histochemistry 92: 149–152

Kinsel L B, Szabo E, Green G L et al 1989 Immunocytochemical analysis of oestrogen receptors as a predictor of prognosis in breast cancer patients: comparison with quantitative biochemical methods. Cancer Research 49: 1052–1056

McClelland R A, Berger U, Miller L S et al 1986 Immunocytochemical assay for oestrogen receptors in patients with breast cancer. Relationship to a biochemical assay and to outcome of therapy. Journal of Clinical Oncology 4: 1171–1176

Parham D M, Baker P R, Robertson A J et al 1989 Breast carcinoma cellularity and its relation to oestrogen receptor content. Journal of Clinical Pathology 42: 1166–1168

Perrot-Applanat M, Groyer-Picard M T, Vu Hai M T et al 1989 Immunocytochemical staining of progesterone receptor in paraffin sections of human breast cancers. American Journal of Pathology 135: 457–468

Pertschuk L P, Feldman J G, Eisenberg K B et al 1988 Immunocytochemical detection of progesterone receptor in breast cancer with monoclonal antibody: relation to biochemical assay, disease-free survival and clinical endocrine response. Cancer 62: 342–349

Poulsen H S, Ozzello L, King W J, Green G L 1985 The use of monoclonal antibodies to estrogen receptors (ER) for immunoperoxidase detection of ER in paraffin sections of human breast cancer tissue. Journal of Histochemistry and Cytochemistry 33: 87–92

Reiner A, Spona J, Reiner G et al 1986 Estrogen receptor analysis on biopsies and fine-needle aspirates from human breast carcinoma: correlation of biochemical and immunohistochemical methods using monoclonal anti-receptor antibodies. American Journal of Pathology 125: 443–449

Rubens R D, Hayward J L 1980 Oestrogen receptors and response to endocrine therapy and cytotoxic chemotherapy in advanced breast cancer. Cancer 46: 2922–2924

Shimada A, Kimura S, Abe K et al 1985 Immunocytochemical staining of oestrogen receptor in paraffin sections of human breast cancer by use of monoclonal antibody: comparison with that in frozen sections. Proceedings of National Academy of Sciences USA 82: 4803–4807

Shintaku I P, Said J W 1987 Detection of oestrogen receptors with monoclonal antibodies in routinely processed formalin-fixed paraffin sections of breast carcinoma. Use of DNase pretreatment to enhance sensitivity of the reaction. American Journal of Clinical Pathology 87: 161–167

Singhakowinta A, Saunders D E, Brooks S C et al 1980 Clinical application of oestrogen receptor in breast cancer. Cancer 46: 2932–2938

**Markers of cell proliferative activity**

Baisch H, Gerdes J 1987 Simultaneous staining of exponentially growing versus plateau phase cells with the proliferation-associated antibody Ki-67 and propidium iodide: analysis by flow cytometry. Cell Tissue Kinetics 20: 387–391

Braun N, Papadopoulos T, Muller-Hermelink H K 1988 Cell cycle dependent distribution of the proliferation associated Ki-67 antigen in human embryonic lung cells. Virchows Archiv. B, Cell Pathology 56: 25–33

Brown D C, Gatter K C 1990 Monoclonal antibody Ki-67: its use in histopathology. Histopathology 17: 489–503

Dean P N, Dolbeare F, Gratznerlt et al 1984 Cell-cycle analysis using a monoclonal antibody to BrdUrd. Cell Tissue Kinetics 17: 427–436

Guillaud P, du Manoir S, Seigneurin D 1989 Quantitation and topographical description of Ki-67 antibody labelling during the cell cycle of normal fibroblastic (MRC-5) and mammary tumour cell lines (MCF-7). Analytical Cellular Pathology 1: 25–39

Hall P A, Levison D A, Woods A L et al 1991 Proliferating cell nuclear antigen (PCNA) immunolocalization in paraffin sections: an index of cell proliferation with evidence of deregulated expression in some neoplasms. Journal of Pathology 162: 285–294

Malaise E P, Chavaudra N, Tubiana M 1973 The

relationship between growth rate, labelling index and histological type of human solid tumours. European Journal of Cancer 9: 305

Matthews M B, Bernstein R M, Franza B R, Garrels J I 1984 Identity of the proliferating cell nuclear antigen and cyclin. Nature 309: 374–376

Moretti S, Massobrio R, Brogelli L et al 1990 Ki-67 antigen expression correlates with tumor progression and HLA-DR antigen expression in melanocytic lesions. Journal of Investigative Dermatology 95: 320–324

Ostmeiser H, Suter L 1989 The Ki-67 antigen in primary human melanomas – its relationship to mitotic rate and tumour thickness and its stability. Archives of Dermatology Research 282: 173–177

Quirke, P, Dyson J E D 1986 Flow cytometry: methodology and applications in pathology. Journal of Pathology 149: 79

Shapiro H M 1989 Flow cytometry of DNA content and other indicators of proliferative activity. Archives of Pathological Laboratory Medicine 113: 591–597

Thaler J, Denz H, Gattringer C et al 1987 Diagnostic and prognostic value of immunohistological bone marrow examination: results in 212 patients with lymphoproliferative disorders. Blut 54: 213–222

Toubiana M, Courdi A 1989 Cell proliferation kinetics in human solid tumours: relation to probability of metastatic dissemination and long-term survival. Radiotherapy & Oncology 15: 1–18

Ueda T, Aozasa K, Tsujimoto M et al 1989 Prognostic significance of Ki-67 reactivity in soft tissue sarcomas. Cancer 63: 1607–1611

Verheijen R, Kuijpers H J H, van Driel R et al 1989 Ki-67 detects a nuclear matrix-associated proliferation-related antigen. II. Localization in mitotic cells and association with chromosomes. Journal of Cell Science 92: 531–540

Wright N A 1984 Cell proliferation in health and disease. In: Anthony P P, MacSween R N M (eds) Recent advances in histopathology. Churchill Livingstone, Edinburgh, p 12–17

**Carcinoembryonic antigen in colorectal cancer**

Bordes M, Michiels R, Martin F 1973 Detection by immunofluorescence of carcinoembryonic antigen in colonic carcinoma, other malignant or benign tumors, and non cancerous tissues. Digestion 9: 106–112

Denk H, Tappeiner G, Eckersdorfer R, Holzner J H 1972 Carcinoembryonic antigen (CEA) in gastrointestinal and extragastrointesinal tumors and its relationship to tumor differentiation. International Journal of Cancer 10: 262–272

Gold P, Freedman S O 1965 Specific carcinoembryonic antigen of the human digestive system. Journal of Experimental Medicine 121: 439–462

Hamada Y, Yamamura M, Hioki K, Yamamoto M, Nagura H, Watanabe K 1985 Immunohistochemical study of carcinoembryonic antigen in patients with colorectal cancer. Cancer 55: 136–144

Midiri G, Amanti C, Benedetti M 1985 CEA tissue staining in colorectal cancer patients. A way to improve the usefulness of serial serum CEA evaluations. Cancer 55: 2624–2629

Minton J P, Martin E W Jr 1978 The use of serial CEA determinations to predict recurrence of colon cancer and when to do a second-look operation. Cancer 42: 1422–1427

Minton J P et al 1985 Result of a 400-patient carcinoembryonic antigen second-look colorectal cancer study. Cancer 55: 1284–1290

Phil E, McNaughtan S, Ma J, Ward H A, Nairn R C 1980 Immunohistologic pattern of carcinoembryonic antigen in colorectal carcinoma. Correlation with staging and blood levels. Pathology 12: 7–13

Rognum T O, Brandtzaeg P, Orjasaeter H, Elgjo K, Hegnestad J 1980 Immunohistochemical study of secretory component, secretory IgA and carcinoembryonic antigen in large bowel carcinomas. Pathology Research and Practice 170: 126–145

Rognum T O, Thorud E, Elgjo K, Brandtzaeg P, Orjasaeter H, Nygaard K K 1982 Large bowel carcinomas with different ploidy, related to secretory component, IgA and CEA in epithelium and plasma. British Journal of Cancer 45: 921–934

Schmid K W, Puelacher C, Riedler L, Stoss F, Marth C 1989 Measuring of immunoreactivity of carcinoembryonic antigen (CEA) in colorectal cancer by microdensitometry. Pathology Research and Practice 184: 382–389

Wagener C, Czaszar H, Totović V, Breuer H 1978 A highly sensitive method for the demonstration of carcinoembryonic antigen in normal and neoplastic colonic tissue. Histochemistry 58: 1–11

Wagener C, Müller-Wallraff R, Nisson S, Groner J, Breuer H 1981 Localization and concentration of carcinoembryonic antigen (CEA) in gastrointestinal tumours: correlation with CEA levels in the plasma. Journal of the National Cancer Institute 67: 593–597

Zamcheck N, Kupchick H Z 1979 Carcinoembryonic antigen (CEA). In: Compendium of assays in immunodiagnosis of human cancer. Developments in Cancer Research 1: 27–38

# PART III

# Immunocytochemistry in diagnosis of non-neoplastic diseases

# 12. Immunologically-mediated renal disorders

## INTRODUCTION

The role of immunocytochemistry in the diagnosis of non-neoplastic conditions is principally restricted to resolving clinically and histopathologically occult or closely similar inflammatory and degenerative diseases. The most common applications are concerned with diagnostic and prognostic typing of immunologically mediated renal and skin disorders. Immunocytochemistry is also useful in resolution of the various types of amyloid depositions and certain other forms of degenerative disorders, and identification of histologically occult infections.

In the four chapters which follow, the salient contributions of immunocytochemistry in these areas of diagnostic histopathological inquiry are presented together with the relevant clinical and morphological features of the relevant disease entities.

Immunologically mediated renal diseases are divisible into two main categories according to the character of their clinical presentation:

1. Proteinuria/nephrotic syndrome which is characterized by heavy loss of protein in the urine (>2 g/d) with the resultant oedema, hypoproteinaemia and or hyperlipidaemia. It is most commonly of primary (idiopathic) type, and occasionally, especially in adults, it may be secondary to glandular dysfunction caused by systemic disease processes such as systemic lupus erythematosus (SLE), diabetes mellitus and amyloidosis.

2. Haematuria/nephritis syndrome which is characterized by haematuria, proteinuria, hypertension and renal dysfunction including sometimes oliguria. Again, this may be due to either primary renal disease or secondary to extrarenal disease processes.

## DIAGNOSTIC CRITERIA

The diagnosis in each of these situations is based on histological, immunocytochemical and ultrastructural analyses performed on renal biopsy material. In the vast majority of cases the most important diagnostic features are found associated with the glomerulus apparatus (see Fig. 12.1) including the walls of the efferent and afferent arterioles, the capillary loops and the subendothelial space, the mesangium, and the epithelial cells forming the parietal and visceral membranes of the Bowman's capsule.

The extraglomerular lesions relate mainly to the tubular epithelial cells and basement membrane and the intima of the small and larger renal arteries.

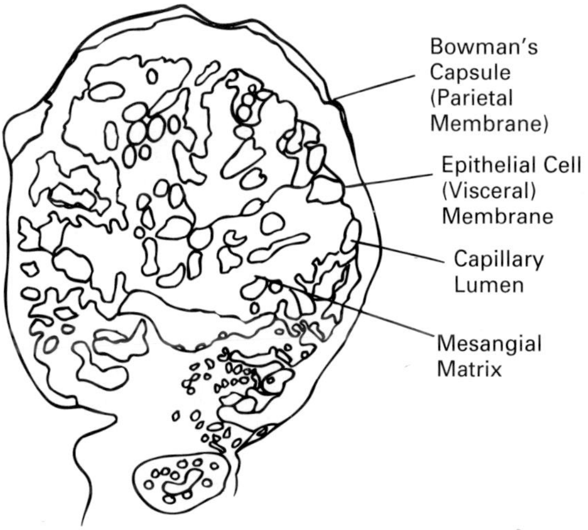

PROXIMAL TUBULAR POLE

Bowman's
Capsule
(Parietal
Membrane)

Epithelial Cell
(Visceral)
Membrane

Capillary
Lumen

Mesangial
Matrix

VASCULAR/DISTAL TUBULAR HILUM

**Fig. 12.1** Schematic representation of glomerular apparatus as seen in a tissue section.

The changes within the glomerulus are described as segmental or global according to whether a part or whole of the glomerulus is affected, respectively. They are also described as focal or diffuse depending on the proportion of glomeruli visibly affected by the disorder. Finally, the actual pattern of distribution of the immunocytochemically definable elements deposited within the glomerulus is described as either globular, finely or coarsely granular, or smooth and linear. These are also described according to their location within the glomerulus such as glomerular basement membrane (GBM), subendothelial, mesangial, subepithelial, crescentic (within the Bowman's capsule), and/or intraluminal.

## IMMUNOCYTOCHEMISTRY

The immunocytochemically definable elements relevant to diagnostic and prognostic analysis of non-neoplastic renal disorders include immunoglobulins typed according to their light chain isotypes and heavy chain classes, complement components, MHC Class II, T lymphocyte surface antigens, fibrin, albumin, and certain amyloid-specific antigens. These are listed in Table 12.1 in terms of the target antigen localized and the broad categories of disorders for which they are most frequently used as markers of the underlying disease process. A more detailed summary of their use is given in Table 12.2 in relation to the individual clinicomorphological category of renal disorder and according to their main diagnostic and/or prognostic significance in typing these disorders. The use of ultrastructural analysis based on conventional transmission electron microscopy as an adjunct to immunocytochemical analysis is also highlighted wherever appropriate. The collective value of these techniques in the diagnosis of immunological renal disorders is illustrated photomicrographically in Figure 12.2.

## Techniques in renal biopsy analysis

Direct immunofluorescence remains the technique of choice for analysing renal disorders. This is mainly because of its long-established use in this field. More recently, however, the indirect immunoperoxidase method has been cited by several authorities to be both reliable and capable of giving high-resolution results.

The analysis also continues to be conducted along the traditional lines with respect to its reliance upon separate segments of the renal biopsy for conventional histopathology on formalin-fixed, paraffin-embedded tissue, immunocytochemistry on frozen tissue sections and electron microscopy on plastic-embedded material. These analyses are often performed in three separate units requiring the services of a specialist renal histopathologist and expert medical laboratory staff trained in the use of the immunofluorescence technique and conventional ultrastructural analysis and the use of a transmission electron microscope.

Attempts are being made to rationalize and streamline the analysis through the use of tissue fixed, processed and embedded using a single technique which is routinely applicable and capable of producing high-quality histopathological, immunocytochemical and ultrastructural information. The use of the LR White resin by Newman and colleagues, and Lowicryl by Davies and co-workers, represents the best achievements so far towards establishing a unified and simplified approach. Nevertheless, diagnostic typing and prognostic classification of immunologically mediated renal disorders is likely to remain the remit of specialist centres.

**Table 12.1** Immunocytochemical markers of immunologically mediated renal disorders

| Marker | Diagnostic/prognostic use |
| --- | --- |
| Kappa (κ), lambda (λ) light chains | Amyloidosis; mixed cryoglobulinaemia |
| IgG, IgA, IgM heavy chains | Variety of glomerulonephritis, tubulointestinal nephritis and vasculitides |
| Complement components, C3 and C1q | Variety of glomerulonephritis, tubulointestinal nephritis and vasculitides |
| Albumin and fibrin | Non-specific markers of gross glomerular injury, e.g. crescentic glomerulonephritis |
| MHC Class II and T lymphocyte surface antigens | Renal allograft rejection; graft-versus-host disease |

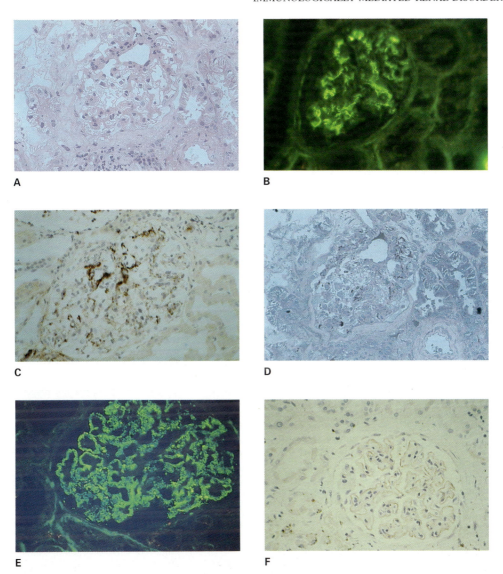

**Fig. 12.2** Illustration of the collective value of conventional histology, immunocytochemistry and immunolabelling under transmission electron microscopy in diagnosis of immunological renal disorders. (**A**) Histological (H&E) appearances of IgA nephropathy. (**B**) and (**C**) Immunofluorescence and immunoperoxidase staining reactions of IgA deposits in the expanded mesangium as in frozen and formalin-fixed, paraffin-embedded renal biopsy sections, respectively. (**D**) Immunocolloidal gold–silver staining (IGSS) of the IgA deposits in an LR White resin semithin (350 nm) section (H&E counterstain). (**E**) and (**F**) Immunofluorescence and immunoperoxidase staining of IgG in membranous glomerulonephritis using sections taken from frozen and formalin-fixed, paraffin-embedded renal biopsy material, respectively. (Courtesy of Dr David Griffiths, Department of Pathology and Dr G. R. Newman, EM Unit, University of Wales College of Medicine, Cardiff, Wales, UK.)

**Table 12.2**    Immunocytochemical features and their diagnostic/prognostic significance in immunologically mediated renal disorders

| Disorder/clinicomorphological entity (incidence) | Main immunocytochemical findings | Diagnostic/prognostic significance |
|---|---|---|
| 1. Primary nephrotic syndrome | | |
| a. Mesangio-proliferative glomerulonephritis/mesangial sclerosis (15% older children; 10% adults) | Diffuse, relatively global immunoglobulin and complement granular deposits in the mesangium dominated by: | |
| | i.  IgM, C3 (75% cases) | IgM disease; differential diagnosis subacute infective endocarditis or malarial nephropathy; small electron-dense mesangial deposits in 50% of cases |
| | ii. CIq with minor amounts of IgG, IgM and C3 | CIq nephropathy; quite prominent electron-dense deposits in the mesangium |
| | iii. IgA, C3 | Berger's IgA disease; deposits in glomerular basement membrane indicative of worse prognosis; differential diagnosis cirrhosis, Henoch–Schönlein syndrome, or systemic lupus erythematosus |
| b. Membranous glomerulonephritis (80% adults; < 10% children) | Diffuse, global, granular immunoglobulin and complement deposits in glomerular basement membrane almost exclusively composed of IgG, C3 | Differential diagnosis mesangio-capillary glomerulonephritis Type III, systemic lupus erythematosus, systemic neoplastic disease or infection if multiple Ig classes found; lack of deposits indicative of advanced disease requiring confirmation by electron microscopy |
| c. Mesangio-capillary glomerulonephritis Type I (10% children; 15% adults) | Diffuse, global, granular deposits of immunoglobulin to complement in glomerular basement membrane dominated by: IgG, C3, CIq located mainly in mesangial and subendothelial space | Localization by electron microscopy of the mesangial and subendothelial deposits needed to confirm the diagnosis; clinical features similar to mixed cryoglobulinaemia but distinguished by the latter's globular, monotypic IgM clumps within glomerular capillary lumen |
| Type II (1% children and adults) | Mainly C3 distributed in coarse granules | Presence of multiple Ig subclasses implies systemic lupus erythematosus, lack of deposits indicates advanced disease |
| Type III | IgG, C3 in subepithelial space | Needs confirmation by precise identification of the deposits by electron microscopy |
| d. Focal segmental glomerulosclerosis | Focal, segmental sclerotic glomerular lesions near the hilum with irregular globular deposits of IgM, C3 and C1q | Pattern of sclerosis is pathognomonic; also otherwise similar lesions also seen in several types of immunological and non-immunological renal disorders |
| e. Minimal-change nephropathy (90% children; 15–20% adults) | Very slight mesangial or hilar IgM, C3 staining; heavy proteinuria indicated by staining of albumin in proximal tubules | Needs confirmation by electron microscopy which shows mainly effacement of visceral epithelial cell foot processes; generally good prognosis |
| 2. Secondary nephrotic syndrome | | |
| a. Diabetic glomerulosclerosis (most common type) | Diffuse, linear staining of glomerular basement membrane (GBM), Bowman's capsule and tubular basement membrane (TBM) for IgG, kappa and lambda light chains | Differential diagnosis relates to linear anti-GBM staining seen in anti-GBM glomerulonephritis and light chain nephropathy |
| b. Amyloidosis | Staining of amyloid with anti-light chain, antiamyloid substance A or P | Ultrastructural confirmation of amyloid pathognomonic; use of anti-immunoglobulin and complement to differentiate from light chain nephropathy; diabetic glomerulosclerosis |

**Table 12.2** (*cont.*)

| Disorder/clinicomorphological entity (incidence) | Main immunocytochemical findings | Diagnostic/prognostic significance |
|---|---|---|
| c. Light chain nephropathy (50% cases with multiple myeloma) | Pathognomonic linear monotypic kappa or lambda immunostaining of glomerular and tubular basement membranes, and Bowman's capsule | Morphologically similar to diabetic glomerulosclerosis especially kappa light chain glomerulosclerosis |
| **3. Haematuria/nephritis syndrome** | | |
| a. Infective mainly poststreptococcal pharyngitis (group A β-haemolytic) infection | Global, coarsely granular mesangial and capillary wall staining with anti-C3 | Intense IgG staining indicative of the very early course of the disease: numerous variably sized subepithelial, subendothelial and mesangial electron-dense deposits typical of the disease-associated lesion |
| b. Systemic lupus erythematosus (SLE) | Focal/diffuse intense staining with anti-C1q with variable amounts of IgG, IgM, IgA immunostaining | Picture virtually identical to membranous glomerulonephritis associated with primary nephrotic syndrome but SLE shows much greater frequency and intensity of C1q immunostaining |
| c. IgA nephropathy | Diffuse, global mesangial deposits intensely staining with anti-IgA and anti-C3; minor amounts of IgG and IgM immunostaining | Henoch–Schönlein syndrome may present with indistinguishable clinicopathological features (see below); lack of CIq immunostaining helpful in distinction from SLE-associated nephritis |
| d. Anti-GBM nephritis (30% cases associated with Goodpasture's syndrome) | Diffuse, global linear staining of glomerular basement membrane (GBM) with anti-immunoglobulin reagents; IgG-dominant immunoglobulin type; 50% cases also show linear tubular basement membrane immunostaining for IgG | Demonstration of anti-basement membrane autoantibodies in pulmonary tissue biopsies confirms diagnosis of Goodpasture's syndrome |
| e. Vasculitic nephritis (main examples: Henoch–Schönlein purpura, Wegener's arteritis, polyarteritis nodosa) | Crescentic hypercellularity and fibrin deposition in Bowman's capsule associated with a general lack of immunoglobulin to complement immunostaining | Detection of antineutrophil cytoplasmic autoantibodies (ANCA) in circulation helpful towards diagnosis of Wegener's arteritis and polyarteritis nodosa |
| f. Mixed cryoglobulinaemia | Globular monotypic IgM-positive clumps in glomerular lumen | Clinicopathological features similar to Type I membrano-proliferative glomerulonephritis |
| g. Crescentic glomerulonephritis (a non-specific indicator of gross glomerular injury) | Antifibrin-positive deposits in Bowman's space; pattern of glomerular immunoglobulin and complement immunostaining according to the underlying cause of glomerular injury | Most commonly (over 90% cases) found in anti-GBM glomerulonephritis as well as vasculitic nephritis |
| **4. Extraglomerular renal disorder** | | |
| a. Ischaemic arteriosclerosis | C3 and to a lesser extent IgM immunostaining in sclerotic renal vessel walls | Lack of glomerular immune deposits confirms the diagnosis |
| b. Intravascular coagulation | Fibrinogen, IgM and complement immunostaining of capillary subendothelial space and arteriolar walls and arterial intima | Scattered intravascular luminal and fibrin-positive microthrombi confirms the diagnosis |
| c. Tubulointestinal inflammation (main example: renal graft rejection) | Ectopic expression of MHC Class II antigens on renal allograft parenchymal cells; pan T cell marker positive mononuclear cell infiltrate with increased ratio of CD8:CD4 positive cells | Expression of MHC Class II antigens in face of immunosuppressive treatment indicative of early signs of allograft rejection or graft-versus-host disease; lowered CD4:CD8 ratio also observed in progressive form of membranous glomerulonephritis |

REFERENCES AND FURTHER READING

**Introduction**

Morel-Maroger L 1982 The value of renal biopsy. American Journal of Kidney Diseases 1: 244–248

Turner M W, Hutchinson T A, Barre P E et al 1986 A prospective study on the impact of the renal biopsy in clinical management. Clinical Nephrology 26: 217–221

**Immunoperoxidase method**

Elias J M, Miller F 1975 A comparison of the unlabeled enzyme method with immunofluorescence for the evaluation of human immunologic renal disease. American Journal of Clinical Pathology 64: 464–471

MacIver A G, Mephram B L 1982 Immunoperoxidase techniques in human renal biopsy. Histopathology 6: 249–267

Sinclair R A, Burns J, Dunhill M S 1980 Immunoperoxidase staining of formalin-fixed, paraffin-embedded, human renal biopsies with a comparison of the peroxidase–anti-peroxidase (PAP) and indirect methods. Journal of Clinical Pathology 34: 859–865

Turner D R, Wilson D M, Lake A et al 1979 An evaluation of immunoperoxidase technique in renal biopsy diagnosis. Clinical Nephrology 11: 13–17

**Immunofluorescence method**

Fligiel S, Hannah J B, Cheng L et al 1983 Direct immunofluorescence of renal biopsy specimens using a liquid fixative: comparison with a rapid freezing method. American Journal of Clinical Pathology 79: 108–111

Habib R, Levy M 1979 Contribution of immuno-fluorescence microscopy to classification of glomerular diseases. In: Kincaid-Smith P (ed) Progress in glomerulonephritis. Wiley Medical Publications, New York, p 119–144

**Plastic embedding of renal biopsies**

Al-Nawab M D, Davies D R 1989 Light and electron microscopic demonstration of extra-cellular immunoglobulin deposition in renal tissue. Journal of Clinical Pathology 42: 1104–1108

Bowdler A L, Griffiths D F R, Newman G R 1989 The morphological and immunohistochemical analysis of renal biopsies by light and electron microscopy using a single processing method. Histochemical Journal 21: 393–402

# 13. Immunologically-mediated skin disorders

## INTRODUCTION

The term immunological skin disorders collectively refers to multiple lesions in the skin and/or mucous membranes which are consistently associated with immune complex depositions in the epidermal or dermal regions. The potential immunological targets in the skin are schematically represented in Figure 13.1.

The immune complex deposits consist of immunoglobulins and/or complement components, and their pattern of distribution and composition is considered to be more or less disease specific when taken in conjunction with other clinicopathological information. Immunocytochemistry plays an important role in determining the pattern of distribution and the composition of immune complex deposition.

The object of this chapter is to describe briefly the methods and reagents which are most commonly used in immunocytochemical analysis of immunological skin disorders, and provide a summary of the salient findings relating to individual skin disorders which are helpful in making the overall diagnosis.

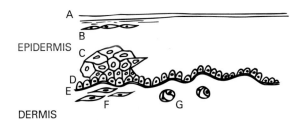

**Fig 13.1** Schematic representation of potential immunological targets in the skin. A = keratin layer; B = granular cell layer; C = keratinocyte layer; D = basal cell layer; E = basement membrane zone; F = dermal fibroblast/collagen matrix; G = dermal small vessels.

## IMMUNOCYTOCHEMICAL METHODS: REAGENTS

Two types of immunocytochemical methods are used in the analysis of immunological skin disorders: direct immunofluorescence and indirect immunofluorescence. Both these methods make use of freshly frozen tissue sections.

Direct immunofluorescence involves the use of commercially available and standardized fluorescein-labelled antihuman IgG-, IgM-, IgA- and/or complement (mainly C3)-specific conjugates. These are used to identify the in vivo pattern and the composition of immune deposition. For analysis of immune complex deposition relating to the basement membrane zone (BMZ) defining the epidermal–dermal junction, the frozen sections are taken from skin biopsies pretreated with 1.0 M sodium chloride solution for 72 to 96 h at 4°C. This has the effect of separating the epidermis from the dermis through the lamina lucida. Frozen sections taken from such biopsy material allow one to determine more precisely whether the immune deposition is epidermally or dermally oriented.

The indirect immunofluorescence method is used for detecting circulating antiskin tissue-specific autoantibodies. For this, frozen sections taken from normal human or guinea pig skin biopsies, of both the salt pretreated and non-pretreated varieties, are most commonly used. The patient's serum, diluted in a series of doubling dilutions, is first incubated with a series of such sections. The sections are then washed with buffer medium to remove excess unbound serum components and incubated individually with either fluorescein-labelled anti-IgG, –IgM, –IgA or –complement component conjugates to reveal

**Table 13.1**   Diagnostically important immunocytochemical features of predominantly epidermal skin disorders

| Disorder (predilection/relative incidence) | Immunocytochemical findings | |
| --- | --- | --- |
| | Direct immunofluorescence | Indirect immunofluorescence |
| **1. Primary vesiculobullous** | | |
| i.  Bullous pemphigoid (50+ years old/ common) | Continuous linear deposits of IgG (80–90% cases) and C3 (90–95% cases) at the BMZ with epidermal orientation in lesional and perilesional skin and mucous membranes; IgA and/or IgM found in 25% of cases | Low- to very high-titre anti-BMZ antibodies exclusively of IgG class (70% cases) with epidermal orientation; differential diagnosis— herpes gestationis and cicatricial pemphigoid |
| ii.  Cicatricial pemphigoid | Disrupted IgG/C3 deposits prominently located within healed scars in mucous membrane lesions | Low-titre anti-BMZ IgG class autoantibodies found in fewer than 20% cases with epidermal orientation; differential diagnosis—bullous pemphigoid and herpes gestationis |
| iii.  Herpes gestationis (pregnant and postpartum women/uncommon) | Continuous, linear deposits restricted to lesional skin with C3 (100% cases) and IgG (50% cases) as the main components | Low-titre (1/20 to 1/40) IgG anti-BMZ autoantibodies in small proportion of cases, with epidermal orientation of binding; indirect C3 binding demonstrable in 50% of cases, with epidermal orientation; differential diagnosis—bullous and cicatricial pemphigoid |
| iv.  Linear IgA bullous disease | Continuous IgA deposits at the BMZ with epidermal and/or dermal orientation in lesional and perilesional skin | Low- to high-titre (1/20 to 1/40) IgA anti-BMZ autoantibodies (50% cases) mainly with epidermal orientation binding; differential diagnosis—bullous and cicatricial pemphigoid and herpes gestationis |
| v.  Pemphigus bullous disease Pemphigus vulgaris (most common variety) Pemphigus vegetans (rare) Pemphigus foliaceous (uncommon) Pemphigus erythemadoides: (uncommon) | Continuous perikeratinocyte predominantly IgG-bearing immune deposits in lesional and perilesional skin, with C3 deposition restricted to lesional skin | High titres of exclusively IgG autoantibodies (>80% cases) giving keratinocyte surface staining throughout the epidermis; differential diagnosis—Darier's disease and bullous impetigo |
| vi.  Dermatitis herpetiformis (mainly in 20- to 30-year-olds with B8 and DR3 HLA phenotype) | Disrupted, granular or fibrillar IgA deposits best seen in perilesional skin over the tip and along the sides of dermal papillae; C3 in 50% of cases | Antiskin autoantibodies absent; differential diagnosis—systemic lupus erythematosus (SLE) with IgA predominance in immune complex deposits |
| **2. Secondary vesiculobullous** | | |
| i.  Epidermolysis bullosa aquisita, EBA (minor trauma related in adults/uncommon) | Continuous linear band of IgG/C3 deposition at the BMZ in trauma-susceptible extensor perilesional skin with dermal orientation; less intense IgA/IgM deposits in lesional skin in 25% of cases | Low to high titres of IgG anti-BMZ autoantibodies in 20–80% of cases with dermal orientation of binding; differential diagnosis—bullous and cicatricial pemphigoid |
| Bullous eruption of systemic lupus erythematosus (BESLE) (secondary to SLE/rare) | Continuous linear granular or fibrillar IgG + IgA/IgM and C3 deposits at the BMZ with dermal orientation in lesional and perilesional sun-exposed skin | Low-titre IgG/IgA/IgM anti-BMZ autoantibodies with dermal orientation of binding; differential diagnosis—SLE with coexisting pemphigoid |
| Cutaneous porphyrias (secondary to acquired or hereditary forms of porphyrin metabolic defects/rare) | Continuous linear IgG granular deposits at the BMZ in lesional and perilesional sun-exposed skin; diffuse blood vessel wall IgG + IgM/IgA and C3 deposition is relatively specific for porphyria-induced skin lesions | Antiskin autoantibodies absent; differential diagnosis—vesiculobullous diseases with linear IgG deposits at the BMZ |

the pattern and composition of the autoantibody binding.

The results of the direct and indirect immuno-fluorescence techniques are correlated with the relevant clinical and histological information to arrive at the appropriate diagnosis as described next. Detailed descriptions of the clinicopathological and immunocytochemical features of immunological skin disorders have been provided recently by Gammon (1989). For an appreciation of the immune mechanisms involved in cutaneous diseases the reader is referred to the excellent text edited by Norris (1989).

## DIAGNOSTICALLY IMPORTANT IMMUNOCYTOCHEMICAL FEATURES

Clinicopathologically distinct immunological skin disorders fall into two major categories, depending on whether the main target of immune deposition is the epidermis or the dermis.

The epidermal and dermal skin disorders are in turn divisible into the primary and the secondary types. The primary variety relates to disorders in which the skin is the main site of both the disease and immune deposition, while the secondary variety relates to disorders arising subsequent to the development of certain systemic diseases and in which the skin is usually only one of several sites of immune complex deposition in the body.

The pattern of distribution and composition of the immune deposition are often characteristic of the underlying disease and are described according to the following features.

### Distribution patterns of immune complex deposition

The pattern is described according to the main site of the immune complex deposition, e.g. the epidermis, the BMZ or the dermis. Within each of these sites the distribution of the staining is described as for example, perikeratinocyte, BMZ with epidermal or dermal orientation, upper, mid or lower or papillary dermis. Within the dermis the distribution is further emphasized according to the character of any blood vessel involvement.

The distribution of the staining is also described

Table 13.2   Diagnostically important immunocytochemical features of predominantly dermal skin disorders

| Disorder (predilection/relative incidence) | Direct immunofluorescence | Indirect immunofluorescence |
|---|---|---|
| 1. Mixed connective tissue disorders a. Systemic lupus erythematosus SLE (common in young black women) | Continuous band-like globular granular or stippled IgG/IgM + C3 deposits in the upper dermis just below the BMZ in lesional and perilesional skin; deposits of IgG/IgM + C3 also in dermal vessel walls; additional speckled keratinocyte nuclear staining with anti-IgG or – IgM fluorescein conjugate characteristic of mixed connective tissue disorders | Antiskin autoantibodies absent |
| b. Lupus-like skin lesions (e.g. seen occasionally in leprosy, rheumatoid arthritis, dermatomyositis, drug reactions, etc.) | Disrupted band-like IgM alone deposits in the upper dermis restricted to lesional skin | Antiskin autoantibodies absent |
| 2. Necrotizing venulitis a. Skin-oriented disease (e.g. Henoch–Schönlein purpura, urticarial vasculitis, etc.) | IgG, IgA, IgM and/or IgE +C3 deposits predominantly in the walls of postcapillary venules of mid- and upper-dermis in lesional (70–80% cases) and perilesional (< 50% cases) skin | Antiskin autoantibodies absent |
| b. Systemic disease with skin involvement (e.g. Wegener's granulomatosus, polyarteritis nodosa, etc.) | Same as above but with additional involvement of arterioles and other other vessel walls throughout the dermis | Antiskin autoantibodies absent, but presence of antineutrophil cytoplasmic antigen autoantibodies of diagnostic and prognostic significance |

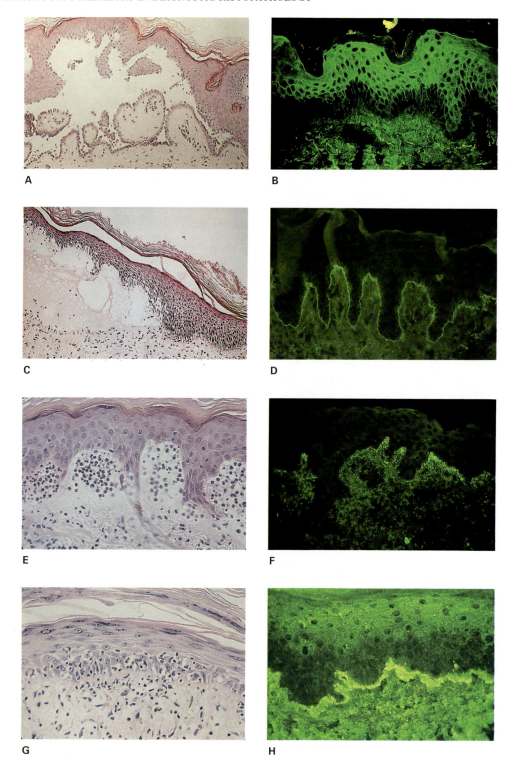

**Fig. 13.2**  Illustration of the correlation of conventional histological appearances and immunofluorescence staining patterns pertaining to various immunological skin disorders: (**A**) and (**B**) H&E and IgG immunofluorescence appearances of pemphigus vulgaris respectively—note the continuous perikeratinocyte-immune deposition; (**C**) and (**D**) results of similar studies in bulbous pemphigoid—note the continuous linear deposition of immune complexes; (**E**) and (**F**) H&E and IgG immunofluorescence patterns in dermatitis herpetiformis—note the disrupted, granular/fibrillar immune deposition; (**G**) and (**H**) H&E and IgG immunofluorescence appearances associated with systemic lupus erythematosus (SLE)—note the continuous band-like granular deposit in the upper dermis just below the basement membrane zone (BMZ). (Courtesy of Dr Arthur Knight, Department of Dermatology, University of Wales College of Medicine, Cardiff, Wales, UK.)

according to the relative degree of lesional and perilesional skin and/or mucous membrane involvement, and whether it is continuous, disrupted, granular or smooth.

## Composition of immune depositions

The composition of immune complex deposition, as well as that of any associated circulating anti-skin autoantibodies, is usually also characteristic of the underlying disease. Thus some skin disorders are dominated solely by IgG or IgM or IgA immunoglobulin class-bearing deposition, whilst others show a mixture of immunoglobulin classes within the immune deposits. The presence or absence of various complement components, particularly C3, is taken as an additional confirmatory feature of the disease.

The immunocytochemical features typical of the epidermal and the dermal varieties of immunological skin disorders are summarized in Tables 13.1 and 13.2, respectively, together with their respective predilection and relative incidence. In Figure 13.2 the correlation between conventional histological appearances and immunofluorescence staining patterns of several immunological skin disorders are illustrated photomicrographically.

REFERENCES AND FURTHER READING

Gammon W R 1989 Immunohistology of cutaneous disease. In: Jennette J C (ed) Immunohistology in diagnostic pathology. CRC Press, p 86–117
Jordon R E, Seu S 1989 Humoral immunopathological mechanisms in the skin. In: Norris D A (ed) Immune mechanisms of cutaneous disease. Marcel Dekker, New York
Norris D A 1989 Immune mechanisms in cutaneous disease. In: Norris D A (ed) Immune mechanisms of cutaneous disease. Marcel Dekker, New York

# 14. Amyloid and other degenerative disorders

## INTRODUCTION

A cell's metabolism is seen biochemically as an algebraic sum of numerous catabolic and anabolic processes continuously in progress to maintain the internal milieu of the cell at a steady state against changes imposed by its microenvironment. These events are finely balanced such that any disturbance in metabolism due to injury is likely to produce a biochemically registerable deleterious effect on the cellular integrity. If persistent, the injury may lead further to development of a morphologically demonstrable lesion.

The biochemical/morphological lesions resulting from a persistent form of imbalance in metabolic activity are usually due to some sublethal form of injury. Such injuries may be associated with either acquired or inheritable defects in metabolism. The associated lesion(s) may be localized or systemically distributed. Furthermore, they may result in a lesser or greater degree of circumscribed cell death. The overall process of development of such lesions is referred to as cell or tissue degeneration with or without necrosis.

There are many varieties of cell degeneration/necrosis depending on the specific subcomponent or type of the metabolism affected by the injury. The importance of such lesions with respect to histopathology lies in the fact that most of them are only readily diagnosable on histological grounds. The histopathologist is therefore in a unique position to recognize the various types of cell degeneration/necrosis according to certain characteristic morphological changes associated with them (see Table 14.1).

It also becomes possible, with limited success, to identify possible causes, predisposing factors or disease associations of the injury and to assess from these the appropriate treatment and the overall disease outcome.

Morphological features associated with a diverse variety of cell degeneration/necrosis, however, do overlap or resemble each other, making it somewhat difficult for the histopathologist to diagnose a given type of metabolic defect with accuracy. Special histological stains and immunocytochemical markers are therefore commonly employed as aids to diagnosis and prognostic analysis of such disorders.

The aim of this chapter is to describe metabolic disorders for which immunocytochemical markers have exhibited either a proven or potential usefulness.

Disorders belonging to the proven category include:

1. Various forms of amyloidosis
2. Alpha-l-antitrypsin deficiency state

whilst those belonging to the potential category include:

1. Copper accumulation states
2. Early myocardial infarction.

## IMMUNOCYTOCHEMICAL MARKERS HELPFUL IN THE DIAGNOSIS OF AMYLOIDOSES

Amyloidosis represents a heterogeneous group of what are primarily degenerative disorders characterized by extracellular deposits of amyloid fibrils defined by their unique blend of tinctorial, optical, ultrastructural and X-ray diffraction pattern properties. Thus:

1. When exposed to the Congo red dye they have a tendency to produce apple-green birefring-

147

ence under polarized light or red fluorescence under green light.

2. Ultrastructurally they consist of randomly oriented aggregates of approximately 10 mm diameter linear non-branching type fibrils with electron-lucent cores.

3. They give cross-$\beta$ pattern on X-ray diffraction.

The unique tinctorial property seems to be associated with a high representation in them of the $\beta$-pleated sheet form of secondary protein structural elements and glycosaminoglycans of the heparin or the heparin sulphate variety. The name amyloid was given by Virchow in 1855 because the fibrillary material behaved like cellulose in an iodine–sulphuric acid test.

Despite these universally shared properties,

amyloid fibrils associated with different diseases have different protein compositions. They seem to reflect either a primary defect in the metabolism of cells around which these fibrils are found deposited or some systemically circulating qualitatively or quantitatively abnormal variety of protein capable of producing such deposits in any part of the body. The identification of the amyloid-associated abnormal protein component has been found to be of value in determining the cause of the amyloid deposition and its more proper management as discussed briefly below.

Not all amyloid-associated abnormal protein components have been worked out in terms of the molecular identities as related to their individual disease associations. But where the appropriate knowledge does exist, immunocytochemistry promises to be more effective than the histological

**Table 14.1**  Amyloidoses with known clinical and abnormal fibrillary protein associations

| Distribution | Clinical association | Fibrillary protein |
| --- | --- | --- |
| Systemic | Plasma cell dyscrasia (e.g. myelomas and monoclonal gammopathies leading to systemic and local amyloid deposition) | AL fibrils from monoclonal immunoglobulin light chains mainly of the lambda variety |
| | Chronic active disease (inflammatory/infectious) (including rheumatoid arthritis) | AA fibrils derived from serum amyloid A protein (SAA) |
| | Hereditary syndromes | |
| i. | Types I and II predominantly neuropathic variety | Genetic variants of prealbumin (e.g. Met 30; Gly 49/Ile 33; Ser 84) |
| ii. | Predominantly nephropathic variety of the familial Mediterranean fever type Typical amyloidosis A | AA fibrils derived from serum amyloid A (SAA) |
| iii. | Predominantly cardiomyopathic variety of the Appalachian type | Prealbumin fibrils of the Ala 60 genetic variant |
| iv. | Cerebral haemorrhage-associated amyloidosis | Cystatin C fibrils comprising Glu 58 genetic variant |
| | Senile systemic amyloidosis | Prealbumin AScl fibrils derived from serum prealbumin |
| | Chronic haemodialysis-associated systemic and local variants | $\beta_2$-microglobulin derived from its raised serum levels ASC1 related to prealbumin; |
| Localized | Senile amyloidosis of the heart; atrial amyloidosis | ASC2 related to atrial natriuretic peptide-related fibrils, respectively |
| | Cerebral amyloidosis comprising amyloid angiopathy and intracortical plaques associated with Alzheimer's disease, senile dementia and Down's syndrome | B-protein (4.2 kDa) fibrils derived from a precursor protein encoded by Ch 21; most probably structurally derived from the paired helical proteins, e.g. 'tau' and 'ubiquitin' |
| | Endocrine amyloidosis | Precalcitonin-related fibrils in medullary carcinoma of thyroid; islet amyloid polypeptide fibrils in pancreatic endocrine neoplasia and maturity onset diabetes |
| | Prions mediated transmissible encephalopathies; Creutzfeldt–Jakob disease; kuru; Gerstmann–Straussler syndrome | Protease-resistant protein, P&P, e.g. sialoglycoprotein P&P 27–30 (isolated from scrapie sheep) |

dye method at unravelling their presence, their identity and their prognostic significance. Table 14.1 lists the systemic and localized varieties of amyloidoses in which the molecular identity of the abnormal fibrillary protein component(s) is well worked out. Systemic amyloidosis is divisible into the primary and the secondary varieties which differ in terms of their respective prognostic significance and approach to their therapeutic management, making it important to differentiate them from each other with accuracy. Figure 14.1 is included to illustrate photomicrographically the collective value of conventional histological and light and electron microscopic immunolabelling techniques in the diagnosis of renal amyloidosis using semithin and ultrathin formalin-fixed, LR White-embedded tissue sections.

## USEFULNESS OF IMMUNOCYTOCHEMICAL MARKERS IN RELATION TO TINCTORIAL STAINING OF AMYLOID SUBSTANCE

The Congo red birefringence, although pathognomonic of amyloid desposition, has several drawbacks. Thus:

1. Birefringence is seen only when the polarizer and analyser are accurately crossed and when the section thickness is 5–10 µm; optimal demonstration requires a polarization microscope equipped with strain-free objectives, well-aligned high-quality Nicol prisms or Polaroid polarizing filters and a 100-watt quartz halide light source.

2. Though a sensitive detector of amyloid, it

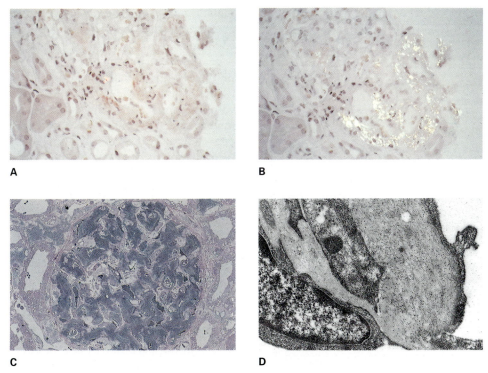

**Fig. 14.1** Illustration of the collective value of conventional histological and light and electron microscopic immunolabelling techniques in the diagnosis of renal amyloidosis: (**A**) Congo red staining (semithin section); (**B**) Congo red lemon-green birefringence under polarized light (semithin section); (**C**) and (**D**) antiserum amyloid protein (SAP) immunoperoxidase and immunocolloidal gold staining of semithin and ultrathin sections, respectively (formalin-fixed, LR White resin-embedded renal biopsy sections. (Courtesy of Dr G. R. Newman, Director of EM Unit, University of Wales College of Medicine, Cardiff, Wales, UK.)

lacks in specificity since it also reacts and produces the green birefringence with alveolar and young haversian bone, neural tissue, collagen, exogenous polysaccharide materials such as plant cell walls, starch and cotton fibres, and fungi.

3. Its staining efficiency is adversely affected by formalin fixation to the point of extinction at times giving rise to false-negative results.

4. It is unable to subclassify amyloidoses accurately despite the availability of the differentiation method based on the use of trypsin, potassium permanganate, or alkaline guanidine treatment.

These difficulties have led to gradual emergence of immunocytochemical markers. The development of antibodies to different amyloid protein constituents has been found helpful in the identification and subclassification of amyloid fibrils in tissue sections.

## IMMUNOCYTOCHEMICAL MARKERS HELPFUL IN IDENTIFICATION AND SUBCLASSIFICATION OF AMYLOID FIBRILS

1. *Antiserum amyloid P (anti-SAP)*: Virtually all types of amyloid fibrils except the intracortical plaques- and neurofibrillary tangles-associated amyloid fibrils of Alzheimer's and other cerebral diseases have SAP bound to them, most probably through their glycosaminoglycan subcomponent. Thus anti-SAP can be used as a pan-amyloid immunocytochemical marker as an adjunct to the Congo red staining when in doubt.

2. *Antiamyloid A (anti-AA)*: This has been used for the identification of secondary amyloidoses-type amyloid fibrils. Since protein AA has been found to be nearly identical in virtually all the patients with secondary amyloidoses it has been possible to produce a reliable monoclonal reagent. A further advantage of immunocytochemical detection of AA fibrils has been their apparent robustness in formalin-fixed, paraffin-embedded tissues.

3. *Antiamyloid L (anti-AL)*: Routine immunocytochemical detection of this type of amyloid fibril poses some special difficulties. Firstly, the AL protein components have a tendency to become denatured in formalin-fixed tissues thus altering its antigenic properties. Secondly, protein AL consists mainly of the N-terminal variable region of a homologous light chain which differs in each patient. Therefore, antibodies against protein AL from one patient show little cross-reactivity with AL protein from other patients, and a battery of antibodies is needed to identify amyloid AL in tissues. For this reason antibodies commonly used against amyloid lambda or amyloid kappa, or those against light chain isotypes are liable to produce highly inconsistent results.

4. Antiprealbumin. Like the amyloid AL, the prealbumin amyloid fibrils are susceptible to denaturation in formalin fixation. As for its specificity for the various genetic variants of prealbumin associated with various forms of hereditary or familial (AF) and cardiomyopathic amyloid (AScI), the antibody of prealbumin shows complete cross-reactivity between these varieties of prealbumins. Thus, immunocytochemical methods based on the antiprealbumin are not usually helpful in differentiating amyloid fibril depositions due to these conditions.

5. Miscellaneous markers. Anti-$\beta_2$-microglobulin works on formalin-fixed, paraffin-embedded tissue sections provided they have been pretreated with trypsin. Caution needs to be exercised in interpreting the results since this protein is expressed by all cells expressing the Class 1 major histocompatibility complex (MHC) antigens. Also, the deposition of this protein in the amyloid fibrillary form is due to a quantitative increase in its circulatory level rather than due to any specific change in its structural property.

An observation of an anticalcitonin immunostaining of amyloid associated with medullary carcinoma of the thyroid is useful confirmatory evidence of the presence of the amyloid substance in the stroma surrounding the tumour cells. A similar observation of islet amyloid polypeptide immunostaining in association with a secondary carcinoma suspected to be arising from pancreatic islet cells may be of value in difficult cases (cf. Toshimori et al 1991).

A more detailed practical account of histochemical and immunohistochemical analysis of amyloid is given by Elias (1990), and some recent advances are described by Pepys (1988).

## IMMUNOCYTOCHEMISTRY AS AN AID IN THE STUDY OF ALPHA-1-PROTEASE INHIBITOR (A1PI)-ASSOCIATED LIVER DISEASE

Alpha-1-antitrypsin inhibitor, recently rechristened more aptly as alpha-1-protease inhibitor (A1PI) (Brantly et al 1988), is a 52 kDa, 394 amino acid residues long, single-chain glycoprotein encoded by Ch 14 (segment 14 q 31–32.3). Its physiological function is associated with its capacity to inhibit any neutrophil lysosomal elastase released into the circulation and/or interstitial space, and thereby prevent tissue damage by this enzyme. It does so apparently through an active site centered around its surface Met 358 residue.

A1PI is a highly polymorphic protein with more than 75 phenotypic/genetic variants. But amongst all these, there are two important salt bridges (Glu 342–Lys 290 and Glu 263–Lys 387, respectively), disruption of either of which due to a mutation in the A1PI gene is likely to lead to its abnormal metabolism and thereby its relative or absolute deficiency in the circulation . In normal individuals the A1PI genes are represented as autosomal codominant alleles referred to as M alleles. Both the alleles have to develop the critical mutations before a deficiency state can manifest itself. A1PI deficiency therefore presents itself in the main as an inheritable autosomal recessive trait.

The major mutation disrupting the critical Glu 342–Lys 290 salt bridge involves the conversion of residue Glu 342 in exon V to Lys 342. This is referred to as the Z mutation and leads to the Z variant of either homozygous or heterozygous inheritable A1PI deficiency state. The major mutation disrupting the second critical salt bridge involves the conversion of Glu 264 in exon III to Val 264. This results in the S form of either homozygous or heterozygous inheritable A1PI deficiency state.

The molecular basis of the deficiency associated with the Z mutation is generally well understood. Both the transcription and the translation of the Z gene variant are normal even in the homozygous state. However, since the Glu 342 to Lys 290 salt bridge cannot form as a result of a Lys instead of Glu residue occupying the 342 position, the nascent Z variant A1PI molecules on the polysome complex are unable to fold rapidly into their normal globular form. This leads, within the cisterna of the rough endoplasmic reticulum of the hepatocytes (their main site of synthesis), for any such unfolded A1PI molecules to aggregate and accumulate as histologically discernible globules instead of being secreted into the circulation.

The S-type mutation involving the Glu 264 to Val 264 replacement is not associated with intracellular accumulation. It seems from X-ray crystallographic studies that the amino acid substitution disrupts the salt bridge associated with this position and thereby renders the S protein less stable and more susceptible to proteolysis.

The engorgement of hepatocytes, typically in the periportal region, with A1PI globules due to the Z mutation is associated with neonatal cholestasis in 10% of the ZZ homozygote individuals. Although the majority of the affected individuals recover from this early condition about 20% go on to develop hepatitis, fibrosis and/or cirrhosis which sometimes may progress far enough to develop frank liver failure. The compound ZS heterozygote status is also associated with an accumulation of the globular form A1PI in the hepatocytes and concomitant liver damage, suggesting that the engorgement process causes liver cell damage either by its bulk or some toxic effect.

For this reason, detection of globular form A1PI in the liver by a combination of histological, histochemical and light and electron microscopic immunocytochemical methods has proved to be of value in predicting or diagnosing cryptogenic forms of hepatitis and/or cirrhosis. (See Figure 14.2 for a photomicrographic illustration.)

The globular A1PI inclusion bodies can be identified histologically as eosinophilic droplets over 3 μm in diameter. A1PI accumulation is also typable by periodic acid–Schiff reagent after treatment with diastase to exclude glycogen. These PAS-positive globules have been shown to be biochemically and immunologically similar to A1PI (Eriksson & Larsson 1975).

This has opened up the possibility of using immunocytochemistry as a more specific and sensitive method for in situ identification of A1PI in liver biopsy material. Polyclonal antiserum to A1PI has been used successfully for this purpose

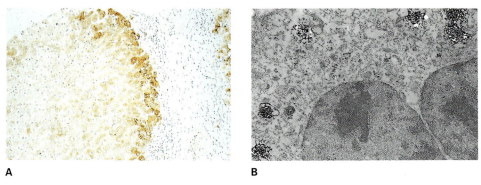

**A**                                                              **B**

**Fig. 14.2**    Illustration of the accumulation of A1PI globules in (**A**) a case with liver cirrhosis (simple two-step immunoperoxidase technique and haematoxylin counterstain); and (**B**) in COS cells transfected with a mutated form of A1PI gene transfectant (pre-embedding immunoperoxidase DAB–silver enhancement followed by EM viewing of an LR White-embedded ultrathin section). See Scobie et al 1990 for further details.

in formalin-fixed, paraffin-embedded tissue sections pretreated with trypsin for gaining access to the antigenic epitopes. The A1PI immunocytochemistry also obviates the use of the rather complicated protocol of 'digestion–Schmorl reaction–PAS', otherwise necessary to exclude interference from lipofuscin- and copper-associated protein deposits often present in addition in the periportal hepatocytes in cirrhotic livers.

## METALLOTHIONEIN IMMUNOCYTOCHEMISTRY AS AN AID IN THE STUDY OF HEPATIC COPPER ACCUMULATION

Metallothionein represents a class of proteins of low molecular weight (less than 10 kDa) polypeptides enriched in cysteinyl residues. These residues act as ligands for binding metal ions such as Zn, Cu and Cd. The structure of mammalian Cd, Zn-metallothionein has been resolved by both X-ray analysis and NMR spectroscopy. According to these data, the molecule exists as a two-domain protein with up to seven metal ions coordinated tetrahedrally in two polynuclear clusters binding respectively three and four metal ions through in all 20 cysteines serving as terminal and bridging ligands.

Information concerning the function of Cu-metallothionein is incomplete but it seems that it is involved in some aspect of Zn and Cu metabolism in addition to its recognized role in metal detoxification. The mammalian metallothionein

appears to bind Cu(I) in a distinct configuration and stoichiometry from Cd(II) and Zn(II). Thus up to 12 Cu ions are able to bind to the apoprotein with a distribution of six ions per cluster. In Cu, Zn hybrid metallothionein the Cu is usually restricted to the B-domain in which it is bound through a trigonal geometry unlike the tetrahedral coordination described for Zn- and Cd, Zn-metallothioneins.

The physiological role of Zn-metallothionein is also still not resolved but it seems likely that it is involved in mammalian Zn and Cu metabolism at the cellular and molecular level. One hypothesis views metallothionein (Mt) as a passive store of Zn, which releases metal to other apo-Zn proteins. Chemical studies indicate that Zn-Mt is indeed unusually reactive in ligand substitution and metal exchange reactions. The interesting aspect of Zn-Mt to apo-Zn protein transfer reaction is that the resultant apo-Mt is very unstable and is very rapidly biodegraded. Thus the level of Mt at any given time and place is very nearly equal to the level of Zn-Mt under physiological conditions. Increase in free Zn is therefore liable to transient increases in Zn-Mt, whilst induction of metallothionein synthesis by chemical mediators of physical, psychological or inflammatory stress (e.g. glucocorticoid hormones, glucagon, epinephrine or interleukin-1, respectively) is associated with a transient fall in the free Zn levels.

In striking contrast, the binding of Cu(I) to Mt is very avid, rendering the Cu-Mt complex very stable, causing it to accumulate, especially at the main sites of Mt synthesis, viz. hepatocytes and the proximal renal tubules. This point is of great relevance and importance in studies of various Cu accumulation states.

Routine pathological diagnosis of hepatic copper accumulation has depended on histochemical stains for copper such as rubeanic acid and rhodanine, and for copper-associated protein using orcein. Analysis of total hepatic copper using atomic absorption spectrophotometry or neutron activation analysis of carefully taken biopsies is also available but is destructive of the specimen.

As discussed above, a proportion of hepatic copper under physiological conditions is likely to be bound to metallothionein because of its very high avidity for this protein. The resultant Cu-Mt is likely to be the most major component of persistent Mt in the hepatocytes. This notion is supported by the following main observation.

Bile is the major excretory route for excess bodily copper, a blockage of the bile duct system is therefore likely to lead to an increase in the hepatocyte Cu-Mt content. This appears to be the case since in primary biliary cirrhosis a linear correlation has been found to exist between the total hepatic copper and cytosolic Mt. The latter is presumably almost entirely Cu-Mt as indicated by our histological, histochemical and immunocytochemical studies on normal human fetal and adult liver specimens and liver biopsies obtained from patients with various conditions associated with hepatic copper retention. We have substantiated

this work recently with correlative atomic absorption spectrophotometric, X-ray microanalysis, histological, histochemical and immunocytochemical studies on rat liver tissue specimens taken from rats given normal and varyingly high levels of dietary copper. The findings of these animal and human studies have helped to identify the following, potentially most helpful application of Mt immunocytochemistry in histopathological analysis of hepatic copper accumulation states.

Mt immunocytochemistry is able to detect selectively cytosolic Cu(I) in addition to orcein which detects mainly the coarsely granular copper-associated protein (CAP—presumably polymerized Mt) sequestered within the lysosomes (see Figure 14.3 for a photomicrographic illustration), or rubeanic acid which is apparently exclusively reactive with Cu(II).

Thus Mt immunocytochemistry is able to detect the evenly distributed cytosolic, probably nascent, Zn/Cu(I)-associated Mt, in contradistinction to the polymerized Mt sequestered within the lysosomal compartment presumably in the process of being degraded and discarded. The latter is most probably equivalent to the orcein-positive copper-associated protein (CAP). The lack of immunocytochemical reactivity of CAP is probably related to the inaccessibility of its epitopes to anti-Mt. The Mt immunocytochemistry also fails to detect Cu associated with the rubeanic acid-positive Cu(II)-rich granular deposits since these most probably represent lipofuscin-associated

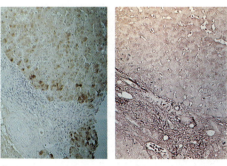
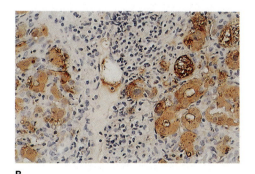

A        B

**Fig. 14.3** Illustration of (**A**) an overall correlation between the typically coarsely granular orcein-positing copper-associated protein (CAP) and smooth cytosolic MT accumulation in a liver biopsy of a case with primary biliary cirrhosis; (**B**) accumulation of immunoreactive MT in large degenerate/necrotic hepatocytes in a liver biopsy taken from a case with Wilson's disease. (MT immunostaining using a simple two-step indirect immunoperoxidase technique with haematoxylin counterstain.)

material arising from any cellular damage caused by the toxic effects of free Cu(II).

The nascent Mt which is presumed to become rapidly associated with either Zn or Cu(I) is mostly induced by dietary Zn metal ions but could also result from stress-related endogenous factors including glucocorticoid hormones and cytokines such as interleukin-1. The metal and the stress-inducible forms of Mt are biochemically distinguishable to be Mt I and Mt II isoforms, respectively. Unfortunately both these isoforms seem to possess virtually the same immunochemical structure, thus disallowing any possibility of differentiating them on immunocytochemical grounds. It is important therefore to bear in mind that any increased presence of immunocytochemically detectable Mt in human liver may be due to either increased Zn metal ion load or acute or chronic stress or both. Hence a careful correlation with clinical and biochemical information is important in the final interpretation and reporting of any such findings.

In a normal adult liver the Mt immunocytochemical positivity is generally weak or negative depending on the overall detection sensitivity of the technique used. The positivity, if present, is associated mainly with individual hepatocytes scattered in and around the central venous zone. This is visible as evenly distributed and finely spicular cytoplasmic staining. Some nuclei are also seen to be positive. Also the bile and the bile duct epithelium are occasionally seen to be positive presumably due to in transit excretory form of Mt. An increase in Mt expression/accumulation leads to an increase in the intensity of Mt immunostaining as well as a much wider distribution of positively stained cells until at some stage virtually all the hepatocytes in all three zones of the liver lobules are intensely Mt immunopositive. Beyond this stage, if liver damage becomes established, then usually the central parts of the liver lobules begin to lose their staining, leaving behind only a few intensely positive degenerate or necrotic hepatocytes in the peripheral regions of the surviving or regenerative lobules (see Fig. 14.3b).

A detailed account of immunocytochemistry of metallothionein in normal, experimental and pathological states has been recently provided by Jasani & Elmes (1991).

## IMMUNOCYTOCHEMICAL MARKERS HELPFUL IN HISTOPATHOLOGICAL ANALYSIS OF EARLY MYOCARDIAL ISCHAEMIA/INFARCTION

Metabolic defects or injuries, apart from causing abnormally high and persistent accumulation of proteins and other metabolites, are also associated with molecular losses often resulting from circumscribed cell death and loss of vital function. The commonest form of injury responsible for such accumulations or losses is ischaemic injury arising from inadequate supply of blood-borne oxygen. From the viewpoint of preventable causes of mortality and morbidity, ischaemic injury to the heart represents the single most common cause encountered by the histopathologist, especially when dealing with a case of sudden death. The death of a person with an episode of myocardial ischaemia/infarction is often so rapid in onset that very little time is available for the tell-tale signs of histological damage and reaction to develop prior to death.

For this reason, special tinctorial and histochemical staining techniques have been developed to detect the earliest biochemical changes associated with heart muscle showing ultrastructural evidence of irreversible cell damage. Recently we have examined the role of immunocytochemistry in assessing these changes and compared its efficiency with the established conventional histological methods. The results obtained correlate very well with recently published experimental animal data from other centres. As discussed below, the human and animal data collectively suggest that the loss of immunocytochemical staining of myoglobin provides the most sensitive marker of early myocardial infarction.

### Biochemical events associated with early myocardial ischaemic injury

The earliest effects of limitation of oxygen supply to energetically active cells is a rapid drop in the ATP pool. This leads to a fall in efficiency, among other cellular reactions, in the sodium membrane pump activity. The result of this, depending on the severity and duration of ischaemia, varies from minor to major water accumulation within various organelles of individual cells. The injury may progress next to an extent that the cell membrane can no longer maintain its semipermeable character and thereby begins to allow the diffusion of macromolecules out of the cell. Beyond this stage the cell's integrity may be compromised to an extent that it can no longer maintain its internal pH neutrality. As a consequence the pH drops to a level at which proteins begin to become denatured as well as activated in an autodestructive manner (e.g. lysosomal hydrolytic enzymes). By this stage the cell is well beyond the point of recovery and essentially dead with the development of pyknosis, karyorrhexis and karyolysis, the cardinal morphological features of cell death. The latter changes appear to arise about 6 h after the onset of ischaemia. Hence the time-scale of early myocardial injury in terms of its unambiguous detection with the routine light microscopical histological technique is set around a period of several hours.

At the clinical level, the time-scale of death resulting from myocardial ischaemia/infarction is such as to be well within this period in at least 25% (and maybe up to 50%) of the cases. This means that postmortem examination of the heart muscle in these patients is likely to yield no positive routine histological evidence of myocardial infarction. In terms of serological detection of protein released from the injured myocardial cells, there is apparently no significant rise in the serum level detectable unless at least 3 h have elapsed since the heart attack prior to death. Thus the long-established serological markers of myocardial infarction such as creatinine kinase (CPK), lactic dehydrogenase (LDH), or glutamic-oxalo-acetic transaminase (GOT) are unable to detect early myocardial ischaemia/infarction of less than about 3 h duration. As a result of ventricular fibrillation at least up to 25% of the afflicted individuals are likely to die within 1 hour of the onset of myocardial injury. As shown by experimental and human data, it has been found that in such cases even the direct macro or macroenzyme histochemical assessment of enzyme loss is unlikely to reveal any significant evidence of the early ischaemic injury.

In the light of the limitations of these markers of an established myocardial infarction a search for a more sensitive marker for the early phase of myocardial infarction has been made necessary.

The development of highly sensitive serological and immunocytochemical techniques for detection of myoglobin offers a potential solution.

## Use of myoglobin as a marker of early myocardial ischaemia/infarction

With the development of sensitive radioimmunoassay techniques, it has become possible to determine fairly easily and rapidly the serum levels of myoglobin, thus allowing its use as a marker in the monitoring of the early-phase of myocardial infarction. This has led to the basic observation that in the early-phase myocardial infarction patients, the serum myoglobin levels are raised well before any rise in the serum levels of the conventionally accepted markers. This important finding has since been confirmed in the dog and the rat models of myocardial ischaemia using both serological and immunocytochemical methods. The latter method in each case was clearly able to show a diffusional loss of myoglobin (molecular weight 17 kDa) selectively from the injured areas of the heart as early as 30 min from the onset of ischaemia.

Quite independently of these studies we had initiated a search for immunocytochemical markers capable of giving either a consistent positive or negative staining in established myocardial infarct specimens taken from a selected series of postmortem cases. Using the information obtained in this manner we then proceeded to look at myocardial blocks taken from patients dying with and without any history and antemortem or postmortem evidence of coronary artery disease and/or myocardial ischaemic disturbances. In each case the results of the immunocytochemical analyses were compared with parallel studies using H&E, phosphotungstic acid haematoxylin (PTAH) and haematoxylin basic fuchsin picric (HBFP) stains.

The following immunocytochemical markers were tested: rabbit antimyoglobin (Miles Scientific), rabbit antimyosin (Miles Scientific), rabbit anticaeruloplasmin (Miles Scientific), rabbit anti-C-reactive protein (CRP) (Dakopatts), rabbit antiprealbumin (Dakopatts), rabbit anti-alpha-1-antitrypsin (A1AT) (Dakopatts), goat anti-C3b (Dakopatts). Of these, the antimyoglobin was found to be the most efficient negative marker and

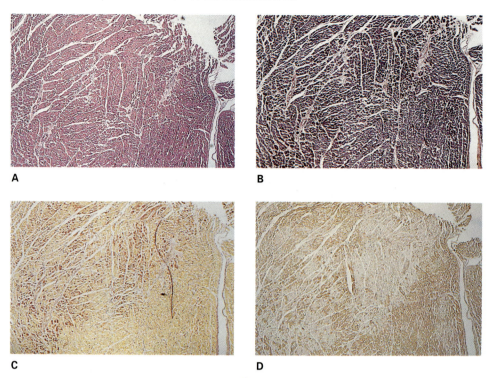

**Fig. 14.4**    Illustration of the sensitivity of myoglobin immunostaining in the detection of loss of myoglobin in the early phase of injury due to myocardial ischaemia/infarction. Staining in serial sections of a left ventricular biopsy taken from a case dying suddenly of natural causes: (**A**) conventional H&E appearances failing to show any signs of injury; (**B**) similarly negative result with PTAH staining; (**C**) the HBFPA technique showing positive red staining indicative of the injured myocardium; (**D**) immunoperoxidase staining (DHSS technique) of myoglobin showing a parallel loss of staining. (Courtesy of Dr Steve Leadbeatter, Department of Forensic Pathology, University of Wales College of Medicine, Cardiff, Wales, UK.)

anti-A1AT a strong positive marker of established myocardial infarction. As far as the early phase of myocardial ischaemia/infarction was concerned myoglobin proved to be the only effective (negative) marker. A follow-up of this with many more cases in each category was able to substantiate the preliminary observations confirming the value of myoglobin immunocytochemistry as a sensitive and reliable method for identification of early myocardial ischaemia/infarction. In fact the overall sensitivity of the method is such that even the agonal reflex myocardial ischaemic changes expected in patients dying of acute asphyxiation have been fairly consistently well detected by this method. This is in a paradoxical sense a drawback of the method for early myocardial infarction. Nevertheless, it also means that myocardial tissue showing no significant loss of myoglobin immunostaining can at least be confidently typed with this method as not having undergone any significant antemortem myocardial ischaemia. The potential value of myoglobin is illustrated photomicrographically in Figure 14.4.

It is noteworthy that amongst the three histological stains used in these studies the HBFP stain was found to be almost equally as valuable as antimyoglobin in the detection of early myocardial ischaemic changes.

REFERENCES AND FURTHER READING

**Amyloid disease**

Elghentany M T, Saleem A 1988 Methods for staining amyloid tissues. A review. Stain Technology 63: 201–212
Elias J M 1990 Histochemical and immunohistochemical analysis of amyloid. Immunohistopathology: a practical

approach to diagnosis. American Society of Clinical Pathologists Press, Chicago, p 441–448

Pepys M B 1988 Amyloidosis: some recent developments. Quarterly Journal of Medicine 67: 283–298

Toshimori H, Narita R, Nakazato M et al 1991 Islet amyloid polypeptide in insulinoma and in the islets of the pancreas of non-diabetic and diabetic subjects. Virchows Archiv. A, Pathological Anatomy & Histopathology 418: 411–417

Virchow R 1855 Ueber den Gang der Amyloiden Degeneration. Archives of Pathological Anatomy and Physiology 8: 364–369

**Alpha-1-antitrypsin deficiency**

Brantly M, Nukiwa T, Crystal R G 1988 Molecular basis of alpha-1-antitrypsin deficiency. American Journal of Medicine 84: 13–31

Eriksson S, Larsson C 1975 Purification and partial characterisation of PAS-positive inclusion bodies from the liver in alpha-1-antitrypsin deficiency. New England Journal of Medicine 292: 176–180

Scobie G, Jasani B, James V, Newman G R, Kalshekar N 1990 Transfection of cos cells by normal and mutant alpha 1 antitrypsin cDNA constructs: biochemical and immunocytochemical findings. Biochemical Society Transaction 18: 998–999

**Metallothionein immunocytochemistry in copper retention**

Elmes E, Clarkson J P, Mahy N J, Jasani B 1989 Metallothionein and copper in liver disease with copper retention: a histopathological study. Journal of Pathology 158: 131–137

Elmes E, Clarkson J P, Jasani B 1989 Role of metallothionein in copper accumulation in man – a histopathological study. In: Chazot G, Abdulla E, Arnaud P (eds) Current trends in trace elements research. Smith-Gordon, Nishimura, p 55–59

Jasani B, Elmes M E 1991 Immunohistochemical detection of metallothionein. Methods in Enzymology 205: 95–107

**Myocardial ischaemia/infarction**

Leadbeatter S, Wawman H M, Jasani B 1989 Immunocytochemical diagnosis of early myocardial ischaemic/hypoxic damage. Forensic Science International 40: 171–180

Leadbeatter S, Waxman H M, Jasani B 1990 Further evaluation of immunocytochemical staining in the diagnosis of early myocardial ischaemic/hypoxic damage. Forensic Science International 45: 135–141

Nomoto K-I, Mori N, Shoji T, Nakamura K 1987 Early loss of myocardial myoglobin detected immunohistochemically following occlusion of the coronary artery in rats. Experimental and Molecular Pathology 47: 390–402

# 15. Histologically-occult infections

## INTRODUCTION

The need for immunological identification of infectious agents in pathological specimens has been instrumental in the development and advances of three widely used immunocytochemical techniques in diagnostic pathology.

Thus, the advent as well as the development of direct and indirect immunofluorescence techniques by Albert Coons and colleagues were both evidently precipitated by the necessity of accurate identification of pathogenic bacteria and viruses in infected tissues (Coons & Kaplan 1950, Coons et al 1950, Weller & Coons 1954). Also, subsequent introduction by Riggs of the more stable derivative of fluorescein, fluorescein isothiocyanate, which ultimately popularized the use of the immunofluorescence technique (see Smith et al (1962) for a review), depended upon the detection of viral antigens in postmortem pathological specimens (Riggs et al 1958, Riggs & Brown 1960). Similarly, Sternberger found spirochaetes a useful difficult target to demonstrate in tissue biopsies, in order to illustrate the power of his improved version of the indirect immunoperoxidase method, the peroxidase–antiperoxidase (PAP) technique (Sternberger et al 1970). Finally, as with the immunofluorescence method, the popularization of the immunoperoxidase technology in diagnostic histopathology was at least in part triggered and propagated by the need to seek and correlate the presence of viral antigens in formalin-fixed, paraffin-embedded tissue specimens (Nayak & Sachdeva 1975, Huang et al 1976).

However, despite the pivotal role played by infectious disorders in promoting the development of immunocytochemical technology, immunocytochemical detection of infectious or parasitic agents has failed to become an established adjunct to diagnosis of infectious diseases in diagnostic histopathology (Chandler 1987).

There are several reasons for this failure:

1. The bulk of the microbiological analysis requiring immuncytochemistry relates to cytological specimens which usually fall outside the remit of histopathological analysis.

2. Immunocytochemistry is unable to type the infectious agent beyond its species of origin and its serotype. Thus in the case of bacteria, for example, it is unable to identify their individual strains or phage types, or analyse their respective growth characteristics or antibiotic sensitivities.

3. Several histological staining techniques are currently available that are quite capable of identifying the species of the pathogenic organisms.

4. The majority of the antimicrobial antibody reagents developed for immunocytochemical application have been designed to work on unfixed tissue preparations in conjunction with direct immunofluorescence technique to provide rapid results. Hence, the choice of commercially available antibodies which work well on formalin-fixed, paraffin-embedded tissue sections in association with the immunoperoxidase method has continued to remain rather limited.

5. The recent great surge of interest in the application of in situ hybridization (ISH) technology, as a more powerful and more precise means of typing microbial infections and infestations, has further diminished the role of immunocytochemistry.

Nevertheless, the advent of the hybrid mono-clonal antibody technology and the general surge of commercial interest in the sale and distribution of diagnostically useful immunocytochemical reagents have helped to balance the situation somewhat. The main purpose of this chapter is to catalogue antibody reagents known to be capable of detecting bacteria, viruses, fungi, protozoa and other related infectious agents, in formalin-fixed, paraffin-embedded tissue sections, with the aim of highlighting their potential usefulness as adjuncts to conventional histological analysis and ISH analysis.

For a general account of the role played by immunocytochemistry in diagnostic analysis of microbiological disorder, the reader is recommended to follow the excellent reviews by Chandler (1987), Kaye (1988), Shapiro & Walker (1989) and Lee & Hallsworth (1990). A practically useful account of the role of ISH in detection of viruses has been recently compiled by Elias (1990). For photomicrographic illustration two of the immunocytochemical stains currently in use in the diagnosis of infectious disease, see Figures 15.1 and 15.2.

## HISTOPATHOLOGICALLY USEFUL ANTIBODY REAGENTS IN DIAGNOSIS OF INFECTIOUS DISEASES

### Bacterial infections

Haematoxylin and eosin (H&E) staining is sufficient for identifying the site of bacterial colonization and analysing the nature of tissue reaction to the infection. It also has the capacity to allow recognition of a few bacterial species according to their morphology and tinctorial properties. Where the numbers of bacteria present in tissue are very low or sparsely distributed, silver impregnation methods (e.g. Dieterle, Steiner & Steiner, or Warthin–Starry) are necessary especially for very small and slender varieties of Gram-negative bacteria. Truant's auramine rhodamine, a fluorescence probe, is useful for sensitive localization of mycobacterial organisms.

Once the microorganisms have been located it is usually necessary to stain them with modified Gram stains (e.g. Brown & Brenn, Brown–Hopps, MacCallum–Goodpasture) or acid fast stains (e.g. Ziehl–Neelsen, Fite's) to identify their species according to their Gram-positive or -negative status, or their acid-fast or acid-non-fast status. These reactions, taken together with basic morphology of the individual members of the bacterial population, allow one to identify the main species of the respective infective agent, e.g. Gram-positive cocci, or Gram-negative bacilli, etc.

Histological stains, however, are unable to type the bacteria according to their serotype, phage type, culture characteristics, or antibiotic sensitivity. All of these except the serotyping demand the use of live bacteria. Serotyping, on the other hand, involves the characterization of the bacterial species according to the variety of surface antigens associated with them. For this, dead but suitably preserved bacteria are usually sufficient. Immunocytochemical staining therefore offers an ideal approach to in situ serotyping of bacteria.

A wide variety of antibody reagents is available for serotyping of bacteria present in smears prepared from body secretions or fluids, or tissue aspirates (Chandler 1987). However, the choice of antibodies which work on formalin-fixed, paraffin-embedded tissue sections is somewhat limited (see Table 15.1) and even these have been used only infrequently as referenced in Table 15.1. Both immunofluorescence and immunoenzyme techniques have been used reliably well for this purpose usually without the need of any special pretreatment (see TECHNICAL CONSIDERATIONS at the end of this chapter).

In situ hybridization offers an important alternative means of analysing bacteria associated with infective lesions according to their genotypic traits (Pollice & Yang 1985).

### Viral, rickettsial and chlamydial infections

Morphological and tinctorial methods for recognition of these microorganisms are available but

**Table 15.1** Histopathologically useful antibody reagents in diagnosis of bacterial infections

| Infective agent | Key reference |
| --- | --- |
| *Mycobacterium leprae* | Alonso et al 1978 |
| *Mycobacterium tuberculosis* | Polin 1984 |
| *Treponema pallidum* | Beckett & Bigbee 1979 |
| *Pseudomonas aeruginosa* | Brownstein 1978 |
| *Legionella pneumophila* | Boyd & McWilliams 1982 |
| *Helicobacter pylori* | Cartun et al 1990 |

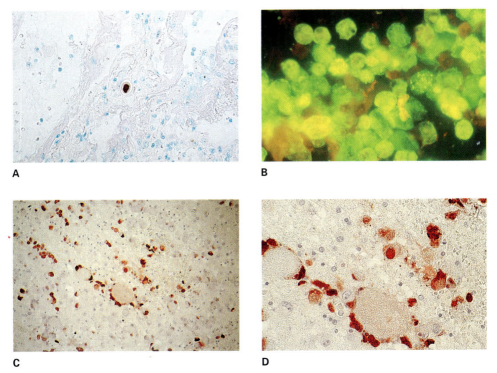

**Fig. 15.1** Illustration of the value of an anti-CMV reagent (CCH2, Dakopatts) in the identification of infected cell nuclei in: (**A**) and (**B**) a case dying of CMV pneumonia—postmortem lung tissue; (**C**) and (**D**) a case dying of CMV encephalitis—postmortem brain tissue (simple two-step indirect immunoperoxidase method and haematoxylin counterstain; and APAAP technique and haematoxylin counterstain, respectively). (**C** and **D** courtesy of Dr Gill Cole, Neuropathology Unit, Department of Pathology, University of Wales College of Medicine, Cardiff, Wales, UK.)

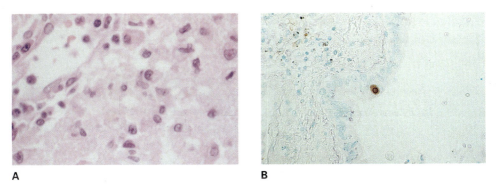

**Fig. 15.2** Illustration of the value of immunofluorescence in the detection of herpes simplex virus (HSV) using the cell culture technique: (**A**) non-specific appearances of viral infection revealed using conventional H&E staining; (**B**) confirmation of HSV infection via culturing of the virus in susceptible cells followed by direct immunofluorescence technique. (Courtesy of Dr Gill Cole, Neuropathology Unit, Department of Pathology, University of Wales College of Medicine, Cardiff, Wales, UK.)

demand fixation of tissues in special fixatives (e.g. Zenker's acetic acid or Bouin's fluid) in order to recognize the characteristic nuclear inclusions when using either H&E or special stains for viral inclusion bodies such as Lendrum's phloxine tartrazine, haematoxylin–Shorr 53, or Masson's trichrome. However, even when this approach is adopted, an experienced pathologist is able to make a presumptive diagnosis of viral infection with a high degree of accuracy in only about 50% of the cases (Straus 1976, Chandler 1987).

Hence, for identification of viruses and other smaller microorganisms in routinely fixed tissue sections immunocytochemistry does offer a more reliable alternative. For this reason a number of antibody reagents directed against viral and other microbial antigens have been developed recently which are suitable for application in a diagnostic histopathological setting (see Table 15.2). The antibodies nevertheless suffer from two basic drawbacks:

1. Largely because of the very small size of the target microorganisms, the formalin-fixed, paraffin-embedded tissue sections have to be treated with proteolytic enzymes in order to make the infective particles more accessible to the antibody reagents (see TECHNICAL CONSIDERATIONS at the end of this chapter).

2. Antibodies are capable of distinguishing only the major viral strains and type, and not their specific substrains and subtypes.

On the other hand, in situ hybridization does offer the potential of subtyping viruses in routine histopathological material as described by Brigati et al (1983), Blum et al (1984), Syrjanen & Syrjanen (1986), and most recently by Elias (1990).

## Fungal, protothecal, protozoal and helminthic infections

These infections are usually quite adequately identifiable with H&E staining alone. For easier recognition of the protozoa and helminths Giemsa stains such as May–Grünwald and Wolbach's Stains may be used. Wilder's reticulum stain is useful for detecting the bar-like intracytoplasmic kinetoplast and nucleus of leishmaniasis and amastigote stages of *Trypanosoma cruzi* (Chandler 1987). Similarly, Masson's trichrome, iron haematoxylin and periodic and Schiff (PAS) stains may be used to make the identification of the trophozoites of *Entamoeba histolytica* easier. As for the fungi and protothecae, Gomori's methenamine silver, PAS and Grindley's stains may be used in combination with the H&E staining to simultaneously demonstrate the profile and character of fungi against the background tissue detail.

With the all-round capability of the morphological and tinctorial approach in recognizing the above variety of microorganisms the diagnostic role played by immunocytochemical staining is limited to the rare circumstance where both the morphological and tinctorial character of the infective or parasitic agents is ambiguous or badly distorted, for example by tissue necrosis or postmortem autolysis. The majority of the antibodies available are used mainly for cell surface antigen analysis either in tissue sections or sera more for the purpose of investigating the natural history and pathogenesis of the disease than for helping with diagnosis in histopathological context. The few antibodies which have been used on diagnostic material are listed and referenced in Table 15.3.

## TECHNICAL CONSIDERATIONS

For the larger microorganism such as the protozoa, helminths, fungi, protothecae and the larger variety of bacteria, formalin-fixed, paraffin-embedded tissue sections can be used without any

**Table 15.2** Histopathologically useful antibody reagents in diagnosis of viral, rickettsial and chlamydial infections

| Infective agent | Key references |
| --- | --- |
| Hepatitis A | Shimizu et al 1978 |
| Hepatitis B | Clausen & Thomsen 1978 |
| Herpes simplex | Vernon 1982, Esiri 1982, Feiden et al 1984 |
| Mumps | Maltseva et al 1979 |
| Measles | Esiri et al 1979, Sata et al 1986 |
| Rabies | Budka & Popow-Kraupp 1982 |
| JC (polyoma virus) | Itoyama et al 1982 |
| Human papillomavirus | Lack et al 1980, Morin et al 1981 |
| Cytomegalovirus | Niedobitek et al 1988, Porter et al 1990 |
| Varicella zoster virus | Maltseva et al 1979 |
| *Mycoplasma pneumoniae* | Hill 1978 |
| *Chlamydia trachomatis* | Patton et al 1983 |
| *Chlamydia psittaci* | Finalyson et al 1985 |

**Table 15.3** Histopathologically useful antibody reagents in diagnosis of fungi, protothecae, protozoa and helminth infections/infestations

| Infective agent | Key references |
| --- | --- |
| *Cryptococcus neoformans* | Russell et al 1979 |
| *Sporothix schenckii* | Russell et al 1979 |
| *Entamoeba histolytica* | Culberston & Harper 1977 |
| *Toxoplasma gondii* | Conley et al 1981 |
| *Trichomonas vaginalis* | Bennett et al 1980 |
| Fungi | Moskowitz et al 1986 |

pretreatment for adequate intensity and quality of immunocytochemical staining. However, for the smaller bacteria and all types of viruses, rickettsiae and chlamydiae, it is necessary to pretreat the dewaxed and rehydrated sections with a proteolytic enzyme solution (e.g. 0.05 to 0.25% trypsin in 0.4% calcium chloride solution in distilled $H_2O$ adjusted to pH 7.8 with either 0.2 NaOH or Tris) for an optimum period varying from 1 to 3.5 h at 37 °C in order to bring out the maximum immunoreactivity (Chandler 1987). The immunoreactivity of certain viruses such as herpes simplex seems to benefit more from digestion with pepsin rather than trypsin whilst the rabies virus has been found to demand sequential digestion with 0.4% pepsin and 0.25% trypsin for maximum immunostaining efficiency (Reid et al 1983).

It is also to be noted that some species of virus (e.g. the herpes family) and bacteria (e.g. *Staphylococcus aureus*) have the capacity to express 'Fc' binding protein capable of binding IgG molecules via the 'Fc' region. The resulting non-specific binding is, however, likely to pose a serious problem only in lightly or unfixed frozen tissue sections or fresh cell preparations. Formalin fixation followed by paraffin embedding of tissues is generally deleterious to Fc receptors and therefore obviates this problem in routine diagnostic immunocytochemical analysis of these organisms.

As for the detection method, although direct immunofluorescence represents the method of choice for rapid diagnosis on fresh unfixed or lightly fixed specimens, the two-layer or three-layer indirect immunoperoxidase method is preferred for most of the work conducted on formalin-fixed, paraffin-embedded tissue sections. There are two main reasons for this preference. Firstly, the indirect method has greater intrinsic detection sensitivity associated with it and, secondly, the immunoperoxidase methods deposits a coloured stain which permits counterstaining with haematoxylin and permanent mounting in a xylene-based mountant. The latter two provide for clear viewing of the infectious or parasitic agent against the background tissue details (Chandler 1987).

The technical considerations of the ISH approach to analysis of infectious microorganisms have been reviewed recently in detail by Elias (1990).

REFERENCES AND FURTHER READING

**Introduction**

Chandler F W 1987 Invasive micro-organisms In: Spicer S S (ed) Histochemistry in Pathologic Diagnosis. Marcel Dekker, New York, p 78–101

Coons A H, Kaplan M H 1950 Localisation of antigen in tissue cells II. Improvements in a method for the detection of antigen by means of fluorescent antibody. Journal of Experimental Medicine 91: 1–13

Coons A H, Snyder J C, Cheevers F S, Murray E S 1950 Localisation of antigen in tissue cells IV. Antigens of rickettsiae and mumps virus. Journal of Experimental Medicine 91: 31–38

Elias J M 1990 Nonradioactive in situ hybridization for viral detection. In: Elias J M (ed) Immunohistopathology – a practical approach to diagnosis. American Society of Clinical Pathologists Press, Chicago, p 404–440

Huang S N, Minassian H, Moore J D 1976 Application of immunofluorescence staining of paraffin sections improved by trypsin digestion. Laboratory Investigation 35: 383–390

Kaplan M H, Coons A H, Deans H W 1950 Localisation of antigen in tissue cells III. Cellular distribution of pneumococcal polysaccharides Types II and III in the mouse. Journal of Experimental Medicine 91: 15–30

Kaye V N 1988 Monoclonal antibodies to microbial antigens in diagnostic pathology. In: Wick M R, Siegal G P (eds) Monoclonal antibodies in diagnostic immunohistochemistry. Marcel Dekker, New York, p 623–630

Lee P C, Hallsworth P 1990 Rapid viral diagnosis in perspective. British Medical Journal 300: 1413–1418

Nayak N C, Sachdeva R 1975 Localisation of hepatitis B surface antigen in conventional paraffin sections of the liver. American Journal of Pathology 81: 479–492

Riggs J L, Siewald R J, Burckhatter J H et al 1958 Isothiocyanate compounds as fluorescent labelling agents for immune serum. American Journal of Pathology 34: 1081–1097

Riggs J L, Brown G C 1960 Demonstration of virus antigen for human post-mortem tissue by fluorescent antibody technique. Federation Proceedings 19: 402

Shapiro H L, Walker D H 1989 Diagnosis of infectious diseases by immunohistology, immunocytology, and in situ hybridization. In: Jennette J C (ed) Immunohistology in diagnostic pathology. CRS Press, p 258–292

Smith C W, Metzger J F, Hoggan M D 1962 Immunofluorescence as applied to pathology. American Journal of Pathology 38: 26–42

Sternberger L A, Hardy P H Jr, Cuculis J J, Meyer H G 1970 The unlabelled antibody–enzyme method of immunohistochemistry. Preparation and properties of soluble antigen–antibody complex (horseradish peroxidase–anti horseradish peroxidase) and its use in identification of spirochetes. Journal of Histochemistry and Cytochemistry 18: 315–333

Weller T H, Coons A H 1954 Fluorescent antibody studies with agents of varicellar and herpes zoster propagated in vitro. Proceedings of Society for Experimental Biology and Medicine 86: 789–794

**Bacterial infections**

Alonso J M, Mangiaterra M L, Szarfman A 1978 Indirect immunoperoxidase reaction applied to human leprosy. Medicira (B Aires) 38: 541–544

Beckett J H, Bigbee J W 1979 Immunoperoxidase localisation of *Treponema pallidum*. Its use in formaldehyde-fixed and paraffin-embedded tissue sections. Archives of Pathological and Laboratory Medicine 103: 135–138

Boyd J F, McWilliams E 1982 Immunoperoxidase staining of *Legionella pneumophilia*. Histopathology 6: 191

Brownstein D G 1978 Pathogenesis of bacteraemia due to *Pseudomonas aeruginosa* in cyclophosphamide-treated mice and potentiation of virulence of endogenous streptococci. Journal of Infectious Diseases 137: 795–801

Cartun R W, Pederson C A, Krzymowski G A, Berman M M 1990 Immunocytochemical detection of *Helicobacter pylori* in formalin-fixed tissue biopsy specimens. Journal of Clinical Pathology 43: 518

Polin R A 1984 Monoclonal antibodies against micro-organisms. European Journal of Clinical Microbiology 3: 387–398

**Viral, rickettsial and chlamydial infections**

Blum H E, Haase A T, Vyas F N 1983 Molecular pathogenesis of hepatitis B virus infection: simultaneous detection of viral DNA and antigens in paraffin-embedded liver sections. Lancet 2: 771–775

Brigati D J, Myerson D, Leary J J et al 1983 Detection of viral genomes in cultured cells and paraffin-embedded tissue sections using biotin-labelled hybridization probes. Virology 126: 32–50

Budka H, Popow-Kraupp T 1981 Rabies and herpes simplex virus encephalitis. An immunohistological study on site and distribution of viral antigens. Virchows Archiv. A, Pathologic Anatomy 390: 353–364

Chandler F W 1987 Invasive micro-organisms. In: Spicer S S (ed) Histochemistry in Pathologic Diagnosis. Marcel Dekker, New York, p 78–101

Clausen P P, Thomsen P 1978 Demonstration of hepatitis B-surface antigen in liver biopsies. A comparative investigation of immunoperoxidase and orcein staining on identical sections of formalin fixed, paraffin embedded tissue. Acta Pathologica Microbiologica Scandinava (A) 86A: 383–388

Esiri M M 1982 Herpes simplex encephalitis. An immunohistological study of the distribution of viral antigen within the brain. Journal of Neurological Science 54: 209–226

Esiri M M, Oppeneheimer D R, Brownell B, Haire M 1982 Distribution of measles antigen and immunoglobulin-containing cells in the CNS in subacute sclerosing panencephalitis (SSPE) and atypical measles encephalitis. Journal of Neurological Sciences 53: 29–43

Feiden W, Borchard F, Burrig K F, Pfitzer P 1984 Herpes oesophagitis. I. Light microscopical and immunohistochemical investigations. Virchows Archiv. A, Pathological Anatomy & Physiology 404: 167

Itoyama Y, Webster H D, Sternberger N H et al 1982 Distribution of papovavirus, myelin-associated glycoprotein, and myelin basic protein in progressive multifocal leukoencephalopathy lesions. Annals of Neurology 11: 396–407

Lack E E, Jervon A B, Smith H G et al 1980 Immunoperoxidase localisation of human papillomavirus in laryngeal papillomas. Intervirology 14: 148–154

Maltseva N, Manovich Z, Seletskaya T et al 1979 Rapid diagnosis of viral neuroinfections by immunofluorescent and immunoperoxidase techniques. Journal of Neurology 220: 125–130

Morin C, Braun L, Casas Cordero M et al 1981 Confirmation of the papillomavirus aetiology of condylomatous cervix lesions by the peroxidase antiperoxidase technique. Journal of National Cancer Institute 66: 831–835

Niedobitek G, Finn T, Herbst H et al 1988 Detection of cytomegalovirus by in situ hybridisation and immunohistochemistry using a new monoclonal antibody CCH2: a comparison of methods. Journal of Clinical Pathology 41: 1005–1009

Pollice M, Yang H L 1985 Use of nonradioactive DNA probes for the detection of infectious bacteria. Clinical Laboratory Medicine 5: 463–473

Sata T, Kurata T, Aoyama Y et al 1986 Analysis of viral antigens in giant cells of measles pneumonia by immunoperoxidase method. Virchows Archiv. A, Pathologic Anatomy 410: 133–138

Shimizu Y K, Mathiesen L R, Lorenz D et al 1978 Localisation of hepatitis A antigen in liver tissue by peroxidase-conjugated antibody method. Light and electron microscopic studies. Journal of Immunology 121: 1671–1679

Straus A J 1976 Light microscopy of selected viral diseases (morphology of viral inclusion bodies). In: Sommers S C (ed) Pathology annual, Vol II. Appleton–Century–Crofts, New York, p 53–75

Syrjanen S, Syrjanen K 1986 An improved in situ DNA hybridization protocol for detection of human papillomavirus (HPV) DNA sequences in paraffin-embedded biopsies. Journal of Virological Methods 14: 293–304

Vernon S E 1982 Herpetic tracheobronchitis: immunohistologic demonstration of herpes simplex virus antigen. Human Pathology 13: 683–686

**Fungal, protothecal, protozoal and helminthic infections**

Bennett B D, Bailey J, Gardner W A Jr 1980 Immunocytochemical identification of trichomonads.

Archives of Pathological and Laboratory Medicine 104: 247

Chandler F W 1987 Invasive micro-organisms. In: Spicer S S (ed) Histochemistry in pathologic diagnosis. Marcel Dekker, New York, p 78–101

Conley F K, Jenkins K A, Remington J S 1981 *Toxoplasma gondii* infection of the central nervous system: use of the peroxidase – antiperoxidase method to demonstrate *Toxoplasma* in formalin fixed, paraffin embedded tissue sections. Human Pathology 12: 690

Culbertson C G, Harper K 1977 Immunoperoxidase staining of *E. histolytica* and soil amebas in formalin fixed tissue. American Journal of Clinical Pathology 68: 529–530

Moskowitz L B, Ganjei P, Ziegels-Weissman et al 1986 Immunohistologic identification of fungi in systemic and cutaneous mycoses. Archives of Pathological and Laboratory Medicine 110: 433

Russell B, Beckett J H, Jacobs P H 1979 Immunoperoxidase localization of *Sporothrix schenckii* and *Cryptococcus neoformans*. Staining of tissue sections fixed in 4% formaldehyde solution and embedded in paraffin. Archives of Dermatology 115: 433–435

**Technical Considerations**

Chandler F W 1987 Invasive micro-organisms. In: Spicer S S (ed) Histochemistry in pathologic diagnosis. Marcel Dekker, New York, p 78–101

Elias J M 1990 Nonradioactive in situ hybridization for viral detection In: Elias J M 1990 Immunohistopathology: a practical approach to diagnosis. ASCP Press, Chicago, p 404–440

Reid F L, Hall N H, Smith J S et al 1983 Increased immunofluorescent staining of rabies-infected, formalin-fixed brain tissue after pepsin and trypsin digestion. Journal of Clinical Microbiology 18: 968–971

# PART IV

# Organization of a routine immunocytochemical service

# 16. Analysis, interpretation and reporting of immunocytochemical requests

## INTRODUCTION

Given the choice of the best primary antibody reagents, an exquisitely sensitive secondary detection system and the most pertinent clinicopathological background information, the work based on these can only produce reliable and meaningful results on a routine basis provided it is conducted in a systematic manner by a team of well-trained and well-motivated staff in a properly organized and well-resourced laboratory. The object of this chapter is to outline the basic requirements for establishing and running such a laboratory.

Like all diagnostic systems, routine immunocytochemical analysis as applied to diagnostic histopathology is divisible into three distinct phases of operation. These are referred to as preanalysis, analysis and postanalysis stages. Each has its unique and essential requirements. These are summarized below under the respective headings. A detailed review of some the key issues has been given recently by Elias (1990).

## PREANALYSIS

This phase is essentially concerned with efficient handling of requests sent for routine immunocytochemical examination of surgical specimens—from the time of receipt to the stage of their analysis. It is also concerned with the organization and regulation of the system adopted for making and accepting immunocytochemical requests. Thus, there are four essential issues which need to be discussed with respect to the preanalysis phase. These are:

1. basis for authorization of immunocytochemical requests
2. request form and its format
3. reception and recording of the requests
4. preparation of tissue specimens for immunocytochemical analysis.

### Authorization of immunocytochemical requests

Immunocytochemical analysis should be requested in principle only when all routine histological and histochemical effort has failed to yield the required diagnostic information. In order to achieve this ideal it is necessary that the request is made, or at least vetted, by an experienced histopathologist. Thus, in general, requests should not be accepted directly from clinicians other than a senior registrar or a consultant-grade histopathologist. This policy, though rather stringent, is likely to save resources otherwise wasted on inappropriate or redundant requests.

### Request form

This should have the standard format of a diagnostic request form with space allocated for recording the relevant personal and hospitalization details of the patient as well as the most pertinent clinical and histopathological findings. The form should also have space designated for entering information regarding the nature of the specimen sent for analysis and the type of immunocytochemical markers requested, as well as for recording and reporting the immunocytochemical results observed. A specimen copy of a request form, with a list of routinely applicable markers, is included in Appendix I. In addition, algorithms for commonly made requests in case of neoplastic

disorders are included in Appendix I as a further
guide for making the appropriate requests.

A specimen copy of a request form similar to
the one which has been used successfully, on a
regional basis over the past 10 years in Wales, is
included to illustrate these points.

## Reception of request

On the arrival of the request, the person in charge
of the immunocytochemistry service unit should
take immediate action to enter the time and date
of arrival of the specimen, the number and the
nature of the specimens received (e.g. 12 spare
sections; or a single formalin-fixed paraffin-
embedded tissue block). A note should then be
made of the marker studies requested and their
suitability for the kind of request made. If there
are any queries about these the requesting pathologist should be contacted for further clarification.
Occasionally the immunocytochemical request
may be accompanied with a request for a second
opinion on the histopathological diagnosis itself.
In such a case it is advisable to show the case first
to the duty histopathologist and enlist his or her
help and advice prior to engaging upon any immunocytochemical analysis.

## Preparation of tissue sections

This involves preparing the required number of
sections from each of the blocks needing analysis.
The sections are cut on to either plain high-quality
or specially coated glass slides. For marker studies
requiring proteolytic enzyme treatment it is essential that the sections are cut on to either very
clean plain glass slides (e.g. Gold Star glass slides)
or slides coated with a special adhesive such as
aminopropylethoxysilane (APES). It should be
noted that any specimens sent as spare sections on
chrom-gel or albumin-coated glass slides should
not be used for this purpose.

It is important to cut all the required sections
(including some spares for repeat or additional
studies) at a single sitting and by the same opera-
tor. This approach has the advantage of avoiding
repeated trimming of the usually precious tissue
block. It also allows mounting of the sections
in the same orientation in a contiguous series,

making any detailed comparison between sections
both easier and more meaningful.

For each marker study requested, it is necessary
to include positive and negative control studies.
These should be based on surgical tissue material
which has been tested previously to be repro-
ducibly and reliably positive or negative for the
marker in question. For formalin-fixed, paraffin
wax-embedded material it is convenient to cut
spare sections from the control tissue and keep
them stored in a dust-free slide filing cabinet,
ready for use whenever required. In the case of
fresh frozen tissue section studies it is possible to
cut spare sections, air-dry them overnight at
ambient temperature and store them at $-20\,°C$ or
$-70\,°F$ in slide boxes for at least 3 months,
without any significant deterioration of tissue
morphology or immunoreactivity.

## ANALYSIS

This includes various necessary pretreatments of
tissue sections, application of the appropriate primary antibody reagents followed by the respective
set of secondary detection system reagents, and
the development of the colour reaction followed
by counterstaining and mounting of the sections.
The salient points regarding these steps are described below under separate headings.

### Pretreatments

*Dewaxing of formalin-fixed, paraffin wax-embedded
sections*

The sections are first of all taken through a series
of absolute xylene and absolute alcohol (ethanol)
changes in order to dewax them thoroughly. Any
residual wax is likely seriously to impair immunocytochemical staining. Hence, every care should
be taken to ensure that the dewaxing is complete.
Five 5-min changes in xylene followed by five 5-
min changes in alcohol at room temperature are
considered to be sufficient for this purpose.

*Endogenous enzyme blocking*

Preblocking of any interfering endogenous enzyme activity constitutes a necessary step for im-
munoperoxidose studies on both formalin-fixed,

paraffin wax-embedded and fresh frozen tissue sections. For the former, the simplest and most reliable method is provided by incubation for 30 min of freshly dewaxed sections in a bath of a freshly prepared mixture of methanol/hydrogen peroxide ($H_2O_2$) (e.g. 47.2 ml absolute methanol + 0.8 ml of 30% v/v $H_2O_2$). For the frozen sections, a less deleterious regimen is necessary, such as that recommended by Andrew & Jasani (1988). It involves the use of azide in combination with nascent $H_2O_2$ produced by glucose oxidase action on glucose included as the substrate in the incubation medium.

*Proteolytic enzyme treatment*

This is a compulsory requirement for a limited set of antigens listed in Table 16.1. Wherever possible, antibody markers not demanding the proteolytic treatment should be used in preference to those which do, since the enzyme treatment is not wholly reliable and is also liable to produce overdigestion of tissue sections derived from inadequately fixed tissue blocks.

The most popular proteolytic enzyme used is trypsin. It is used in concentrations varying from 0.05 to 0.4% (w/v) in calcium chloride solution (0.1%; pH 7.8), and applied for 5–60 min, or even several hours, at 37°C. For some antigens, particularly viral antigens, pepsin is recommended in preference to trypsin. Such variable use of proteolytic enzyme treatment demands that the recommended conditions are strictly adhered to so that any potentially gross variations in the overall staining efficiency are avoided.

Following the enzyme treatment, it is important to remove thoroughly the residual enzyme on the sections by washing them in running cold tap

**Table 16.1** Markers requiring proteolytic enzyme pretreatment

1. Immunoglobulin heavy and light chain-related antigens including ichotypic markers
2. Polypeptide hormones, e.g. ACTH and HCG
3. Cytoskeletal proteins, e.g. desmin, vimentin and α-SMA
4. Extracellular matrix proteins, e.g. laminin and Type IV collagen
5. Miscellaneous antigens such as F-VIII-RAG, KP1 (CD68), Ki-1 (CD30), polyclonal CD3, α-antitrypsin (AAT)

water for at least 15 min. The sections are then equilibrated with the staining buffer medium, viz. phosphate-buffered saline (PBS; 0.01 M phosphate; pH 7.2; 0.15 M sodium chloride).

**Staining procedure**

Three principal operations are involved in an indirect immunoperoxidase procedure. These include: the primary antibody reagent incubation step, the addition of secondary detection reagent(s), and the development of peroxidase-based colour reaction. Before and after each of these steps the sections are washed with PBS to remove any excess unbound reagents. Protocols of four routinely applicable indirect immunoperoxidase techniques are listed in Appendix II in Tables 1–4, respectively.

*Primary reagent step*

This is best organized on an overnight basis at 4°C (e.g. in a fridge). Several advantages accrue from this approach as compared to a shorter incubation regimen applied at ambient temperature. Thus in general the longer incubation period permits the use of much higher dilutions of the primary antibody reagent. This results in more economical use of usually expensive or precious primary reagents, and a greater signal-to-background ratio in the final staining. The staining is also more reproducible since a steady end-point is reached in each run. Furthermore it provides a psychologically convenient break for the staff after what is usually a long-winded and a demanding pretreatment staining protocol.

*Secondary detection system step(s)*

This phase of analysis involves the application of one or more reagents in a sequential order culminating in a non-covalent attachment of the enzyme marker to the tissue-bound primary antibody molecules.

**Development of colour reaction**

The colour reaction is most popularly developed

using diaminobenzidine (DAB) as the chromogen, and hydrogen peroxide ($H_2O_2$) as the obligate substrate of peroxidase enzyme.

## Counterstaining and mounting

Haematoxylin is preferred to all other types of counterstains since it helps to reproduce in the immunocytochemically stained section, the same quality of nuclear staining as seen in a standard H&E-stained section.

A xylene-based mountant is similarly preferred to a water-based mountant as it gives the same degree of optical clarity and permanent preservation as the routine histological slides.

The counterstained and mounted slides are labelled legibly and accurately with the essential information relating to the case and the primary and secondary systems used.

## POSTANALYSIS

This involves light microscopic assessment of the reference positive and negative control results followed by examination, interpretation and reporting of the test results.

## Assessment of positive and negative control results

The positive control sections are assessed in terms of the intensity and distribution, of specific and non-specific staining visible at low, medium and high magnification.

Strong or widely distributed specific staining clearly visible at low power is graded and recorded as +++ whilst focal or moderately strong staining clearly visible only at medium power is recorded as ++. Finally, weak or very focal reactions clearly visible only at high powers are accorded a + rating, and any borderline or equivocal staining a ± rating. Staining limited to one side or corner of the section is recorded as zonal in order to indicate its possible artefactual origin from either uneven fixation/processing or a staining mishap such as partial drying out of the section.

Any non-specific staining observed is graded similarly to the specific staining. Any staining arising from endogenous sources is stated as such, and specified as to its origin, if possible, e.g. endogenous peroxidatic activity (EPA), or endogenous pigment (melanin or haemosiderin), etc. All the above information is recorded on the slide label as a prewarning to the reporting pathologist.

The negative control results are thoroughly screened at low, medium and high power for any unexpected or spurious staining and the character of this should be recorded briefly again on the slide label for ready reference when interpreting the test results.

## Assessment of test results

Having ascertained the sensitivity and the specificity of staining obtained in the reference control studies, one is ready to examine and interpret the test results with a measured degree of objectivity and confidence. The test results are graded for the overall intensity and distribution of the staining on exactly the same scale as the positive control slides. In addition the character of the staining is described with respect to the reactions obtained in the normal, reactive and pathological cell or tissue components. The staining quality is also described according to its topographical location (e.g. interstitial, pericellular, cell surface, cytoplasmic, perinuclear and/or nuclear) as well as its consistency (e.g. smooth, granular, punctate, fibrillary or luminal). All these features are recorded on the request form under the respective markers tested.

## Interpretation of test results

Having taken a proper account of any non-specific staining or any lack of staining due to recognized sources of tissue artefacts, the attention is focused upon the residual specific staining for the final interpretation of the results. A number of possible sources of non-specific stain are illustrated photomicrographically in Figure 16.1.

The specific staining is assessed according to whether it is part of the background normal tissue, reactive cell component, or part of the pathological process. The presence of relevant normal or reactive stained components is recorded on the request form as 'R' with the appropriate level of grading. The staining of the disease-associated

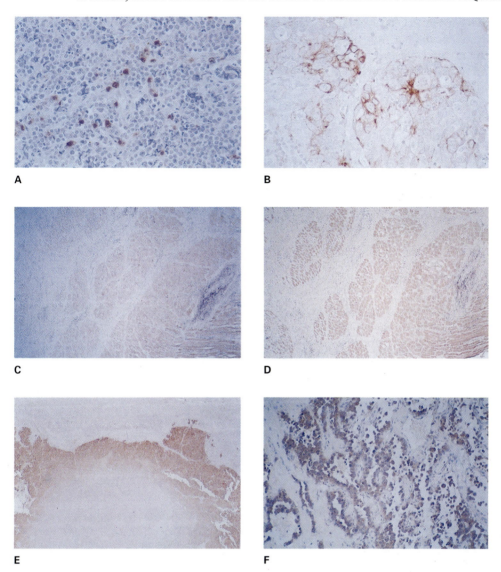

**Fig. 16.1** Illustration of non-specific/artefactual forms of staining causing interpretational difficulties: (**A**) inadequate inhibition of endogenous peroxidatic activity in eosinophils associated with Hodgkin's lymphoma; (**B**) necrotic areas of tumour tissue giving falsely strong CEA positivity; (**C**) and (**D**) false-positive (cross-reactive) staining of skeletal muscle due to MB2 and polyclonal CD3 antibodies, respectively; (**E**) zonal positivity due to inadequate fixation of the tissue; (**F**) false-positivity of a lung carcinoma with anti-VIP antibody due to inadvertent partial dehydration of the section during the primary antibody incubation step.

elements is recorded in terms of its grading and any other qualifications. All separate test results relevant to a single case are systematically assessed and recorded in this manner. The overall immunocytochemical findings observed are then summarized in relation to the available clinicopathological information in the form of a report described below.

## Reporting of the results

In keeping with the clinicopathological information provided, the immunocytochemical findings are reported as being either confirmatory or not confirmatory, or consistent or inconsistent, or helpful or not unhelpful, with respect to the most favoured diagnosis or differential diagnosis. If the results have proved inconsistent or unhelpful, further tests may be recommended to resolve the situation. These recommendations should be stated clearly in the report with the reasons given for their possible usefulness. Alternatively, it may be necessary to discuss the case with the relevant clinicians before proceeding to further studies or writing up the concluding report. Diagnostic algorithms with the expected results for commonly made requests in relation to neoplastic diseases are included in Appendix III for the reader's interest.

The final report, once written, is typed, checked and authorized prior to its despatch to the clinician and/or pathologist in charge of the case. A copy of the final report, as well as the interim reports, including the original request forms, are all filed safely and systematically in yearly report files according to their allocated immunocytochemistry case numbers. Similarly, the control and the test slides are also filed in their proper order in slide-safe filing cabinets.

It is mandatory that this is done for every case and every run, whether reported or not, since both the forms and/or the slides are likely to be needed for any future referral of the patient, internal quality control, audit assessments, or research and development projects as discussed in the next chapter.

REFERENCES AND FURTHER READING

Andrew S, Jasani B 1987 An improved method for the inhibition of endogenous peroxidase non-deleterious to lymphocyte surface markers. Application of immunoperoxidase studies on eosinophil-rich tissue preparations. Histochemical Journal 19: 426–430
Elias J M 1990 Immunohistochemical methods. In: Immunohistopathology – a practical approach to diagnosis. American Society of Clinical Pathologists, Chicago, p 1–90
Gatter K C, Mason D Y, Heyderman E et al 1987 Which antibodies for diagnostic pathology? Histopathology 11: 661–664

# 17. Staff requirements, quality assurance and research and development

## INTRODUCTION

The improvement in the quality and commercialization of primary antibody reagents and the standardization of secondary detection systems have helped to make immunocytochemistry an increasingly widely applicable and helpful adjunct to histopathological analysis of diseased tissue.

However, the basic immunocytochemical reagents comprise complex proteinaceous reagents applied in multistep procedures. Hence, in order to maintain adequate standards, it is necessary on the one hand to have well-trained and well-motivated staff who are routinely engaged in the application of the immunocytochemical technique, and on the other to have internal standards regularly included in immunocytochemical analysis to ensure internal quality control. There is also a need to participate in a well-run external quality assurance scheme for comparison and improvement in overall standards of practice. Finally, whilst new primary antibody reagents of value to histopathological analysis continue to emerge, it is necessary for the routine laboratory to maintain an active interest in research and development with the view to adopting the new reagents as soon as they become commercially available. These issues are discussed more fully below.

## STAFF REQUIREMENTS

### Technical staff

The staff performing immunocytochemical tests must be fully trained in histological techniques. This is because virtually all the skills related to histological tissue preparation, processing, sectioning and staining form an essential basis for proper immunocytochemical analysis of histopathological tissue specimens. In addition it is necessary for the staff to have a sufficient grasp of histochemical techniques and a working knowledge of antibodies and their properties.

The more specialist knowledge and expertise pertaining to the maintenance of high standards of practice may be acquired through continuing work experience, reading of technical texts, in-house training and/or attendance of short courses and technically oriented conferences.

The practice of immunocytochemistry, even at the routine technical level, is a demanding exercise requiring a good blend of histological, histochemical and immunological knowledge, expertise and experience. In addition, because every immunocytochemical analysis involves a multistep and a rather complex procedure it is essential that at least one senior member of the technical staff and an assistant are deployed on a full-time basis for routine immunocytochemical work. In order to support these staff, e.g. during the periods of work overload or absence due to annual leave or illness, it is necessary to train additional staff on a temporary rotation basis, such that at least one additional fully trained staff member is always available to assist with the routine immunocytochemical workload.

### Scientific staff

The need for continuing research into new immunocytochemical reagents and techniques is very much the remit of a large teaching hospital especially those providing a regional diagnostic immunocytochemistry service.

Immunocytochemistry is still an evolving area of technical expertise and there is a need to keep abreast of new developments in the field in order to maintain high and up-to-date standards of practice. For this it is necessary to employ at least one full-time research or scientific-grade permanent staff member who is fully trained and versed in routine immunocytochemical practice. The research staff may be encouraged to take on original research in order to gain further scientific experience and knowledge. The research unit, if endowed with senior clinical or scientific supervisory staff, may also encourage individuals to undertake project work based on immunocytochemical techniques leading to a thesis for undergraduate or higher degree qualification.

## Clinical staff

Whilst it is feasible for routine technical staff and histopathologists working in small district general hospitals to cope with the demands of immunocytochemistry applied to a small number of the most useful markers, in a large teaching hospital unit using many dozens of primary antibodies in all combinations, the employment of a clinical staff member with specialist interest in diagnostic immunocytochemistry may be desirable. Ideally this specialist staff should be a person with basic or advanced-level training in immunology giving him or her the authority to manage in addition to the routine service requirements, research and development as well as the advanced training needs of the unit itself, and the postgraduate training needs of the parent pathology department and other departments undertaking immunocytochemical research or applications.

## QUALITY ASSURANCE

The quality of immunocytochemical service is governable in four different ways: internal and external quality controls and internal and external audits. The question of the internal quality control has been adequately dealt with in the previous chapter under 'Analysis' and 'Postanalysis'. The aim of this section is to describe briefly the purpose of the other two types of quality control.

## External quality control

This involves assessment of the immunocytochemical marker status of selected sections distributed by an external quality assurance panel organized on a regional or national basis. The results of individual immunocytochemical laboratory units are compared at regular intervals with each other to assess the consistency and the accuracy of the practice. Consistently unreliable performances are noted and the laboratory units concerned are recommended and advised on a confidential and non-punitive basis to improve their standards to adequate levels of performance.

## Internal and external audits

These are concerned with the assessment of laboratory performance on the basis of its time and cost-effectiveness with a view to maintaining economical but adequate standards of patient care.

The average turnover times of individual technical procedures are estimated and costed and given regionally or nationally agreed reference units, e.g. the Welcan UK unit. The number of units with respect to number of patient requests received is used as an index of the level of efficiency and adequacy of the service with respect to individual tests.

The internal audit provides a useful way of judging the overall efficiency with which immunocytochemical requests are dealt with. The external audit, on the other hand, has the merit of providing useful information for organization of better and more appropriate service and training facilities on a regional or nationwide basis.

## RESEARCH AND DEVELOPMENT (R&D)

Because of high costs, labour intensiveness and expertise requirements of developing new diagnostically useful immunocytochemical markers or techniques, it is best to restrict any such R&D practices to centres of excellence with the relevant resources. Thus, for example, for assessing or developing new markers for lymphoma diagnosis it is best to conduct the exploratory work in a centre with a well-resourced technological base backed up by a large bank of well-characterized lymphoma cases and a resident lymphoma expert.

The other aspect of R&D work relates to adaptation of any new commercially available markers. The most important point to establish at the outset is whether the marker is suitable for use on routinely fixed and processed tissue sections. Secondly, it is necessary to follow the manufacturer's recommendations as closely as possible in terms of the conditions of application and the type of positive and negative control specimens selected for the initial assessment. After successful results have been achieved the conditions may be modified to suit the local immunocytochemical approach. Every attempt should be made to resist any radical change in the standardized protocol established for the bulk of the daily routine work.

## Establishment of specificity and sensitivity ranges of new immunocytochemical markers

Before a primary antibody reagent can qualify as a generally reliable diagnostic marker, it is necessary to establish its target specificity and sensitivity with respect to a whole range of normal, reactive and disease-associated tissue specimens. This should be achieved preferably with secondary detection systems and incubation conditions relating to both low- and high-efficiency detection of the target antigen. Furthermore, in order to extract the maximum use out of a given marker, its specificity and sensitivity should be assessed both when used alone and as a member of a panel of markers.

For prognostic markers there is the additional need to include accurate clinical follow-up data of sufficiently long duration, in order to assess their long-term, clinically more useful predictive indices.

For unusual or rare cases, a multicentre trial should be conducted to acquire a large enough number of cases to provide reliable indices of marker specificity and sensitivity. Also it is important to ensure that the cases which are entered into the trial are accurately diagnosed in the first place.

FURTHER READING

Wold L E, Corwin D J, Rickert R R et al 1989 Interlaboratory variability of immunohistochemical stains: results of the cell markers survey of the College of American Pathologists. Archives of Pathological and Laboratory Medicine 113: 680–683

# Appendix I
# Specimen request/report form with a list of routinely requested immunocytochemical marker studies

Patient's Particulars: Name     *Address*     *Date of Birth*
       Sex

Hospital Unit No.     Pathology No.     Immunocytochemistry No.
*Requesting Pathologist*     *Reporting Pathologist*
Hospital
Specimen Details:    Date Sent     *Clinical Findings*
         Date Received     *Histopathological Diagnosis*

*Marker Studies/Results*

| | | | | | | |
|---|---|---|---|---|---|---|
| Lymphoreticular | Pan-leucocyte (CD45) | | | | | |
| | Pan T cell | CD3 (poly) | MT1 (CD43) | | | |
| | Pan B cell | L26 (CD20) | MB2 | | | |
| | Restricted T cell | UCHL-1 (CD45RO) | | | | |
| | Restricted B cell | MT2 | λ | κ | IgG | IgA | IgM |
| | Hodgkin's cell | LeuMI (CD15) | Ki-1 (Ber-H2) (CD30) | | | |
| | Mononuclear/ Phagocytic cells | KP1 (CD68) | S-100 | Factor XIIIa | | |
| Epithelial | Pan-epithelial | Cytokeratin | CEA | EMA | HMFGII | |
| | Prostate | PSA | PAPh | | | |
| Soft tissue | Pan-mesenchyme | Vimentin | | | | |
| | Muscle | Desmin | Myoglobin | α-smooth muscle actin | | |
| | Myoepithelial cell | S-100 | | | | |
| | Schwann cell | S-100 | Leu7 (CD57) | | | |
| Neuroendocrine/ Neuroectodermal | Pan-neural | NSE | ChA | SYNP | GFAP | NF |
| | Diffuse | Gastrin | VIP | Bombesin | 5HT | |
| | Thyroid | Thyroglobulin | Calcitonin | CGRP | ChA | CEA |
| | Pituitary | GH | PRL | LH FSH TSH | ACTH | α-HCG |
| | Islet cell | Insulin | Glucagon | Somatostatin PP | VIP | Gastrin α-HCG |
| | Melanoma | S-100 | HMB45 | | | |
| Miscellaneous | Germ cell | PLAP | βHCG | AFP | AAT | |
| | Inflammation/ Degeneration | C3b | Fibrinogen | SAP | SAA | MT |

Key: +++ Strong, ++ moderately strong, + weak ± borderline, − negative, R=reactive cell component.
REPORT

# Appendix II
# Diagnostic algorithms for commonly-made requests for neoplastic diseases

**Diagnostic Request 1:** Lymphoma ? Carcinoma ?

| Principal markers | Expected results | |
|---|---|---|
| | *Lymphoma* | *Carcinoma* |
| WBC | WBC+ | WBC– |
| CK | CK– | CK+ |
| HMFGII | HMFGII –/+ | HMFGII+ |

**Diagnostic Request 2:** Melanoma ? Carcinoma ?

| Principal markers | Expected results | |
|---|---|---|
| | *Melanoma* | *Carcinoma* |
| CK | CK– | CK+ |
| S-100 | S-100+ | S-100–/(+) |
| M3080 | M3080+ | M3080– |
| HMFGII | HMFGII– | HMFGII+ |
| CEA | CEA– | CEA+/– |

**Diagnostic Request 3:** Mesothelioma ? Carcinoma ?

| Principal markers | Expected results | |
|---|---|---|
| | *Mesothelioma* | *Carcinoma* |
| CEA | CEA– | CEA+ |
| CK | CK+/– | CK+ |
| VIM | VIM+ | VIM–/(+) |

**Diagnostic Request 4:** Lymphoma — T cell ? B cell ?

| Principal markers | Expected results | |
|---|---|---|
| | *T cell* | *B cell* |
| WBC | WBC+ | WBC+/(–) |
| UCHL-1 | UCHL-1 +/(–) | UCHL-1 –/(+) |
| CD3 | CD3+ | CD3– |
| L26 | L26– | L26+ |

**Diagnostic Request 5:** Germ-cell tumour? Seminoma ? Other type ?

| Principal markers | Expected results | |
|---|---|---|
| | *Seminoma* | *Other type* |
| PLAP | PLAP+ | Embryonal carcinoma |
| CK | CK– | PLAP+/CK+/AFP–/HCG– |
| AFP | AFP– | Yolk-sac tumour |
| HCG | HCG– | PLAP+/CK+(–)/AFP+/HCG– |
| | | Choriocarcinoma |
| | | PLAP+/CK+(–)/AFP+(–)/HCG+ |

**Diagnostic Request 6:**   Primitive neuroectodermal tumour ? Glial ? Neuronal differentiation ?

| Principal markers | Expected results | |
| --- | --- | --- |
| | *Glial* | *Neuronal* |
| NSE | NSE+ | NSE+ |
| GFAP | GFAP+ | GFAP– |
| S-100 | S-100+(–) | S-100– |
| NF | NF– | NF+ |
| VIM | VIM+(–) | VIM– |

**Diagnostic Request 7:**   Sarcoma ? Rhabdomyosarcoma ? Other type ?

| Principal markers | Expected results | |
| --- | --- | --- |
| | *Rhabdomyosarcoma* | *Other type* |
| VIM | VIM+ | Leiomyosarcoma VIM+/DES+/ MYG– |
| DES | DES+ | Epithelioid sarcoma |
| MYG | MYG+ | Synovial sarcoma VIM+/DES–/ CK+(–) |
| S-100 | S-100– | Liposarcoma VIM+/DES–/ S-100+(–) |
| CK | CK– | |
| Factor VIII-RAG | F-VIII-RAG– | Angiosarcoma VIM+/DES–/ F-VIII-RAG+ |

**Diagnostic Request 8:**   Carcinoma — Thyroid follicular ? Medullary ?

| Principal markers | Expected results | |
| --- | --- | --- |
| | *Thyroid follicular* | *Medullary* |
| Tg | Tg+ | Tg– |
| CAL | CAL– | CAL+ |
| CGRP | CGRP– | CGRP+ |
| CEA | CEA– | CEA+ |

**Diagnostic Request 9:**   Soft-tissue tumour ? Leiomyoma ? Schwannoma ?

| Principal markers | Expected results | |
| --- | --- | --- |
| | *Leiomyoma* | *Schwannoma* |
| α-SMA | α-SMA+ | α-SMA– |
| S-100 | S-100(+)/– | S-100+/(–) |
| Leu7 | Leu7– | Leu7+ |

**Diagnostic Request 10:**   Carcinoma — Prostate ? Bladder ?

| Principal markers | Expected results | |
| --- | --- | --- |
| | *Prostate* | *Bladder* |
| PSA | PSA+ | PSA– |
| PAPh | PAPh+ | PAPh– |
| CEA | CEA– | CEA+ |

**Diagnostic Request 11:**   Neuroendocrine tumour ?

| Principal markers | Expected results |
| --- | --- |
| NSE | NSE+ |
| ChGA | ChGA+/(–) |
| SYNP | SYNP +/(–) |

**Diagnostic Request 12:**   Sarcoma ? Carcinoma ?

| Principal markers | Expected results | |
| --- | --- | --- |
| | *Sarcoma* | *Carcinoma* |
| VIM | VIM+ | VIM–/(+) |
| CK | CK–/(+) | CK+/– |
| HMFGII | HMFGII(+)/– | HMFGII+ |

**Diagnostic Request 13:**   CNS tumour — Primary ? Secondary ?

| Principal markers | Expected results | |
| --- | --- | --- |
| | *Primary* | *Secondary* |
| WBC | WBC– | WBC+/– |
| CK | CK– | CK+/– |
| NSE | NSE+ | NSE–/(+) |

*Key*: + consistently positive; – consistently negative; +(–) predominantly positive; –(+) predominantly negative

# Appendix III
# Protocols of routinely applicable indirect immunoperoxidase techniques

**Table A.1** Simple indirect immunoperoxidase technique

| Step | Operation | Comment |
|---|---|---|
| 1 | Dewax in a series of xylene and absolute alcohol baths | A necessary step for all paraffin wax-embedded tissue sections |
| 2 | Inhibit endogenous peroxidase with methanol/$H_2O_2$ for 30 min at 17°C (R.T.) | A necessary step in all immunoperoxidase enzyme procedures. The methanol/$H_2O_2$ solution is prepared freshly by adding $H_2O_2$ (30% v/v) into absolute methanol to a final concentration of 0.5% |
| 3 | Rehydrate and equilibrate in the diluent buffer | Usually phosphate-buffered saline (PBS; 0.01 M, pH 7.2) |
| 4 | Incubate in primary mouse monoclonal or rabbit polyclonal antibody ideally for 16 h at 4°C | The primary antibodies are diluted in PBS containing 5–20% normal swine serum or 0.6% bovine serum albumin (BSA) as a blocking agent |
| 5 | Wash in PBS × 3 (1–10 min each time) at 17°C (R.T.) | To remove any unbound primary antibody |
| 6 | Incubate in secondary antirabbit IgG or antimouse Ig peroxidase conjugate for 0.5–1 h at 17°C (R.T.) | The conjugate is usually applied at 1:100 dilution of a commercially available stock solution |
| 7 | Wash as in step 5 | To remove any unbound conjugate |
| 10 | Incubate in diaminobenzidine (DAB)/$H_2O_2$ substrate solution for 5 min at 17°C (R.T.) | Leads to the formation of insoluble polymeric DAB producing amorphous brown colour deposit at the site of tissue-bound primary antibody/bridge antibody/PAP immune complexes. The DAB is stored in a concentrated (5 mg/ml) solution at −20°C. The substrate solution is prepared freshly by diluting the stock solution in 0.1 M PBS 10×, and adding $H_2O_2$ to a final concentration of 0.001% |
| 11 | Counterstain for nuclei, dehydrate in a reversed series of alcohol and xylene baths, and mount under a cover-slip using a permanent mountant | Counterstain usually haematoxylin; mountant usually Terpene(R) |

**Table A.2**  Peroxidase–antiperoxidase (PAP) method

| Step | Operation | Comment |
|------|-----------|---------|
| 1–5 | Same as in Table 1 | Same as in Table 1 |
| 6 | Incubate in secondary bridge antibody (antirabbit or -mouse IgG) 0.5–1 h at 17°C (R.T.) | Polyclonal antirabbit or -mouse IgG prepared in goat, sheep or swine; this is added in excess (usually 1:100 dilution of the stock solution) to allow univalent binding |
| 7 | Wash as in step 5 | To remove any unbound bridge antibody |
| 8 | Incubate in PAP complex (freshly diluted) 0.5–1 h at 17°C (R.T.) | PAP is made up of a stable either mouse or rabbit antiperoxidase–peroxidase immune complex designed to bind to the free valency of the appropriate bridge antibody. It is usually applied at 1:100 dilution of the stock prepared in PBS |
| 9 | Wash as in step 5 | To remove any unbound PAP |
| 10 | Incubate in diaminobenzidine (DAB)/$H_2O_2$ substrate solution | Leads to the formation of insoluble polymeric DAB producing amorphous brown colour deposit at the site of tissue-bound primary antibody/bridge antibody/PAP immune complexes. The DAB is stored in a concentrated (5 mg/ml) solution at −20°C. The substrate solution is prepared freshly by diluting the stock solution in 0.1 M PBS 10×, and adding $H_2O_2$ to a final concentration of 0.001% |
| 11 | Counterstain for nuclei, dehydrate in a reversed series of alcohol and xylene baths, and mount under a cover-slip using a permanent mountant | Counterstain usually haematoxylin; mountant usually Terpene (R) |

**Table A.3**  Avidin–biotin complex (ABC) procedure

| Step | Operation | Comment |
|------|-----------|---------|
| 1–5 | Same as in Table 1 | Same as in Table 1 |
| 6 | Incubate in biotin-labelled antimouse Ig or rabbit IgG 0.5–1 h at 17°C (R.T.) | Commercially available in a kit form through e.g. Vectastain |
| 7 | Wash as in Table 1 | |
| 8 | Incubate in freshly preformed ABC 0.5–1 h at 17°C (R.T.) | Commercially available in a kit form through e.g. Vectastain |
| 9–11 | Same as in Table 1 | Same as in Table 1 |

**Table A.4**  DNP Localization System (DLS) procedure

| Step | Operation | Comment |
|------|-----------|---------|
| 1–5 | Same as in Table 1 | Same as in Table 1 |
| 6 | Incubate in DNP-labelled antirabbit IgG+DNP-labelled antimouse IgG mixture for 30 min at 17°C (R.T.) | DNP Localization System kit obtainable from Bioclinical Services Ltd, Cardiff, UK |
| 7 | Wash as in Table 1 | |
| 8 | Incubate in polyvalent monoclonal IgM anti-DNP bridge antibody for 30 min at 17°C (R.T.) | Ditto |
| 9 | Wash as in Table 1 | |
| 10 | Incubate in DNP-labelled peroxidase conjugate for 30 min at 17°C (R.T.) | Ditto |
| 11 | Wash as in Table 1 | |
| 12 | Incubate in DNP-labelled glucose oxidase 30 min at 17°C (R.T.) | Ditto |
| 13 | Wash as in Table 1 | |
| 14 | Incubate in DAB/glucose solution in PBS 16 h at 17°C (R.T.) | Ditto |
| 15 | Counterstain and mount as per Table 1 | Same as in Table 1 |

# Index